Heart Disease and Pregnancy

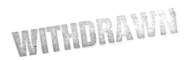
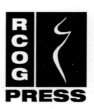
RCOG PRESS

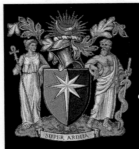

Since 1973 the Royal College of Obstetricians and Gynaecologists has regularly convened Study Groups to address important growth areas within obstetrics and gynaecology. An international group of eminent clinicians and scientists from various disciplines is invited to present the results of recent research and to take part in in-depth discussions. The resulting volume, containing enhanced versions of the papers presented, is published within a few months of the meeting and provides a summary of the subject that is both authoritative and up to date.

SOME PREVIOUS STUDY GROUP PUBLICATIONS AVAILABLE

Infertility
Edited by AA Templeton and JO Drife

Intrapartum Fetal Surveillance
Edited by JAD Spencer and RHT Ward

Early Fetal Growth and Development
Edited by RHT Ward, SK Smith and D Donnai

Ethics in Obstetrics and Gynaecology
Edited by S Bewley and RHT Ward

The Biology of Gynaecological Cancer
Edited by R Leake, M Gore and RHT Ward

Multiple Pregnancy
Edited by RHT Ward and M Whittle

The Prevention of Pelvic Infection
Edited by AA Templeton

**Screening for Down Syndrome in the
First Trimester**
Edited by JG Grudzinskas and RHT Ward

**Problems in Early Pregnancy: Advances
in Diagnosis and Management**
Edited by JG Grudzinskas and PMS O'Brien

**Gene Identification, Manipulation
and Treatment**
Edited by SK Smith, EJ Thomas and
PMS O'Brien

Evidence-based Fertility Treatment
Edited by AA Templeton, ID Cooke and
PMS O'Brien

**Fetal Programming: Influences on
Development and Disease in Later Life**
Edited by PMS O'Brien, T Wheeler
and DJP Barker

Hormones and Cancer
Edited by PMS O'Brien and AB MacLean

**The Placenta: Basic Science and Clinical
Practice**
Edited by JCP Kingdom, ERM Jauniaux
and PMS O'Brien

Disorders of the Menstrual Cycle
Edited by PMS O'Brien, IT Cameron
and AB MacLean

Infection and Pregnancy
Edited by AB MacLean, L Regan and D Carrington

Pain in Obstetrics and Gynaecology
Edited by AB MacLean, RW Stones
and S Thornton

Incontinence in Women
Edited by AB MacLean and L Cardozo

Maternal Morbidity and Mortality
Edited by AB MacLean and J Neilson

Lower Genital Tract Neoplasia
Edited by Allan B MacLean, Albert Singer
and Hilary Critchley

Pre-eclampsia
Edited by Hilary Critchley, Allan MacLean,
Lucilla Poston and James Walker

Preterm Birth
Edited by Hilary Critchley, Phillip Bennett
and Steven Thornton

Menopause and Hormone Replacement
Edited by Hilary Critchley, Ailsa Gebbie
and Valerie Beral

Implantation and Early Development
Edited by Hilary Critchley, Iain Cameron
and Stephen Smith

Multiple Pregnancy
Edited by Mark Kilby, Phil Baker,
Hilary Critchley and David Field

Heart Disease and Pregnancy

Edited by

Philip J Steer, Michael A Gatzoulis
and Philip Baker

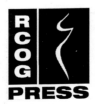

Philip J Steer BSc MB BS MD FRCOG
Professor of Obstetrics and Deputy Head (Teaching) of the Division of Surgery, Oncology, Reproductive Medicine and Anaesthetics, Faculty of Medicine, Imperial College London, and Honorary Consultant Obstetrician, Chelsea and Westminster Hospital, 369 Fulham Road, London SW10 9NH

Michael A Gatzoulis MD PhD FACC FESC
Professor of Cardiology and Congenital Heart Disease and Consultant Cardiologist, Royal Brompton Hospital and the National Heart and Lung Institute, Imperial College London, Sydney Street, London SW3 6NP

Philip Baker DM FRCOG
Professor of Maternal and Fetal Health, Maternal and Fetal Health Research Centre, The University of Manchester, St Mary's Hospital, Hathersage Road, Manchester M13 0JH

Published by the **RCOG Press** at the Royal College of Obstetricians and Gynaecologists, 27 Sussex Place, Regent's Park, London NW1 4RG

www.rcog.org.uk

Registered charity no. 213280

First published 2006

ISBN 1-904752-30-6

Cover image © Philip Steer

RCOG Editor: Andrew Welsh
Design/typesetting by Karl Harrington, FiSH Books, London
Index by Liza Furnival
Printed by Henry Ling Ltd, The Dorchester Press, Dorchester DT1 1HD

Contents

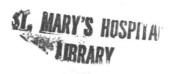

SECTION 3 ANTENATAL CARE – FETAL CONSIDERATIONS

SECTION 4 ANTENATAL CARE – SPECIFIC MATERNAL CONDITIONS

SECTION 5 INTRAPARTUM CARE

SECTION 6 POSTPARTUM CARE

SECTION 7 CONSENSUS VIEWS

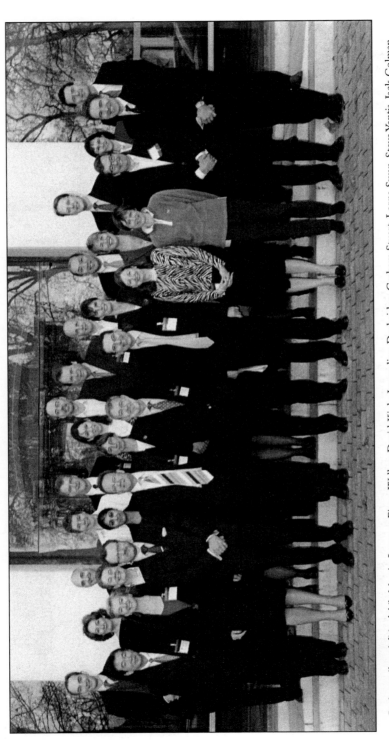

Back row (from left to right): Martin Lupton, Fiona Walker, David Kiely, Jacqueline Durbridge, Graham Stuart, Lorna Swan, Steve Yentis, Jack Colman, Martin Dresner, TG Teoh, Piers Daubeney, Sarah Vause, Pat O'Brien

Middle row (from left to right): Margaret Ramsay, Mandish Dhanjal, Kate Harding, Jolien Roos-Hesselink, Catherine Nelson-Piercy

Front row (from left to right): Koichiro Niwa, Helena Gardiner, Ian Greer, Philip Baker, Philip Steer, Michael Gatzoulis, Carole Warnes, Sara Thorne, David Williams, Mark Johnson

Participants

Philip Baker
Convenor of RCOG Study Groups and Professor of Maternal and Fetal Health, Maternal and Fetal Health Research Centre, The University of Manchester, St Mary's Hospital, Hathersage Road, Manchester M13 0JH, UK.

Jack M Colman
Associate Professor of Medicine (Cardiology), University of Toronto; Toronto Congenital Cardiac Centre for Adults; University of Toronto Cardiac Diseases in Pregnancy Program, Mount Sinai Hospital and Toronto General Hospital/UHN. 600 University Avenue, Suite 1603, Toronto, Ontario, Canada M5G 1X5.

Mandish K Dhanjal
Consultant Obstetrician and Gynaecologist, Queen Charlotte's and Chelsea Hospital, Du Cane Road, London W12 0HS, and Honorary Senior Lecturer, Imperial College London, UK.

Piers Daubeney
Consultant Paediatric and Fetal Cardiologist, Royal Brompton Hospital, Sydney Street, London SW3 6NP and Chelsea and Westminster Hospital, Fulham Road, London SW10 9NH, UK.

Martin Dresner
Consultant Obstetric Anaesthetist, Department of Anaesthesia, Leeds General Infirmary, Great George Street, Leeds LS1 3EX, UK.

Jacqueline Durbridge
Consultant Anaesthetist, Magill Department of Anaesthesia, Chelsea and Westminster Hospital, 369 Fulham Road, London SW10 9NH, UK.

Helena Gardiner
Senior Lecturer and Director of Perinatal Cardiology, Institute of Reproductive and
Developmental Biology, Faculty of Medicine, Imperial College Queen Charlotte's
and Chelsea Hospital, Du Cane Road, London W12 0NN and Consultant
Paediatric and Fetal Cardiologist and Honorary Senior Lecturer, Department of
Paediatric Cardiology, Royal Brompton and Harefield Hospital NHS Trust, Sydney
Street, London SW3 6NP, UK.

Michael A Gatzoulis
Professor of Cardiology and Congenital Heart Disease and Consultant Cardiologist,
Adult Congenital Heart Centre and Centre for Pulmonary Hypertension, Royal
Brompton Hospital and the National Heart and Lung Institute, Imperial College
London, Sydney Street, London SW3 6NP, UK.

Kate R Harding
Consultant Obstetrician, 10th Floor, North Wing, St Thomas' Hospital, Lambeth
Palace Road, London SE1 7EH, UK.

Mark Johnson
Consultant and Reader in Obstetrics, Academic Department of Obstetrics, Imperial
College Faculty of Medicine, Chelsea and Westminster Hospital, 369 Fulham Road,
London SW10 9NH, UK.

David G Kiely
Director, Sheffield Pulmonary Vascular Disease Unit, Royal Hallamshire Hospital,
Glossop Road, Sheffield S10 2JF, UK.

Martin Lupton
Consultant Obstetrician, Chelsea and Westminster Hospital, 369 Fulham Road,
London SW10 9NH, UK.

Catherine Nelson-Piercy
Consultant Obstetric Physician, Guy's and St Thomas' Hospital, 10th Floor,
Directorate Office, North Wing, St Thomas' Hospital, Lambeth Palace Road,
London SE1 7EH, UK.

Koichiro Niwa
Consultant Cardiologist, Head of Pediatric and Adult Congenital Heart Disease
Unit, Chiba Cardiovascular Center, 575 Tsurumai, Ichihara, Chiba 290-0512, Japan.

Patrick J O'Brien
Obstetric Lead Consultant, University College London Hospitals, Obstetric
Hospital, UCH, Huntley Street, London WC1E 6AU, UK.

Margaret Ramsay
Senior Lecturer in Fetomaternal Medicine, Department of Obstetrics and
Gynaecology, Queen's Medical Centre, Nottingham NG7 2UH, UK.

Jolien W Roos-Hesselink
Cardiologist, Erasmus MC, Thoraxcentrum, Room BA300, Dr Molewaterplein 40, 3015 GD Rotterdam, Netherlands.

Philip J Steer
Professor of Obstetrics and Deputy Head (Teaching) of the Division of Surgery, Oncology, Reproductive Medicine and Anaesthetics, Faculty of Medicine, Imperial College London, and Honorary Consultant Obstetrician, Chelsea and Westminster Hospital, 369 Fulham Road, London SW10 9NH.

Graham Stuart
Consultant Cardiologist (Congenital Heart Disease), Congenital Heart Unit, Level 4, Dolphin House, King Edward Building, Bristol Royal Infirmary, Bristol BS2 8HW, UK.

Lorna Swan
Consultant Cardiologist, Adult Congenital Heart Disease Unit, Royal Brompton and Harefield NHS Trust, London, SW3 6NP, UK.

TG Teoh
Consultant, Fetal Medicine Unit, St Mary's Hospital, London W2 1NY, UK.

Sara Thorne
Consultant Cardiologist, Cardiology Department, University Hospital Birmingham (Queen Elizabeth), Metchley Park Road, Birmingham B15 2TH, UK.

Sarah H Vause
Consultant in Fetomaternal Medicine, St Mary's Hospital, Hathersage Road, Manchester M13 0JH, UK.

Fiona Walker
Consultant Cardiologist, GUCH Unit, The Heart Hospital, 16–18 Westmoreland Street, London W1G 8PH, UK.

Carole A Warnes
Professor of Medicine, Mayo Medical School and Director, Adult Congenital Heart Disease Clinic, Mayo Clinic, 200 First Street SW, Rochester, MN 55905, USA.

David Williams
Consultant in Obstetric Medicine, University College London Hospitals, Obstetric Hospital, UCH, Huntley Street, London WC1E 6AU, UK.

Steve M Yentis
Consultant Anaesthetist, Magill Department of Anaesthesia, Intensive Care and Pain Management, Chelsea and Westminster Hospital, 369 Fulham Road, London SW10 9NH, UK.

Additional contributors

Bernard Clarke
Consultant Cardiologist, The Manchester Heart Centre, Manchester Royal Infirmary, Oxford Road, Manchester M13 9WL, UK.

Charles A Elliot
Clinical Lecturer, Pulmonary Vascular Disease Unit, Respiratory Medicine, Royal Hallamshire Hospital, Glossop Road, Sheffield S10 2JF, UK.

Emily Gelson
Clinical Fellow, Academic Department of Obstetrics, Imperial College Faculty of Medicine, Chelsea and Westminster Hospital, 369 Fulham Road, London SW10 9NH, UK.

Henryk Kafka
Visiting Consultant Cardiologist, Adult Congenital Heart Unit, Royal Brompton Hospital, Sydney Street, London SW3 6NP, UK, and Division of Cardiology, Queen's University Cardiovascular Laboratory, Kingston General Hospital, 76 Stewart Street, Kingston, Ontario, Canada K7L 2V7.

Asma Khalil
Senior Research Fellow in Fetomaternal Medicine, Homerton University Hospital, Homerton Row, London E9 6SR, UK.

Onome Ogueh
Consultant in Obstetrics and Gynaecology, Department of Obstetrics and Gynaecology, Brighton and Sussex University Hospitals NHS Trust, Princess Royal Hospital, Lewes Road, Haywards Heath RH16 4AZ, UK.

Mathew Sermer
Professor of Obstetrics & Gynaecology and Medicine, University of Toronto; Head, Obstetrics and Maternal Fetal Medicine, Mount Sinai Hospital; University of Toronto Cardiac Diseases in Pregnancy Program. 600 University Avenue, Room 1007, Toronto, Ontario, Canada M5G 1X5.

Candice K Silversides
Assistant Professor of Medicine (Cardiology), University of Toronto; Toronto Congenital Cardiac Centre for Adults; University of Toronto Cardiac Diseases in Pregnancy Program, Mount Sinai Hospital and Toronto General Hospital/UHN. 585 University Avenue, 5N-521 North Wing, Toronto, Ontario, Canada M5G 2N2.

Samuel C Siu
Professor of Medicine (Cardiology), University of Toronto; Toronto Congenital Cardiac Centre for Adults; University of Toronto Cardiac Diseases in Pregnancy Program, Mount Sinai Hospital and Toronto General Hospital/UHN. PMCC 3-526, Toronto General Hospital, 200 Elizabeth Street, Toronto, Ontario, Canada M5G 2C4.

Peter Stewart
Consultant Obstetrician, Jessop Wing, Royal Hallamshire Hospital, Tree Root Walk, Sheffield S10 2SF, UK.

Shigeru Tateno
Chief, Electrophysiology, Pediatric and Adult Congenital Heart Disease Unit, Chiba Cardiovascular Center, 575 Tsurumai, Ichihara, Chiba 290-0512, Japan.

Hideki Uemura
Consultant Cardiac Surgeon, Adult Congenital Heart Unit, Royal Brompton Hospital, Sydney Street, London SW3 6NP, UK.

Anselm Uebing
Fellow in Adult Congenital Heart Disease, Royal Brompton Hospital, Sydney Street, London SW3 6NP, UK.

Victoria J Webster
Consultant Anaesthetist, Jessop Wing, Royal Hallamshire Hospital, Tree Root Walk, Sheffield S10 2SF, UK.

Christine KH Yu
Subspecialty Trainee in Maternal and Fetal Medicine, King's College London and St Mary's Hospital, London W2 1NY, UK.

Discussant

Ian A Greer
Regius Professor of Obstetrics and Gynaecology, Division of Developmental Medicine, Maternal and Reproductive Medicine, University of Glasgow, Glasgow, UK.

DECLARATION OF INTEREST

All contributors to the Study Group were invited to make a specific Declaration of Interest in relation to the subject of the Study Group. This was undertaken and all contributors complied with this request. Helena Gardiner is a medical advisor to Echo UK, the fetal heart charity. Kate Harding has shares in GlaxoSmithKline. Martin Lupton is a consultant for the Roman Catholic Archdiocese of Westminster. Philip Baker's department receives financial support from Pfizer UK for a clinical trial. Tommy's, the baby charity, contributes to the funding of the group and to his personal salary. He holds a patent for diagnostic testing for pre-eclampsia. Philip Steer is the Editor-in-Chief of *BJOG – An International Journal of Obstetrics and Gynaecology*. Steve Yentis was Honorary Secretary of the Obstetric Anaesthetists Association until May 2006.

Preface

In the Confidential Enquiry into Maternal Deaths in the United Kingdom 2000–2002, cardiac disease for the first time became the leading medical cause of death in relation to pregnancy. This prompted the Meetings Committee of the Royal College of Obstetricians and Gynaecologists in London to suggest heart disease and pregnancy as an important topic to be addressed as part of the regular series of Study Groups organised and funded by the College. This met with the approval of Philip Baker, Convenor of Study Groups, and so Philip Steer (obstetrician) and Michael Gatzoulis (cardiologist) set about bringing together a distinguished group of obstetricians, maternal medicine specialists, anaesthetists, obstetric physicians and cardiologists (both adult and paediatric) with an interest in care before, during and after pregnancy to consider this vitally important topic. A particular challenge was to gather together the limited amount of scientific data in an area of practice based largely on anecdote and relatively small case series, and from this restricted knowledge base to construct a consensus on issues of diagnosis and management. Accordingly, each participant was asked to prepare a presentation, on which the following chapters are based, on a specified aspect of the topic and subsequently to amend their chapter in the light of the discussions at the meeting, which was held on 13–15 February 2006 at the RCOG in London.

From the perspective of the participants, the meeting itself was a great success. There was an unusual sense of mission because all of those taking part are heavily involved in promoting effective care of women with heart disease who are or who wish to become pregnant, and are working hard to raise the profile of what is becoming almost a subspecialty in its own right. Some may question such a degree of specialisation but, with cardiovascular disease now becoming the leading cause of death in women generally, collaboration between cardiologists and obstetricians is only going to increase in this area in the future.

The chapters are laid out in a way that we hope readers will find intuitive, starting with prepregnancy counselling and contraception, moving through the antenatal period to delivery and the puerperium, and finishing with long-term outcome (about which distressingly little is as yet known – this should be an important focus for future research).

Finally, we list the consensus statements signed up to by all the members of the Study Group. There are a gratifyingly large number of these, which is a tribute to the flexibility and open-mindedness of the participants. It has to be admitted that most are based upon opinion rather than hard data. Nonetheless, we hope that readers will find them a useful basis on which to consider building or modifying their own guidelines for practice, and upon which future more evidence-based guidelines can be constructed.

This volume, which has resulted from the meeting, is much more than the transcript of a fascinating meeting. Because of the way the meeting was designed, it also covers the clinical aspects of heart disease in pregnancy in a more comprehensive way than would have been possible had we produced a traditional meeting report. Indeed, we would like to see this volume as an initial attempt to produce a comprehensive text for those who take on the challenge of caring for this high-risk group of women. It brings together not only the data that we have available but also the considered opinions of many who see it as their life's work to advance knowledge in this area. We thank the participants who gave their time freely to help make the meeting such a success and who have produced a series of outstanding chapters. Outcomes of pregnancy in women with heart disease will not always be good but we hope that the knowledge and opinions documented in this book will help to improve them in the future.

Philip J Steer
Michael A Gatzoulis
Philip Baker

Section 1

Prepregnancy
counselling and
contraception

Chapter 1
Preconceptual counselling for women with cardiac disease

Sarah Vause, Sara Thorne and Bernard Clarke

Introduction

The majority of women want to have children and women with heart disease are no exception. Complex heart disease is no bar to sexual activity. Most women with heart disease do have some awareness of the risks of pregnancy but their ideas are often inaccurate, ranging from overly optimistic to overly pessimistic.[1] They may be equally poorly informed about the prognosis of their heart condition, even in the absence of pregnancy. Many doctors do not have a good understanding of the risks of pregnancy in women with heart disease and thus such women may be deprived of appropriate advice and counselling unless a specialist referral is made. Discussions with a cardiologist and/or an obstetric physician with a specialist interest in pregnancy and heart disease should begin in adolescence. These discussions should cover future pregnancies and their prevention, both to prevent accidental and possibly dangerous pregnancies and to allow them to come to terms with their future childbearing potential. They also need to be able to plan their families in the knowledge of their likely future health and life expectancy.

In the UK, the majority of women seen preconceptually by cardiologists and/or obstetricians will be women with congenital heart disease (CHD). This is because the incidence of CHD (0.8%) in pregnant women in the UK is higher than the incidence of acquired heart disease (0.1%). Furthermore, most women with CHD are already known to the cardiac services. Many women with acquired disease are recent immigrants and are unaware of their condition, which is an important reason why they are at particularly high risk. The diagnosis may be made only when they are pregnant and become symptomatic. For this reason, deaths in pregnancy from acquired heart disease outnumber those from CHD.[2]

Components of preconceptual counselling

Preconceptual counselling should ideally:[3]

- display attitudes and practices that value pregnant women, children and families and respect the diversity of people's lives and experiences
- incorporate informed choice, thus encouraging women and men to understand health issues that may affect conception and pregnancy

■ encourage women and men to prepare actively for pregnancy, and enable them to be as healthy as possible

■ attempt to identify couples who are at increased risk of producing babies with a congenital abnormality and provide them with sufficient knowledge to make informed decisions.

These four components will be discussed below in relation to cardiac disease in pregnancy.

Valuing pregnant women, children and families and respecting diversity

Preconceptual counselling should display attitudes and practices that value pregnant women, children and families and respect the diversity of people's lives and experiences. All women have a cultural context within a multicultural society. For some women, issues related to culture may need specific attention, including:

■ their religious beliefs (particularly in relation to contraception and termination of pregnancy)

■ the role of the partner and extended family in pregnancy decisions

■ communication, where English is not the first language.

Assumptions are often made about the anticipated views of certain racial, cultural or religious groups and this may consciously or subconsciously affect the way in which doctors counsel women. Addressing these overtly helps one to compensate for any unintentional bias.

All people have a social and emotional context and when women and their partners seek advice this context must be considered. Their attitudes and expectations are likely to have been influenced by their previous experiences and those of their family. These may include:

■ the anxieties of over-protective parents

■ worries relating to their inability to embark on, or continue, a meaningful relationship if pregnancy is contraindicated

■ wanting to fulfil their partner's desire for a child, or guilt if they cannot do so

■ 'I'm lucky to be alive – am I pushing my luck or being greedy? Do I deserve a child?'

While it is important to explore and respect the context of her previous experiences, preconceptual counselling should promote the autonomy of the woman. It should enable her to determine her personal priorities and support her decision making.

Informed choice and understanding

Preconceptual counselling should incorporate informed choice, thus encouraging women and men to understand health issues that may affect conception and pregnancy. The counselling should provide information in a frank, honest and understandable way so as to give the woman a realistic estimate of both maternal and fetal risk and allow her to make an informed decision as to whether to embark on a pregnancy. The counselling should include information on:

■ the effects of cardiac disease on pregnancy, in terms of both maternal and fetal risks

■ the effects of pregnancy on cardiac disease, including the risk of dying or long-term deterioration

■ whether these effects will change with time or treatment

■ the other options that are available, such as contraception, surrogacy or adoption

■ the long-term outlook – a woman with a short life expectancy may feel that neither pregnancy nor surrogacy nor adoption is appropriate, as a child may then have to deal with the terminal illness and death of the mother

The risk of maternal death during pregnancy is often difficult to quantify but it is important to give the woman, her partner and her family as accurate an assessment of risk as is possible within our current state of knowledge.[4] Although for the majority of women the risk will be less than 1%, for some conditions the risk may be considerably higher. Such high-risk cardiac conditions, where the risk is greater than 1% and in some cases up to 50%, include:

■ any form of cyanotic CHD, for example Eisenmenger syndrome

■ pulmonary hypertension

■ poor systemic ventricular function, for example a systemic right ventricle

■ severe left heart obstructive lesions, for example mitral and aortic stenosis

■ Marfan syndrome, especially if the aortic root is dilated

■ previous repair of a coarctation with a Dacron™ (polyethylene terephthalate) patch

■ previous peripartum cardiomyopathy

■ poor cardiac function for any reason at the time of conception.

The risks to the fetus include the following:

■ intrauterine growth restriction with cyanotic heart disease

■ iatrogenic prematurity

■ fetal abnormality (typical risk of 3%, but this varies with the type of maternal lesion, and is also related to paternal lesions)

■ teratogenesis, for example from warfarin or captopril

■ fetal loss resulting from invasive prenatal testing.

For some complex conditions, there is little or no information available, either because of the rarity of the woman's disease or because they represent a new cohort of survivors to adulthood with surgically modified disease. These women need a thorough assessment of their current cardiac status and appropriate advice based on how their cardiovascular system is likely to adapt to the physiological changes of pregnancy.

One successful pregnancy should not engender complacency. Some conditions, such as peripartum cardiomyopathy, have a high recurrence risk.[5] Other conditions could worsen with age and in each subsequent pregnancy the risks would be higher.

Information about contraception and termination

Facilitating informed choice also means that doctors must provide information relating to the choice of not getting pregnant and thus appropriate contraceptive advice. Informed choice also means that the woman should be aware of the option of termination of pregnancy should she find herself unexpectedly pregnant after deciding that she was not planning to conceive. The assurance that clinicians will be non-judgemental and supportive of a decision to terminate a pregnancy is important. Open discussion of this option and provision of contact numbers to facilitate access to services reinforces that this is an option available to the woman.[2] Termination of pregnancy in women with heart disease is not without risks, and it should be performed in a centre with appropriate anaesthetic and cardiac facilities.

Information about clinical management

During the preconceptual appointment the proposed plan of care for the pregnancy should be outlined. Women with significant cardiac disease should be managed in a centre with appropriate expertise, preferably in a joint obstetric–cardiac clinic, but for some women this may mean travelling long distances. Women should be made aware of how likely it would be that they would need admission antenatally, iatrogenic preterm delivery, lower segment caesarean section (LSCS) or high-dependency care in a hospital that may be many miles from home. However, for most cardiac conditions a normal vaginal delivery with good analgesia and a low threshold for forceps assistance is the safest mode of delivery for the mother, since it is associated with less blood loss and less rapid haemodynamic changes than caesarean section. The few maternal cardiac indications for delivery by caesarean section include Marfan syndrome, aortic aneurysm of any cause, and an acutely unwell mother.

Information in an appropriate language

If the woman and her doctor do not speak the same language, a professional interpreter should be used. Interpreters from within the family, including the husband, should not be used as in the family's desire to help the woman have a successful pregnancy the risks may not be accurately relayed to her.[2]

Preparing for pregnancy

Preconceptual counselling encourages women and men to prepare actively for pregnancy and enables them to be as healthy as possible. The consultations provide the ideal opportunity to minimise risk and optimise cardiac function before pregnancy:[6]

- valvotomy by catheter or surgical intervention before pregnancy – if valve replacement is performed the choice of the type of valve used may be influenced by the desire for a further pregnancy; the use of tissue valves obviates the need for anticoagulation during pregnancy
- treatment of arrhythmias (surgical or medical)
- treatment of underlying medical conditions, such as hypertension or diabetes
- avoidance of teratogens – medication may need to be changed before pregnancy
- discussion re anticoagulation – women using warfarin need to be aware of its teratogenic potential and the risk of fetal intracranial haemorrhage, and they

should understand the need for conversion to heparin once pregnancy is confirmed. Contact numbers should be provided to facilitate this as early as possible in pregnancy. The involvement of haematologists will enable appropriate dosing and monitoring. For women with mechanical valves the risks of warfarin versus the risks of heparin should be discussed with them to enable them to make an informed choice.

- dental treatment – women with complex heart disease may need to be referred to a tertiary dental hospital for dental care; it is better for any dental problems to be resolved before pregnancy
- timing of pregnancy – for those with a systemic right ventricle or univentricular heart, pregnancy is likely to be tolerated better when the woman is in her 20s rather than her late 30s. A woman's life may not allow her the luxury of making this choice but other women may have a choice and should be discouraged from purposely delaying pregnancy because of considerations such as a career.
- contraception – until the above cardiac problems have been appropriately addressed, the provision of appropriate contraception is important
- general pre-pregnancy advice should not be forgotten, for example folic acid
- provision of phone numbers to facilitate prompt contact and reassessment once pregnancy is confirmed.

Women undergoing assisted conception often have additional risk factors such as increased age, and the risk of ovarian hyperstimulation and multiple pregnancy with a concomitant increase in the risk of pre-eclampsia. These conditions can compound the risk of heart disease. In women undergoing assisted conception, it is important that precautions should be taken to avoid hyperstimulated cycles and to minimise the chance of multiple pregnancy by only carrying out single-embryo replacements during *in vitro* fertilisation (IVF) cycles.

Risk of congenital abnormality

Preconceptual counselling attempts to identify couples who are at increased risk of producing babies with a malformation, and should provide them with sufficient knowledge to make informed decisions. Many couples have worries about the recurrence risk to their unborn baby. For the majority of women with CHD, with no family history and no chromosomal abnormality, the risk of recurrence of CHD in the fetus is around 3%. Prenatal fetal echocardiography can be arranged and most couples can be reassured that the most likely outcome is a healthy baby.

For women with a family history of heart disease, or other features to suggest an underlying genetic or chromosomal problem, the preconceptual appointment offers the opportunity to refer a woman to the clinical geneticist or to arrange karyotyping if this has not previously been done. Karyotyping may detect balanced translocations or the 22q11 deletion. While the woman may have previously been seen by a geneticist, she may welcome the opportunity to discuss the risks to the fetus again once she begins to contemplate pregnancy.

Preconceptual care should also include a discussion of the various prenatal tests available, their risks and limitations, the timing of the tests and the way in which they are performed. Information about how to access these tests, including contact numbers, should be provided. Discussion should also include the options available, including termination, should the fetus be found to be affected.

For other women with conditions such as Marfan syndrome the preconceptual appointment offers the opportunity to discuss the recurrence risk, and the need for appropriate follow-up of the infant postnatally to establish a diagnosis and, if needed, to implement long-term surveillance.

Conclusion

Successful preconceptual counselling will empower a woman with cardiac disease to make informed choices relating to pregnancy by providing non-directive counselling and access to the appropriate multidisciplinary specialised services. Optimising her health before pregnancy will improve the likelihood of a successful pregnancy outcome.

References

1. Moons P, De Volder E, Budts W, De Geest S, Elen J, Waeytens K, *et al.* What do adult patients with congenital heart disease know about their disease, treatment and prevention of complications? A call for structured patient education. *Heart* 2001;86:74–80.

2. Drife JO, Lewis G, Clutton-Brock T, editors. *Why Mothers Die: The Sixth Report of the Confidential Enquiries into Maternal Deaths in the United Kingdom 2000–2002.* London: RCOG Press; 2004.

3. Health Canada. *Family-Centred Maternity and Newborn Care: National Guidelines.* Ottawa: Ministry of Public Works and Government Services; 2000 [www.hc-sc.gc.ca].

4. Steer PJ. Pregnancy and contraception. In: Gatzoulis MA, Swan L, Therrien J, Pantely GA, editors. *Adult Congenital Heart Disease – a Practical Guide.* Oxford: Blackwell Publishing; 2005. p. 17.

5. Elkayam U, Tummala PP, Rao K, Akhter MW, Karaalp IS, Wani OR, *et al.* Maternal and fetal outcomes of subsequent pregnancies in women with peripartum cardiomyopathy. *N Engl J Med* 2001;344:1567–71.

6. Thorne SA. Pregnancy in heart disease. *Heart* 2004;90:450–6.

Chapter 2
Contraception in women with heart disease

Mandish K Dhanjal

Introduction

Cardiac disease is the main cause of maternal mortality in the UK, being responsible for 17% of maternal deaths.[1] This is accounted for in approximately equal proportions by those with congenital heart disease reaching childbearing age, cardiomyopathy, ischaemic heart disease, aneurysm or dissection of the thoracic aorta, and pulmonary hypertension.

There are a handful of cardiac conditions where pregnancy is contraindicated because of mortality rates approaching 50%. It is imperative that such women have the most reliable methods of contraception available. However, contraceptive agents may themselves influence heart disease, or may interact with medications used by such women. The World Health Organization (WHO) has classified contraceptive agents into four classes depending on how suitable their use is in medical conditions (Table 2.1).[2]

The WHO classification for an individual agent will vary according to circumstance and concomitant medical illnesses such as cardiac disease, hypertension and diabetes. For example, a woman starting the combined oral contraceptive (COC) pill who has a family history of ischaemic heart disease will be classified as:

- WHO 2 if she is aged under 35 years
- WHO 3 if she is aged over 35 years
- WHO 4 at all ages if she has ischaemic heart disease herself.

Table 2.1. WHO classification and interpretation of medical eligibility for contraceptives

WHO class	Eligibility for contraceptives with medical conditions	'ABCD' classification
1	No restriction for use	**A**lways usable
2	Advantages of method generally outweigh theoretical or proven risk	**B**roadly usable
3	Theoretical or proven risks generally outweigh advantages	**C**aution/counselling
4	Unacceptable health risk	**D**o not use

Table 2.2. Classification of medical illness (e.g. heart disease) according to risk to maternal health if pregnant; adapted with permission from Thorne *et al*.[3]

Class	Risk of maternal morbidity and mortality resulting from pregnancy with medical illness	Counselling required if pregnancy considered
1	No detectable increased risk	No contraindication to pregnancy
2	Slightly increased risk	Can consider pregnancy
3	Significantly increased risk	If pregnancy still desired after counselling, intensive specialist cardiac and obstetric monitoring will be required antenatally, in labour and postnatally
4	Unacceptably high risk	Pregnancy not advisable; offer emergency contraception or termination if pregnancy occurs; if declined care for as class 3

Counselling patients regarding risks of pregnancy

Adolescents with congenital heart disease should have the issue of pregnancy and contraception discussed with them at the age of 12–15 years (depending on individual maturity), ideally in a paediatric cardiology clinic. Suitable contraception should be offered to all women with heart disease who are sexually active and who either do not yet wish to conceive or in whom pregnancy is contraindicated.

All women with heart disease considering pregnancy should be offered preconception counselling. In those women with congenital heart disease, this counselling should be from a specialist in adult congenital heart disease.

The WHO classification for contraceptives can be extended and adapted to cover the risk of maternal morbidity and mortality resulting from pregnancy in women with specific medical conditions, such as heart disease (Table 2.2).[3]

Fetal consequences should also be taken into consideration when discussing whether pregnancy is advisable. Heart diseases causing cyanosis can result in chronic fetal hypoxia that significantly reduces the chances of a live birth. A prepregnancy resting arterial oxygen saturation of 85–90% is associated with a 45% chance of live birth, but this drops to only 12% with oxygen saturation below 85%.[4] Moreover, such low saturation is also associated with high maternal haemoglobin concentration, poor placental perfusion and intrauterine growth restriction (IUGR). A growth-restricted baby often needs to be delivered preterm, compounding the problem.

Classification of cardiac conditions

In general, the most efficacious contraceptives should be used with the most severe heart disease as the consequences of contraceptive failure are far greater for this group of women.

Class 1 cardiac conditions

In class 1 cardiac conditions, such as the following, there are no contraindications to pregnancy:[3]

1. uncomplicated, small or mild lesions, such as

    (a) mitral valve prolapse with no more than trivial mitral regurgitation

    (b) patent ductus arteriosus

    (c) ventricular septal defect

    (d) pulmonary stenosis

2. successfully repaired simple lesions, such as

    (a) patent ductus arteriosus

    (b) ventricular septal defect

    (c) ostium secundum atrial septal defect

    (d) total anomalous pulmonary venous drainage

3. isolated ventricular extrasystoles and atrial ectopic beats

Class 2 and 3 cardiac conditions

Class 2 and 3 cardiac conditions are those with a slightly or significantly increased risk of maternal morbidity and mortality (Table 2.3).[3] Individual specialist assessment is required to establish which class of risk these conditions should be allocated to. Combinations of abnormalities, or additional risk factors, may further increase the risks of pregnancy.

Table 2.3. Cardiac conditions in which pregnancy poses a class 2 or 3 risk; reproduced with permission from Thorne *et al.*[3]

Class 2 if otherwise well and uncomplicated	Class 2–3 depending on individual	Class 3[a]
■ Unoperated atrial septal defect ■ Repaired tetralogy of Fallot ■ Arrhythmias	■ Mild left ventricular impairment ■ Hypertrophic cardiomyopathy ■ Native or tissue valvular heart disease not considered class 4 ■ Congenital heart disease ■ Marfan syndrome without aortic dilatation (with or without a family history of aortic dissection) ■ Heart transplantation	■ Mechanical valve ■ Systemic right ventricle[b] ■ Following Fontan operation (for tricuspid atresia) ■ Cyanotic heart disease ■ Other complex

[a] If there are other risk factors, pregnancy may carry a class 4 risk
[b] Congenital heart disease in which the right ventricle supports the systemic circulation

Class 4 cardiac conditions

Pregnancy is not advisable in Class 4 cardiac conditions, such as the following:[3]

1. pulmonary arterial hypertension of any cause

2. severe systemic ventricular dysfunction with
    (a) NYHA class III–IV (New York Heart Association classification, see Appendix A) or
    (b) ventricular ejection fraction less than 30%

3. previous peripartum cardiomyopathy with any residual impairment of left ventricular function

4. severe left heart obstruction – aortic or mitral stenosis with valve areas less than 1 cm^2

5. Marfan syndrome with aorta dilated more than 4 cm

6. in women with two or more of the following risk factors:
    (a) reduced left ventricular systolic function with ejection fractions less than 40%
    (b) left heart obstruction – aortic or mitral stenosis with valve areas of less than 1.5 cm^2 or less than 2.0 cm^2, respectively
    (c) previous cardiovascular events including heart failure, transient ischaemic attacks or stroke
    (d) reduced functional capacity (a disease of NYHA class II or higher).

Preconception counselling is imperative for women with class 4 cardiac conditions. It is inevitable that some women will decide to go ahead with a pregnancy despite the risks to their own health, and their right to do so must be respected and supported. However, when women do decide they do not want to fall pregnant, it is essential that the most effective of the appropriate contraceptive agents are recommended and supplied. If there is failure of this regular contraception, emergency contraception should be provided promptly. Failing this, termination of pregnancy should be available with a minimum of delay.

Pulmonary arterial hypertension

Pulmonary arterial hypertension[5,6] can be primary or secondary and includes Eisenmenger syndrome. Any form is associated with maternal mortality rates of up to 50%.[7] The mechanism of the disease includes pulmonary vasoconstriction, pulmonary vascular remodelling and thrombosis resulting in an increased pulmonary vascular resistance. The pulmonary blood flow cannot increase in pregnancy. Even mild pulmonary hypertension (pulmonary artery systolic pressure of 36–50 mmHg) is associated with substantial maternal mortality rates. Pregnancy is associated with progression of the disease.[1] Many women with pulmonary hypertension are cyanotic, placing the fetus at risk from chronic hypoxia.[4] There may be a risk of teratogenicity with the vasodilator bosentan, further emphasising the need for adequate contraception.[8]

Specific problems with contraceptive agents include:

■ Thrombosis: oestrogen-containing compounds are contraindicated in this group.

- Drug interactions: patients are usually on warfarin, which interacts with combined hormonal contraceptives. Deep intramuscular injections may lead to haematomas and are best avoided, e.g. medroxyprogesterone acetate (Depo-Provera® (Pharmacia, Surrey)).
- Vasovagal: in one study,[9] insertion of an intrauterine device (IUD) through the cervix led to a vasovagal episode in 1.2% of women. Larger IUDs are associated with an even higher frequency of bradycardia.[10] Bradycardias may be poorly tolerated in pulmonary hypertension and can lead to circulatory collapse.
- General anaesthetic: this can be challenging in a cyanotic patient and carries a high risk of morbidity and mortality

The most suitable method is the subdermal progestogen implant Implanon® (Organon, Cambridge), although the progestogen-only pill (POP) can also be used. Increased doses are required if the patient is on bosentan as this drug is an enzyme inducer that reduces the efficacy of some progestogens.[11] Vasectomy should not be recommended, as the male will usually outlive his partner.

Severe left heart obstruction

In severe left heart obstruction there is an obstruction to the outflow of blood from the heart, resulting in maternal hypotension and a fixed cardiac output. Pregnancy can result in left ventricular dilatation and eventually failure. Valvular heart disease in particular predisposes to infective endocarditis. Contraceptive agents that can cause a bacteraemia such as IUDs at the time of insertion should be covered with antibiotics[12] and have recently been reclassified as WHO 3 in cases of complicated valvular heart disease.[3] Copper devices are associated with a small risk of causing infection (pelvic inflammatory disease) during long-term use, but this risk appears to be lower with newer devices releasing progestogen, such as the levonorgestrel intrauterine system (Mirena® (Schering Health Care, Burgess Hill, West Sussex)).

Marfan syndrome

Aortic dissection is a particular risk in women with Marfan syndrome with aortic root dilatation greater than 4 cm, or a rapidly dilating aorta.[13,14] Type A (ascending) aortic dissection has a 22% mortality rate in pregnancy.[15] Pregnancy should be avoided in such women until an aortic root replacement procedure has been performed. Beta blockers and antihypertensives are the mainstay of treatment and hence any agent potentially causing hypertension should be avoided, for example combined hormonal contraceptives (WHO 3).

Contraceptive agents

There is a range of contraceptive agents suitable for each cardiac condition. The one recommended for use should be tailored according to the individual's particular circumstances. The following points should be considered when deciding on the most appropriate contraceptive agent:

- degree of efficacy of the method
- thrombotic risks of oestrogen-containing contraceptives

- hypertensive risks of oestrogen-containing contraceptives
- infective risks with insertion of an IUD
- vagal stimulation with insertion of an IUD
- bleeding risks with patients on warfarin (copper IUDs, intramuscular injections)
- effects of anaesthesia.

Efficacy of use of contraceptive agents

Very few women use a contraceptive agent perfectly and consistently exactly in accordance with the product instructions. Most women fall into the category of 'typical use', where they occasionally use the method incorrectly.[1] Pregnancy rates for typical users are therefore a better reflection of the efficacy that can be expected from a contraceptive (Table 2.4). There is a paucity of data on pregnancy rates with typical use in the UK and most data are obtained from studies in the USA.[1] Only the most reliable contraceptive methods should be recommended for those with class 3 or 4 risk.

The contraceptive methods that will be considered in detail below are those where fewer than 10% of women conceive in the first year of typical use.

Table 2.5 shows the relative advisability of various contraceptive methods in common or difficult cardiac clinical conditions.

Female sterilisation

Sterilisation used to be considered the most effective form of contraception before the development of newer, safer progestogen-based contraceptive agents.[16,17] It is considered to be permanent but is not without risks, resulting in it being rated as WHO 2. The disadvantages of female sterilisation include:

- usually requires general anaesthetic
- a failure rate of 1:200
- in failures there is a higher risk of ectopic pregnancies, which can rupture and result in severe haemorrhage and pain
- the psychological effect and a risk of regret.

This procedure is usually performed laparoscopically and involves:

- instrumentation of the cervix which may result in a vasovagal response
- creation of a carbon dioxide (CO_2) pneumoperitoneum, which reduces venous return and results in CO_2 being absorbed systemically.

Laparoscopy is thus not appropriate for women with pulmonary vascular disease or a Fontan circulation who do not tolerate a reduction in venous return. A bradycardia may prove fatal in those with pulmonary vascular disease. Those with right to left shunts can develop paradoxical emboli from CO_2 gas.[18] Using regional anaesthesia with a reduced amount of CO_2 may combat some of these problems but requires skilled operators.[19] A safer method for high-risk individuals is probably a mini-laparotomy, which can be performed under regional block.

Sterilisation at the time of caesarean section should definitely be considered for those women who are at grave risk from a future pregnancy, such as those with peripartum cardiomyopathy, or those who have completed their families and in whom a

Table 2.4. Efficacy of contraceptive methods with typical and perfect use; adapted with permission from WHO[2]

Contraceptive method	% of women experiencing an unintended pregnancy within first year of use	
	Typical use	Perfect use
No method	85	85
Spermicides	29	18
Withdrawal	27	4
Periodic abstinence	25	
Calendar		9
Ovulation method		3
Symptothermal		2
Post-ovulation		1
Cap		
Parous women	32	26
Nulliparous women	16	9
Sponge		
Parous women	32	20
Nulliparous women	16	9
Diaphragm	16	6
Condom		
Female	21	5
Male	15	2
COC and POP	8	0.3
Combined hormonal patch (Evra®)	8	0.3
Combined hormonal ring (NuvaRing®)	8	0.3
Depo-Provera®	3	0.3
Combined injectable (Lunelle™)	3	0.05
IUD		
Copper T	0.8	0.6
Mirena® IUS	0.1	0.1
Implanon®	0.05	0.05
Female sterilisation	0.5	0.5
Male sterilisation	0.15	0.15

The shaded area indicates that the contraceptive methods are not reliable for women with heart disease in class 2–4
COC = combined oral contraceptive; IUD = intrauterine device; IUS = intrauterine system; POP = progestogen-only pill

future pregnancy would be at least class 3. The conventionally performed bilateral tubal ligation is associated with a higher failure rate than an interval procedure.[17] Bilateral salpingectomy is a more secure method of contraception and one that cannot be reversed.

ESSURE is a newer sterilisation method in which intra-tubal stents are inserted into the proximal section of the fallopian tube hysteroscopically, requiring only oral analgesia.[20] They rely on mechanical obstruction and stimulation of tissue ingrowth by an inflammatory process to effect tubal occlusion within 3 months. The insertion

Table 2.5. WHO class for contraceptive methods in specific clinical conditions; reproduced with permission from Thorne et al.[3]

Clinical condition[a] WHO class	Combined hormonal methods (oestrogen-containing)	POP ('minipill')	Cerazette®	Implanon®	Depo-Provera®	Mirena® IUS	Standard IUCD	Emergency hormonal contraception
Physiological murmur	1	1	1	1	1	1	1	1
Paroxysmal atrial fibrillation (even on warfarin[b]) with structurally normal heart	3	1	1	1	1 (3 on warfarin[b])	1	1	1
Repaired tetralogy of Fallot without complications	1	1	1	1	1	1	2	1
Unoperated atrial septal defect	3	1	1	1	1	1	1	1
Dilated cardiomyopathy	4	(1)[c]	1	1	1 (3 on warfarin[b])	1	1	1
Moderate aortic stenosis	2	1	1	1	1	2	3	1
Bjork–Shiley mitral valve replacement[c]	4	1	1	1	3	3	4	1
Bileaflet mitral valve replacement[c]	3	1	1	1	3	3	4	1
Cyanotic heart disease without pulmonary hypertension	4	(1)[c]	1	1	2 (3 on warfarin[b])	2	3	1
Eisenmenger syndrome and pulmonary hypertension of any cause	4	(1)[c]	1	1	1	4 (3[d])	4	1
Fontan circulation even on warfarin[c]	4	(1)[c]	1	1	3	4 (3[d])	4	1

a Refer to sections on specific contraceptive methods for more information

b Warfarin: requires care with monitoring internationalised normalised ratio (INR), which may alter with both oestrogen and progestogen hormone therapy; with Depo-Provera there is a specific risk of local haematoma (see text)

c Although safe, the limited efficacy of the POP limits its use in women in whom pregnancy carries a particular risk (class 3 or 4, as in Tables 2.2 and 2.3)

d May be used if no other method is suitable and the risk of pregnancy outweighs the risk of insertion

IUCD = intrauterine contraceptive device; IUS = intrauterine system; POP = progestogen-only pill of the hysteroscope requires a greater degree of cervical dilatation than with coil insertion, accounting for the slightly higher risk of vasovagal attacks (1.85%).[21]

Male sterilisation

A vasectomy is clearly the safest method of contraception for the woman as well as being more efficacious than female sterilisation. It should, however, be considered very carefully if it is to be used as contraception in the partner of a woman with severe heart disease. Her lifespan will be significantly reduced and he may wish to father children in the future with a new partner.

Combined hormonal contraceptives

These are combinations of oestradiol and a progestogen which inhibit ovulation and are therefore very effective contraceptives. The three types are:

■ the combined oral contraceptive (COC) pill
■ the combined contraceptive skin patch (Evra®; Janssen-Cilag, High Wycombe, Bucks), which contains ethinyl oestradiol and norelgestromin.
■ the combined contraceptive vaginal ring (NuvaRing®; Organon, Cambridge), which contains ethinyl oestradiol and etonogestrel (licensed in other countries but not yet available in the UK).

Table 2.6 shows the WHO risk classification for combined hormonal contraceptive use in various cardiac conditions.[3] The main risks in heart disease are due to the thrombogenic potential, both arterial and venous, because of the oestrogen component:

■ Arterial thrombosis: the risks of ischaemic stroke[22] and ischaemic heart disease are increased if there are additional risk factors such as smoking, hypertension, diabetes and obesity.[23,24] Migraine, particularly if focal or associated with an aura, is an additional risk factor for ischaemic stroke.[24]
■ Cardiac thrombosis: with atrial fibrillation, dilated cardiomyopathy, mechanical heart valves. Anticoagulation may not protect fully if combined hormonal contraception is used.[3]
■ Venous thrombosis:[22] deep vein thrombosis (DVT) can result in paradoxical emboli causing stroke in those with pulmonary arteriovenous malformations, cyanotic heart disease due to right to left shunts or patent foramen ovale (PFO).[25]

There is also a risk from the interaction with warfarin metabolism of both oestrogens and progestogens: the internationalised normalised ratio (INR) needs to be monitored more frequently when initiating treatment.

Patent foramen ovale is associated with embolic stroke.[26] It occurs in 10–20% of the population, who usually remain asymptomatic and are thus often undiagnosed.[27] In PFO there is a theoretical risk of paradoxical embolism. An expert group has recommended that combined hormonal contraceptives be graded WHO 2 in such circumstances.[3] Those in whom PFO was diagnosed following an embolic stroke or neurological decompression sickness after diving are WHO 4.

Table 2.6. WHO risk classification for the use of combined hormonal contraceptives (combined oral contraceptive (COC) pill, Evra® and NuvaRing®) in women with various cardiac conditions; reproduced with permission from Thorne et al.[3]

WHO 1 Always usable	WHO 2 Broadly usable	WHO 3 Caution in use[a]	WHO 4 Do not use
■ Physiological murmurs in the absence of heart disease	■ Most arrhythmias other than atrial fibrillation or flutter	■ Atrial fibrillation or flutter on warfarin[b]	■ Atrial fibrillation or flutter, if not anticoagulated
■ Mitral valve prolapse with only trivial mitral regurgitation	■ Uncomplicated mild native mitral and aortic valve disease	■ Bileaflet mechanical valve in mitral or aortic position if taking warfarin[b]	■ Bjork–Shiley or Starr–Edwards valves even if taking warfarin
■ Bicuspid aortic valve with normal function	■ Tissue prosthetic valve lacking any of the features noted in WHO 3 and 4 columns	■ Atrial septal defect with left to right shunt that may reverse with physiological stress, e.g. Valsalva manoeuvre	■ Pulmonary hypertension or pulmonary vascular disease, e.g. Eisenmenger syndrome
■ Mild pulmonary stenosis	■ Surgically corrected congenital heart disease lacking any of the features noted in WHO 3 and 4 columns	■ Repaired coarctation with aneurysm and/or hypertension	■ Dilated left atrium > 4 cm
■ Repaired aortic coarctation with no hypertension or aneurysm	■ Small left to right shunt not reversible with physiological manoeuvres, e.g. small ventricular septal defect, small patent ductus arteriosus	■ Marfan syndrome with unoperated aortic dilatation	■ The Fontan heart[c] even if taking warfarin
■ Other simple lesions successfully repaired in childhood and with no sequelae, such as ostium secundum atrial septal defect, ventricular septal defect, patent ductus arteriosus or total anomalous pulmonary venous drainage	■ Uncomplicated Marfan syndrome	■ Past thromboembolic event if taking warfarin[b]	■ Cyanotic heart disease even if taking warfarin
	■ Hypertrophic cardiomyopathy lacking any of the features noted in the WHO 3 and 4 columns		■ Pulmonary arteriovenous malformation
	■ Past cardiomyopathy, fully recovered, including peripartum cardiomyopathy		■ Past thromboembolic event (venous or arterial), not taking warfarin
			■ Poor left ventricular function of any cause, e.g. dilated cardiomyopathy (ejection fraction <30%)
			■ Coronary artery disease
			■ Coronary arteritis, e.g. previous Kawasaki disease with coronary involvement

[a] WHO 3: carefully consider all alternatives, which are usually preferable first; exceptions if (i) the patient accepts the risks and rejects the alternatives, or (ii) the risk of pregnancy is very high and the only acceptable alternative methods are less effective

[b] Warfarin: requires care with monitoring internationalised normalised ratio (INR), which may alter with both oestrogen and progestogen hormone therapy

[c] Fontan operation for tricuspid atresia and other conditions where there is only one functional ventricle; the single ventricle is used to support the systemic circulation; this results in a low cardiac output and hypercoagulable circulation

NB. In the presence of any feature listed in columns 3 or 4, the more exclusive category should be applied; for example, mitral valve disease with dilated left atrium moves to WHO 4; furthermore, the presence of two or more features in the WHO 2 or 3 columns or the addition of an independent risk factor such as smoking or hypertension generally contraindicates COC use (i.e. WHO 4)

Progestogen-only methods

The progestogen-only methods include:

- progestogen-only pills (POP)
- Depo-Provera (medroxyprogesterone acetate)
- Mirena intrauterine system (IUS) (levonorgestrel)
- Implanon subcutaneous progestogen implant (etonogestrel)

Progestogen-only contraceptive methods are far safer for women with heart disease than methods using oestrogens as they are not associated with an increase in arterial or venous thrombosis.[28-30] They are often considered the contraceptives of choice in women with severe cardiovascular or pulmonary vascular disease (see Table 2.1). The main problems with these methods are:

- irregular vaginal bleeding for a variable duration
- interaction with warfarin metabolism
- reduced contraceptive efficacy of some types if used with bosentan, which is an enzyme inducer (Table 2.7)[11]
- simple ovarian cysts.

The advantages of these methods include a variable reduction in menstrual loss after continued use, which is helpful to those with cyanotic heart disease who are intolerant of anaemia from menorrhagia, and to those on warfarin, which may itself cause menorrhagia. Table 2.8 shows the safety of various progestogen-only contraceptives in women with heart disease.

Progestogen-only pills

Progestogen-only pills (POP) do not inhibit ovulation and need to be taken at approximately the same time each day. If pill taking is delayed (e.g. forgotten) for longer than 3 hours after the due time, the risk of contraceptive failure starts to rise. This makes them a less reliable method than other progestogen-only contraceptives and they should thus not be used in women with major heart diseases.

Table 2.7. Effect of bosentan on the efficacy of progestogen-only contraceptives

Progestogen-only contraceptive	Efficacy with bosentan	Use in pulmonary vascular disease
Progestogen-only pill (POP)	Reduced	Avoid
Cerazette®	Reduced	Increase dose
Depo-Provera®	Not affected	Avoid if on warfarin
Mirena® intrauterine system (IUS)	Not affected	Avoid
Implanon®	Reduced	Add Cerazette

Table 2.8. Safety of progestogen-only contraceptive methods in women with heart disease; reproduced with permission from Thorne et al.[3]

Progestogen-only contraceptive method[a]	Cardiac condition	Class
Standard POP[b]	All cardiac patients	1
Cerazette® POP[c]	All cardiac patients	1
Medroxyprogesterone acetate (Depo-Provera®)	All cardiac patients not on warfarin	1
	All cardiac patients taking warfarin[d]	3
Implanon®[c]	All cardiac patients	1
Mirena® IUS	Cardiac patients generally, even if taking warfarin[a]	1
	Structural heart disease,[e] except as below 2	
	Prosthetic heart valves[a,e] 3	
	Previous endocarditis 3	
	Pulmonary hypertension, Fontan circulation, or other condition in which vagal reaction at insertion would be poorly tolerated[f]	4 (3)
Emergency contraception (Levonelle®)	All cardiac disease[c]	1

[a] Warfarin: requires care with monitoring internationalised normalised ratio (INR), which may alter after initiation of any progestogen hormone therapy; the effect of the exceptionally low levonorgestrel blood levels with Mirena IUS is unknown, but is likely to be minimal

[b] Although safe, the standard progestogen-only pill is less effective than all the other progestogen-only methods; it should not normally be advised where pregnancy poses a high or unacceptable risk (class 3 and 4 conditions)

[c] Efficacy reduced by bosentan; see text

[d] Risk of large haematoma at site of injection

[e] If used, appropriate parenteral antibiotic cover (see the British National Formulary[®]) is advised to prevent endocarditis following insertion

[f] See text; may be used if no other method is suitable and the risk of pregnancy outweighs the risk of insertion

IUS = intrauterine system; POP = progestogen-only pill

Cerazette

Cerazette® (Organon, Cambridge) (desogestrel 75 μg) is a newer POP causing anovulation with a similar efficacy to the COC.[31] The risk of contraceptive failure does not increase until 12 hours after a due pill has been forgotten, increasing the time when the woman can remember to take the pill and restore contraceptive efficacy. This pill is therefore suitable to be used by women with major heart disease. Cerazette is a prodrug for the etonogestrel used in the Implanon contraceptive implant. It can therefore be used to test a woman's tolerance of the hormone before inserting the implant. Cerazette can be used at high doses in women on bosentan (WHO 3).

Depo-Provera

Depo-Provera is a highly effective deep intramuscular injectable contraceptive that lasts for 12 weeks. Its use is limited in women on anticoagulants who may develop haematomas at the injection site (WHO 3). It is not affected by bosentan but women on this drug are also likely to be on warfarin. Depo-Provera can result in a hypooestrogenic status with long-term use and this may have implications for women with, or women at risk of, ischaemic heart disease.[32]

Mirena IUS

The Mirena IUS is an intrauterine device that is inserted into the uterus (its insertion sometimes requires cervical dilatation). It is more effective than sterilisation.[2] It releases 20 μg/day of levonorgestrel directly into the uterus. This causes endometrial shedding, which can result in light irregular per vaginal bleeding for 3–6 months. This can be problematic for some women but, if tolerated, usually settles resulting in a thin or absent endometrium and hence light or non-existent periods. Progestogenic adverse effects are minimal as only a small amount of the hormone is absorbed systemically.

This is an excellent contraceptive for woman with heart disease except those with peripheral vascular disease or a Fontan circulation, or any other woman who cannot tolerate the vagal response that sometimes accompanies insertion. If used in such women, the insertion should be performed in hospital with an anaesthetist present who can administer atropine if necessary, although this does not guarantee safety if there is a severe bradycardia. The incidence of bradycardia is greater with IUS insertion than with copper intrauterine contraceptive devices (IUCDs). This may be due to the larger size of the IUS.[33] Women should be screened for sexually transmitted infections (STIs) or empirically covered with antibiotics. Those at risk of bacterial endocarditis should be given appropriate antibiotic prophylaxis for insertion. The progestogens actually result in thicker cervical mucus, which tends to prevent infections with long-term use of the Mirena, unlike the copper coils. It requires replacement after 5 years.

Implanon

The Implanon subdermal device is more effective than sterilisation[2] and is the safest form of contraception for those with peripheral vascular disease. It is, like the Mirena IUS, well tolerated in those with major heart disease. It is inserted, by trained operators, into the subdermal tissue of the non-dominant arm under local anaesthetic. There is less risk of haematoma formation than with Depo-Provera and thus it can be inserted in women on warfarin who simply need to apply pressure to the insertion site for 5 minutes to prevent bleeding. Blood levels are also steadier than with Depo-Provera, which leads to fewer progestogenic adverse effects. Twenty percent of women are rendered amenorrhoeic after 2 years but irregular menstrual bleeding can be problematic after insertion and is often the reason why women request removal.[34] Implanon requires removal and replacement after 3 years. In those with peripheral vascular disease on bosentan, Cerazette should be added to improve the efficacy (see Table 2.7).

Copper intrauterine contraceptive devices

Copper-containing coils are an effective form of contraception and are inserted into the uterus after cervical dilatation. The major advantage of banded copper IUCDs is that they only require replacement after 5–10 years. The risks associated with this method of contraception are:

■ infection at the time of insertion and with long-term use

■ a vasovagal response with insertion (less frequent than with the Mirena IUS)
■ menorrhagia.

These devices should therefore be avoided in those with pulmonary vascular disease or previous bacterial endocarditis. Women should be screened for STIs before insertion or empirically treated. They should be used with caution in those with complicated valvular disease, where, if used, insertion should be covered with antibiotics. Caution is also necessary in those taking anticoagulation medication because of the risk of menorrhagia (WHO 3).

Emergency contraception

It is essential that emergency contraception be available for women who fail to take appropriate precautions against unwanted pregnancy, particularly if they have a serious heart condition. It should not be used as a regular form of contraception because of the high annual failure rate associated with such an approach.

There are three methods available (Table 2.9), although levonorgestrel (Levonelle® (Schering Health Care, Burgess Hill, West Sussex)) is better tolerated and more effective than the combined oestrogen–progestogen (Yuzpe) regimen. It has a 1% failure rate if used within 72 hours of unprotected sexual intercourse (UPSI).[35] Common adverse effects are nausea (23%) and vomiting (6%). There is a reported interaction between warfarin and levonorgestrel resulting in an increase in the INR of up to four-fold. The Yuzpe regimen may be more appropriate in women anti-coagulated with warfarin.[36]

Barrier methods

Male and female condoms should not be considered as a very effective method for prevention of pregnancy, but should be encouraged to prevent STIs in combination with a more secure contraceptive method, i.e. as 'dual protection'.[2]

Table 2.9. Emergency contraception for women with heart disease

Emergency contraceptive	Use up to after UPSI	Caution	Additional points
Levonelle® (single-dose levonorgestrel 1.5 mg)	72 hours	Interaction with warfarin	If on bosentan, increase dose to 2.5–3.0 mg
Yuzpe regimen	72 hours	Nil as long as not used repeatedly	Although short-term exposure to oestrogen is unlikely to be harmful, Levonelle is just as effective
Copper IUCD	5 days	Pulmonary vascular disease, Fontan circulation	Cover with antibiotics if at risk of bacterial endocarditis

IUCD = intrauterine contraceptive device; UPSI = unprotected sexual intercourse

Termination of pregnancy

Urgent termination of pregnancy facilities should be readily available and accessible for women with medical conditions where pregnancy places their lives at risk.[37]

Medical termination of pregnancy

Medical termination of pregnancy can be performed throughout gestation. Mifepristone is given orally and is usually followed 1–2 days later with a prostaglandin (misoprostol or gemeprost). The advantages for women with heart disease are:

- if successful, it avoids the need for general anaesthetic that is usually used with surgical procedures
- the drugs used are generally safe for women with cardiac conditions.

The disadvantages of medical termination are:

- the procedure can take several days to complete
- there may be significant bleeding
- the termination may not be complete, requiring a surgical evacuation of the uterus
- the procedure can be painful over a longer duration
- bleeding and pain can cause a tachycardia that may not be tolerated in conditions such as pulmonary vascular disease and severe mitral stenosis
- the expulsion of products of conception or the delivery of the fetus can have unpredictable timing.

Surgical termination of pregnancy

Surgical termination of pregnancy can be performed by suction at up to 14 weeks of gestation, or dilatation and evacuation at more advanced gestations (up to 24 weeks). The procedure may require cervical priming with a prostaglandin. The advantages for women with heart disease are:

- the timing of surgery can be planned
- the analgesia requirements are easily dealt with
- there is less risk of continued bleeding and pain
- it can be performed under regional blockade.

The disadvantages of surgical termination include:

- the risks of surgery include perforation of the uterus, infection and bleeding
- it requires skilled operators
- it involves cervical dilatation.

Conclusion

Women with cardiac disease should be counselled regarding contraception. There is a vast array of contraceptive agents available, which vary in efficacy, risks of thrombosis, hypertension and infection, interactions with other drugs and ease of use. They should be appropriately tailored for each individual, taking into account the severity of the condition and the impact any adverse effects of the contraceptive may have on the disease. Emergency contraception should be offered in the event of unprotected intercourse and urgent termination of pregnancy facilities should be available for medical conditions where pregnancy places a woman's life at risk.

References

1. de Swiet M, Nelson-Piercy C. Cardiac disease. In: Lewis G, editor. *Why Mothers Die 2000–2002: the 6th Report of the Confidential Enquiries into Maternal Deaths in the United Kingdom*. London: RCOG Press; 2004.
2. World Health Organization. *Improving Access to Quality Care in Family Planning: Medical Eligibility Criteria for Contraceptive Use (Revised)*. Geneva: WHO; 2004.
3. Thorne S, Nelson-Piercy C, MacGregor A, Gibbs S, Crowhurst J, Panay N, et al. Pregnancy and contraception in heart disease and pulmonary arterial hypertension. *J Fam Plann Reprod Health Care* 2006;32:75–81.
4. Presbitero P, Somerville J, Stone S, Aruta E, Spiegelhalter D, Rabajoli F. Pregnancy in cyanotic congenital heart disease. *Circulation* 1994;89:2673–6.
5. The Task Force on Diagnosis and Treatment of Pulmonary Arterial Hypertension of the European Society of Cardiology. Guidelines on diagnosis and treatment of pulmonary arterial hypertension. *Eur Heart J* 2004;25:2243–78.
6. McQuillan BM, Picard MH, Leavitt M, Weyman AE. Clinical correlates and reference intervals for pulmonary artery systolic pressure among echocardiographically normal subjects. *Circulation* 2001;104:2797–802.
7. Outcome of pulmonary vascular disease in pregnancy: a systematic overview from 1978 through 1996. *J Am Coll Cardiol* 1998;31:1650–7.
8. Segal ES, Valette C, Oster L, Bouley L, Edfjall C, Herrmann P, et al. Risk management strategies in the postmarketing period: safety experience with the US and European bosentan surveillance programmes. *Drug Saf* 2005;28:971–80.
9. Farmer M, Webb A. Intrauterine device insertion-related complications: can they be predicted? *J Fam Plann Reprod Health Care* 2003;29:227–31.
10. Aznar R, Reynoso L, Ley E, Gamez R, De Leon MD. Electrocardiographic changes induced by insertion of an intrauterine device and other uterine manipulations. *Fertil Steril* 1976;27:92–6.
11. Dingemanse J, van Giersbergen PL. Clinical pharmacology of bosentan, a dual endothelin receptor antagonist. *Clin Pharmacokinet* 2004;43:1089–115.
12. Murray S, Hickey JB, Houang E. Significant bacteremia associated with replacement of intrauterine contraceptive device. *Am J Obstet Gynecol* 1987;156:698–700.
13. Lind J, Wallenburg HC. The Marfan syndrome and pregnancy: a retrospective study in a Dutch population. *Eur J Obstet Gynecol Reprod Biol* 2001;98:28–35.
14. Elkayam U, Ostrzega E, Shotan A, Mehra A. Cardiovascular problems in pregnant women with the Marfan syndrome. *Ann Intern Med* 1995;123:117–22.
15. Weiss BM, von Segesser LK, Alon E, Seifert B, Turina MI. Outcome of cardiovascular surgery and pregnancy: a systematic review of the period 1984–1996. *Am J Obstet Gynecol* 1998;179(6 Pt 1):1643–53.
16. Peterson HB, Xia Z, Hughes JM, Wilcox LS, Tylor LR, Trussell J. The risk of pregnancy after tubal sterilisation: findings from the U.S. Collaborative Review of Sterilisation [CREST study]. *Am J Obstet Gynecol* 1996;174:1161–70.
17. Royal College of Obstetricians and Gynaecologists. *Male and Female Sterilisation. Evidence-based Clinical Guidelines No. 4*. London: RCOG Press; 2003.

18. Sammut MS, Paes ML. Anaesthesia for laparoscopic cholecystectomy in a patient with Eisenmenger's syndrome. *Br J Anaesth* 1997;79:810–12.

19. Snabes MC, Poindexter AN 3rd. Laparoscopic tubal sterilisation under local anaesthesia in women with cyanotic heart disease. *Obstet Gynecol* 1991;78(3 Pt 1):437–40.

20. Duffy S, Marsh F, Rogerson L, Hudson H, Cooper K, Jack S, et al. Female sterilisation: a cohort controlled comparative study of ESSURE versus laparoscopic sterilisation. *BJOG* 2005;112:1522–8.

21. Agostini A, Bretelle F, Ronda I, Roger V, Cravello L, Blanc B. Risk of vasovagal syndrome during outpatient hysteroscopy. *J Am Assoc Gynecol Laparosc* 2004;11:245–7.

22. World Health Organization Collaborative Study of Cardiovascular Disease and Steroid Hormone Contraception. Venous thromboembolic disease and combined oral contraceptives: results of an international multicentre case–control study. *Lancet* 1995;346:1575–82.

23. World Health Organization Collaborative Study of Cardiovascular Disease and Steroid Hormone Contraception. Acute myocardial infarction and combined oral contraceptives: results of an international multicentre case–control study. *Lancet* 1997;349:1202–9.

24. Lidegaard Ø. Oral contraceptives, pregnancy and risk of cerebral thromboembolism: the influence of diabetes, hypertension, migraine and previous thrombotic disease. *Br J Obstet Gynaecol* 1995;102:153–9.

25. de Swiet J. Paradoxical embolism associated with oral contraceptives: an underdiagnosed lesion? *Postgrad Med J* 1979;55:419–20.

26. Lechat P, Mas JL, Lascault G, Loron P, Theard M, Klimczac M, et al. Prevalence of patent foramen ovale in patients with stroke. *N Engl J Med* 1988;318:1148–52.

27. Kerut EK, Norfleet WT, Plotnick GD, Giles TD. Patent foramen ovale: a review of associated conditions and the impact of physiological size. *J Am Coll Cardiol* 2001;38:613–23.

28. Vasilakis C, Jick H, del Mar Melero-Montes M. Risk of idiopathic venous thromboembolism in users of progestogens alone. *Lancet* 1999;354:1610–11.

29. World Health Organization Collaborative Study of Cardiovascular Disease and Steroid Hormone Contraception. Cardiovascular disease and use of oral and injectable progestogen-only contraceptives and combined injectable contraceptives. Results of an international, multicenter, case–control study. *Contraception* 1998;57:315–24.

30. Heinemann LAJ, Assman A, DoMinh T, Garbe E. Oral progestogen-only contraceptives and cardiovascular risk: results from the Transnational Study on Oral Contraceptives and the Health of Young Women. *Eur J Contracept Reprod Health Care* 1999;4:67–73.

31. Korver T, Klipping C, Heger-Mahn D, Duijkers I, van Osta G, Dieben T. Maintenance of ovulation inhibition with the 75-microg desogestrel-only contraceptive pill (Cerazette) after scheduled 12-h delays in tablet intake. *Contraception* 2005;71:8–13.

32. Sorensen MB, Collins P, Ong PJL, Webb CM, Hayward CS, Asbury EA, et al. Long-term use of contraceptive depot medroxyprogesterone acetate in young women impairs arterial endothelial function assessed by cardiovascular magnetic resonance. *Circulation* 2002;106:1646–51.

33. Harrison-Woolrych M, Zhou L, Coulter D. Insertion of intrauterine devices: a comparison of experience with Mirena and Multiload Cu 375 during post-marketing monitoring in New Zealand. *N Z Med J* 2003;116:U538.

34. Funk S, Miller MM, Mishell DR Jr, Archer DF, Poindexter A, Schmidt J, et al. The Implanon US Study Group. Safety and efficacy of Implanon, a single-rod implantable contraceptive containing etonogestrel. *Contraception* 2005;71:319–26.

35. Task Force on Postovulatory Methods of Fertility Regulation. Randomised controlled

trial of levonorgestrel versus the Yuzpe regimen of combined oral contraceptives for emergency contraception. *Lancet* 1998;352:428–33.

36. Ellison J, Thomson AJ, Greer IA. Drug points: apparent interaction between warfarin and levonorgestrel used for emergency contraception. *BMJ* 2000;321:1382.

37. Royal College of Obstetricians and Gynaecologists. *The Care of Women Requesting Induced Abortion. Evidence-based Guideline No. 7.* London: RCOG Press; 2004.

Section 2

Antenatal care general considerations

Chapter 3

Cardiovascular changes in normal pregnancy

Emily Gelson, Onome Ogueh and Mark Johnson

Introduction

Physiological adaptation to pregnancy is the most rapid and profound change that a woman's body will undergo in her lifetime. Cardiac output increases by 50% and blood volume by 25% in association with a considerable increase in the blood flow to the kidneys, skin and uterus. It is assumed that these changes are essential for a normal pregnancy, as women with cardiac and renal disease are less able to sustain a viable pregnancy. We do not understand how these changes are regulated or how they interrelate in early pregnancy in normal women, still less in women with pre-existing heart disease. Such an understanding is essential before reasoned management plans for women with heart disease embarking on pregnancy can be formulated.

Cardiovascular system adaptations

The key elements of the cardiovascular adaptation to pregnancy are changes in peripheral resistance, cardiac output and blood volume. It is probable that the initial step in the cardiovascular adaptation to pregnancy is a fall in peripheral resistance in response to increased circulating levels of oestrogens or vasodilatory peptides and factors such as calcitonin gene-related peptide (CGRP) and nitric oxide (NO).[1,2] Studies of chronically catheterised baboons suggest that arterial and venous dilatation in the first trimester creates a relatively underfilled vascular state associated with a fall in blood pressure.[3] In the human, peripheral resistance falls to 70% of non-pregnant levels by 8 weeks of gestation.[4] This reduction is reflected in the fall in blood pressure that occurs in early pregnancy and which continues until the beginning of the third trimester when the blood pressure starts to rise again. It has been proposed that cardiac output and blood volume increase in response to this state of relative vascular underfill.[5]

Systemic vascular resistance

The systemic vascular resistance (SVR) falls to about 70% of its preconception value by 8 weeks of gestation.[4,6,7] In the study by Robson et al.,[8] there was a progressive fall from a prepregnancy value of 1326 (dyn s)/cm⁵ to 875 (dyn s)/cm⁵ at 20 weeks of gestation (i.e. a 34% fall). During the second half of pregnancy, total peripheral resistance showed a small but statistically significant increase, reaching 996 (dyn s)/cm^5 at 38 weeks of gestation (Figure 3.1). The SVR was estimated from the formula SVR ((dyn s)/cm^5) = 80 × mean arterial blood pressure (mmHg) / cardiac output (l/min).

Cardiac output

Doppler echocardiography is a non-invasive method of assessing haemodynamic changes in maternal circulation during normal gestation.[9] It is safe, does not cause any discomfort, is reproducible and accurate,[10] and has been validated against Fick, dye dilution, thermodilution methods and electromagnetic flow probes. Furthermore, the temporal variability of flow measurements using the non-invasive Doppler method is sufficiently small for it to be useful in serial haemodynamic studies.[10] The aortic site is the most reliable, and the pulsed wave method has the theoretical advantage that the position of the recording is known and can be repeated at approximately the same site.[11]

Spatling and colleagues[7] reported in 1992 an increase in the cardiac output from a median non-pregnant level of 2.6 to 3.8 l/min by 8–11 weeks of gestation, and a peak value of 4.7 l/min at 12–15 weeks. Thereafter, the levels remained more or less the same for the remainder of the pregnancy and puerperium. These values are lower than those reported from earlier studies, with Ueland and Hansen[12] having reported a cardiac output of 5.0 l/min in non-pregnant women, rising to 7.0 l/min at 28–32 weeks of

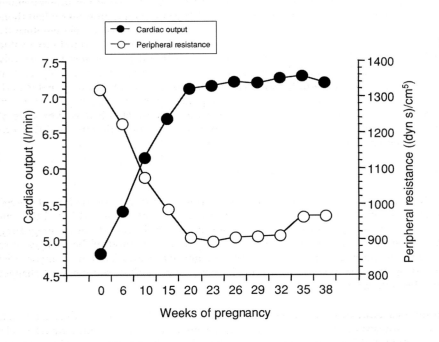

Figure 3.1. Peripheral resistance and cardiac output during pregnancy; data from Robson et al.[8]

the animal work of Davison and Lindheimer,[27] who have shown that renal enlargement during pregnancy in rats is caused by increased water content.

Renal blood flow

Effective renal plasma flow (ERPF), as estimated by the excretion of *para*-aminohippurate (PAH), is raised by 200–250 ml/min above that of non-pregnant women throughout early and mid-pregnancy, but is in the normal range near term.[28] Davison[29] found a 60–80% increase by mid-pregnancy, followed by about a 25% fall towards term. This pattern of change is in agreement with Dunlop,[30] who found an increase of 70–80% between conception and mid-pregnancy and then a decrease during the third trimester to a value still some 50–60% above non-pregnant norms. The terminal fall has been ascribed to the effect of the women being studied in the supine position.[31] However, Ezimokhai *et al.*[32] found a significant reduction in ERPF between the 29th and 39th week of pregnancy in women studied in the lateral recumbent position, suggesting that the late pregnancy decrease cannot be attributed solely to the effect of posture.

The gold standard for estimating renal blood flow is by measurement of PAH clearance. Unfortunately, this is an invasive and time-consuming procedure, making its use during pregnancy impracticable. In non-pregnant humans the clearance of radioactive isotopes can be used to measure renal plasma flow but the use of such substances in pregnancy is contraindicated. Doppler ultrasonography is a non-invasive technique that has been used serially to assess the renal vasculature during pregnancy.[33] In one study,[33] the pulsatility index, resistance index and the A/B (peak systolic waveform amplitude/end-diastolic amplitude) ratio of the Doppler waveform were measured. These indices were chosen because alterations in the vascular resistance are regarded as central to the increased renal blood flow known to occur during normal pregnancy. Indeed, it has been reported that the renal artery A/B ratio correlates significantly with both glomerular filtration rate (GFR) and ERPF, but the relationship was not precise enough to allow estimation of renal haemodynamics.[34] Nevertheless, an index of vascular resistance may be more sensitive to early disease than quantification of flow because pathological changes causing increased resistance may lead initially to increased cardiac contractility, thus maintaining flow until late in the disease process. For example, pulsatility index is increased early in renal allograft rejection because of inflammatory deposits within and around the vessel lumen.[35] The pulsatility index is also significantly increased in acute renal failure for a variety of reasons,[36] and a return to normal values predates the onset of diuresis by 24 to 48 hours.[37] In addition, the resistance index correlates significantly with the prevalence of arteriosclerosis and glomerular sclerosis, with and focal interstitial fibrosis in patients with renal parenchymal disease.[38]

Sturgiss *et al.*[33] did not find any significant difference between waveform indices from renal arteries in non-pregnant women and those women in early, middle or late pregnancy. There was also no significant change in the mean pulsatility index, resistance index or A/B ratio in the right and left, upper and lower, interlobar and interlobular arteries. This lack of significant change is surprising because of the large increase in renal blood flow during pregnancy and it is thought to be the result of reduced renal vascular resistance. It is likely, however, that waveform pulsatility reflects an interaction of several haemodynamic factors, many of which are altered by pregnancy.[33]

The augmentation of renal haemodynamics in pregnancy is difficult to explain. It may be due to an increased secretion of several hormones, including relaxin, placental lactogen, prolactin, progesterone and cortisol, which can alter the renal haemo-dynamics.[39] The current prime candidate is relaxin, which has been shown to increase both ERPF and GFR to levels seen in mid-pregnancy when infused into either non-pregnant women or male rats. Furthermore, the relaxin infusions provoked similar falls in plasma osmolality as seen during pregnancy (reviewed by Conrad and Novak[40]). However, attempts in the human to demonstrate an effect of relaxin have been unsuccessful as human chorionic gonadotrophin (hCG) failed to increase the circulating levels of relaxin to those seen during pregnancy.[41] It is also possible that the alteration of extracellular volume that occurs during pregnancy influences the GFR and ERPF.

Postpartum studies of the renal system have given conflicting results, with some indicating that the renal system returns rapidly to normal following delivery, and others indicating that dilatation persists for up to 3 months. The exact role of the various hormones in augmenting renal haemodynamics during human pregnancy still needs to be defined.

Uterine blood flow

The structure of the vessels of the uterus undergoes considerable modification during pregnancy and this influences the distribution of blood flow. The spiral arteries supplying the placenta dilate owing to physiological alterations in their structure and can reach 30 times their prepregnancy diameter. Before conception, the spiral arteries lie coiled in the myometrium and basal layers of the endometrium that are not shed at menstruation. They are normally muscular vessels, well able to respond to vasoactive stimuli. During pregnancy the majority of the spiral arteries in the placental bed lose this ability and dilate because of trophoblastic invasion destroying the muscular component, with dilatation being greater with increasing proximity to the placenta.[42] A wave of trophoblast invasion with villous trophoblast extending down the lumen of the decidual part of the vessel starts at 10 weeks of gestation and is complete by 16 weeks.[43] A second wave of endovascular trophoblastic invasion occurs at 16–22 weeks and extends more deeply to involve the myometrial portions of the spiral arteries. This increases the capacity of the spiral arteries and reduces or abolishes their capacity to respond to vasoactive stimuli.[44] Uterine blood flow increases progressively during pregnancy and the mean uterine flow in a singleton pregnancy at 34–40 weeks is 500–600 ml/min (Figure 3.3).[45,46]

Cardiac output is thought to peak at 20 weeks of gestation and to remain constant or decline thereafter (Figure 3.1). Thus any increase in uterine blood flow after 28 weeks must be dependent on a reduction in flow to other tissues secondary to an increase in peripheral resistance. Indeed, blood pressure does rise with advancing gestation (Figure 3.2) and it may be responsible for the increase in uterine perfusion. However, given that the perfusion of all organs except the kidney is thought to continue to rise or to remain static (Figure 3.3), it remains unclear which vascular bed constricts. Possible explanations are that the cardiac output continues to increase with advancing gestation, that there is indeed a marked process of vasoconstriction affecting peripheral vascular beds such as the renal and/or the cerebral vasculature, or that the initial fall in peripheral resistance is due to arteriovenous (AV) shunting which is then reversed with advancing gestation. Consistent with the last possibility is the fall in the AV pO_2 difference in early pregnancy, which reverses with advancing gestation (Figure 3.4). However, where these AV shunts are sited is also uncertain given that hand and foot perfusion (taken to reflect total skin perfusion) increase with

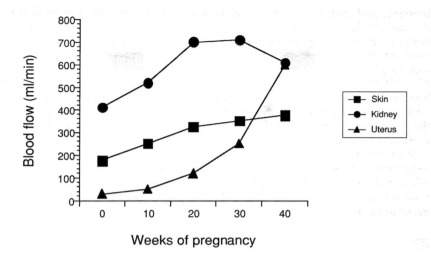

Figure 3.3. Blood flow to peripheral organs before and during pregnancy

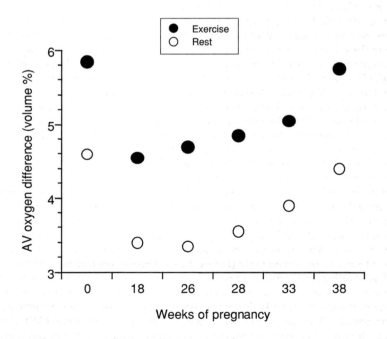

Figure 3.4. Arteriovenous (AV) oxygen difference before and during pregnancy; data from Bader et al.[13]

gestation and limb perfusion (taken to reflect muscle blood flow) is unchanged (Figure 3.5). Whatever mechanism is responsible, the blood pressure rises and this results in an increase in uterine perfusion.

The role of hormonal factors

The endocrine changes of pregnancy have been studied in detail but only rarely have they been correlated to physiological adaptations. Longo[47] suggested in 1983 that hormonal factors may be responsible for at least some of the physiological adaptations to pregnancy, but Spatling *et al.*[7] found no direct relationship between oestrogen and progesterone levels and the cardiac or respiratory changes of pregnancy. However, in support of Longo's hypothesis, relationships have been reported between the circulating levels of oestrogen, progesterone and relaxin and uterine perfusion, and between maternal levels of relaxin and the fetal heart rate.[48,49] The 'unifying hypothesis' suggests that peripheral vasodilation is a primary determinant of body fluid regulation in pregnancy,[5] triggering the haemodynamic and subsequent hormonal responses that result in sodium and water retention. It remains unclear what mediates such changes, although it is likely that the corpus luteum plays a role. This hypothesis is supported by studies of the haemodynamic and hormonal changes in the menstrual cycle and during *in vitro* fertilisation (IVF). Haemodynamic changes during the luteal phase of the

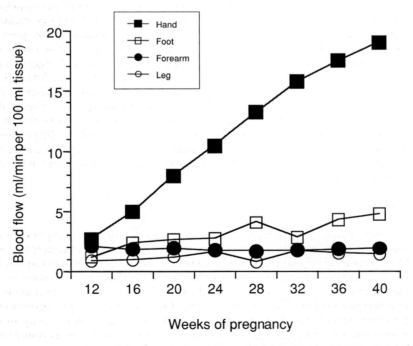

Figure 3.5. Blood flow to hand, foot, arm and leg from the end of the first trimester to 40 weeks of gestation; data from Ginsburg and Duncan[78]

menstrual cycle mimic those of early pregnancy, with arterial vasodilatation, reduced mean arterial pressure and increased cardiac output. These changes coincide with activation of the renin–angiotensin–aldosterone system (RAS). This suggests that changes seen in early pregnancy occur independently of the placenta and may thus be dependent on the corpus luteum. Increased oestrogen during the luteal phase, resulting in an increase in prostacyclin, may account for these haemodynamic changes.[50]

The role of the corpus luteum in circulatory dysfunction has been studied in women undergoing *in vitro* fertilisation. Ovarian hyperstimulation syndrome (OHSS) is a rare complication of ovulation induction, resulting in ascites, pleural effusion, hypo-volaemia, oliguria, electrolyte imbalance, haemoconcentration and hypercoagulability. This syndrome was initially explained by ovarian enlargement and a sudden increase in capillary permeability. However, peripheral arteriolar vasodilatation has since been identified as the initial trigger for the development of this syndrome.[51] Severe OHSS is associated with dramatically increased circulating plasma oestradiol levels. It has therefore been proposed that hyperoestrogenaemia may contribute to the circulatory dysfunction seen. Studies in asymptomatic patients have demonstrated that circulatory dysfunction is in fact a universal event in patients undergoing IVF, with decreasing peripheral vascular resistance, a fall in mean arterial pressure and an increased cardiac output seen following ovulation. These changes are mirrored by an increase in plasma oestradiol, with a delayed increase in plasma renin and aldosterone in one study (although not in an earlier smaller study).[51–54] If this dissociation is real then, given that the RAS seems to be activated from the middle of the luteal phase, perhaps either progesterone or relaxin are involved in inhibiting aldosterone action in the case of progesterone and altering renal haemodynamics in the case of relaxin.[40]

Chapman *et al.*[55] found a significant decrease during pregnancy in SVR associated with an increase in cardiac output at 6 weeks of gestation, well before placentation is completed at 12 weeks.[56] Therefore, they too suggested that maternal factors, possibly related to changes in ovarian function, are responsible for the initial peripheral vasodilatation found in human pregnancy.[55] This view is supported by changes in SVR and blood pressure found in pseudopregnant rats[57] and in women in the luteal phase compared with the follicular phase of the menstrual cycle as alluded to above.[50] It is possible that it is the free rather than the total levels of oestrogen and progesterone that are relevant to the induction of the physiological changes of pregnancy or that other factors are involved. Indeed, giving oestrogen pharmacologically only slightly increases cardiac output and plasma volume.[58] Other hormones such as relaxin, hCG and CGRP or factors such as asymmetric dimethylarginine (ADMA), an endogenous inhibitor of nitric oxide synthase, may also have a role.

Relaxin

During pregnancy, circulating relaxin is derived exclusively from the corpus luteum[59] and is regulated by gonadotrophin concentrations during the cycle of conception and by hCG during early pregnancy.[60] Circulating concentrations rise to a peak towards the end of the first trimester, then decline to a plateau and remain essentially unaltered for the remainder of pregnancy.[61] In the isolated rat atrial preparation, relaxin is the most potent inotrope and chronotrope agent known.[62] In addition, during pregnancy in the rat, it controls plasma osmolality and renal blood flow and reduces reactivity in the mesenteric arteries.[63,64] In humans, relaxin may initiate the fall in plasma osmolality[65] and it has been related to the fetal but not the maternal heart rate.[48]

Human chorionic gonadotrophin

Human chorionic gonadotrophin appears in the maternal circulation within a week of fertilisation and increases rapidly to peak levels by about the ninth week of pregnancy. It then falls rapidly to about one-tenth of the peak levels and stays at this level until the end of pregnancy. Uterine arteries contain hCG receptors.[66,67] The hormone stimulates the production of vasodilatory eicosanoids and decreases the production of vasoconstrictive eicosanoids in the uterine artery,[67] suggesting that hCG could be one of the hormones responsible for increased uterine blood flow during pregnancy. Plasma osmolality falls in early pregnancy following a resetting of the osmotic threshold at which vasopressin is released.[68] It has been suggested that this phenomenon is induced by hCG as its administration to non-pregnant women results in a reduction in plasma osmolality.[69]

Asymmetric dimethylarginine

Asymmetric dimethylarginine is synthesised in endothelial cells and inhibits nitric oxide synthase, thus reducing nitric oxide production. During pregnancy, its circulating levels fall initially but then rise with advancing gestation (Figure 3.6(a)).[70] The similarity in the pattern of change in ADMA levels and peripheral resistance during pregnancy suggests that they are related. Indeed, ADMA levels are related to mean arterial pressure in non-pregnant women, in normotensive pregnant women and in women with pre-eclampsia ($r^2 = 0.41$, $P = 0.0001$).[70] In vitro, endothelial cell production of ADMA declines with increasing oestradiol concentrations (Figure 3.6(b)).[71] This suggests that the initial decline in ADMA levels in early pregnancy may be related to the increase in circulating oestradiol levels, which inhibits endothelial ADMA production. As oestrogen levels increase with advancing gestation, the subsequent increase in ADMA is presumably from another source, possibly the placenta, as trophoblasts have been shown to produce ADMA in culture.[72]

Calcitonin gene-related peptide

Calcitonin gene-related peptide is a potent endogenous vasodilator that is thought to regulate peripheral blood flow. The administration of CGRP to rats in which a pre-eclampsia-like syndrome has been induced by the infusion of L-NAME reverses the pre-eclampsia. Conversely, infusion of a CGRP antagonist to pregnant rats increases blood pressure and induces fetal growth restriction.[73,74] These data suggest that during pregnancy in the rat CGRP may have a role in the regulation of blood pressure.

Flow-mediated dilatation

The vascular endothelium is a single layer of cells that lines blood vessels and is essential for the vasodilatation seen in response to increases in blood flow-associated shear stress. This process is called flow-mediated dilatation (FMD) and may play an important role in the reduction in peripheral resistance observed in pregnancy, since the increased blood flow results in greater shear stress at the vascular endothelial surface. There are multiple mechanisms involved in FMD, including increased NO release, prostacyclin and endothelium-derived hyperpolarisation factor (EDHF). The activity of all three is reported to be enhanced in various vascular beds during pregnancy (reviewed in Parkington et al.[75]). The response seems to be stimulus-

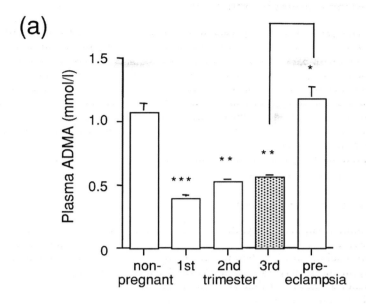

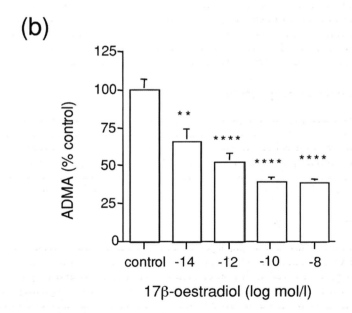

Figure 3.6. (a) Plasma concentrations of asymmetric dimethylarginine (ADMA) in normal pregnancy and pre-eclampsia; (b) effect of increasing oestradiol concentration on endothelial release of ADMA into culture supernatant; adapted with permission from (a) Holden *et al.*[70] and (b) Holden *et al.*[71]

specific, which in experimental models of FMD means the shear stress profile induced by the experimental model. Furthermore, the duration of the response is also important. In radial artery FMD, a brief shear stress stimulus results in an NO-dependent FMD, whereas a more prolonged stimulus of 15 minutes or longer results in FMD which is both NO- and prostaglandin-independent. Clearly, the prolonged stimulus of pregnancy may invoke even more mechanisms of FMD.[76] Indeed, it has been suggested that there is a sequential recruitment of mechanisms in response to flow,[77] but this hypothesis has yet to be tested.

Conclusion

The maternal adaptation to pregnancy described above is believed to be important for the normal outcome of pregnancy, especially given the relationship between blood pressure and fetal growth. Certainly, the outcome data from women with pre-existing heart disease suggests that impairment of cardiac function is associated with a relatively less good outcome of pregnancy. Equally, pregnancy may have a detrimental effect on women with pre-existing heart disease. The challenge now is to establish which cardiovascular changes are associated with normal pregnancy, particularly those that occur at the end of pregnancy and influence uterine blood flow. The impact of pre-existing heart disease on these changes can then be investigated, in the hope of being able to intervene to improve not only the fetal, but also the maternal, outcome of pregnancy.

References

1. Stevenson JC, Macdonald DW, Warren RC, Booker MW, Whitehead MI. Increased concentration of circulating calcitonin gene related peptide during normal human pregnancy. *Br Med J (Clin Res Ed)* 1986;293:1329–30.

2. Williams DJ, Vallance PJ, Neild GH, Spencer JA, Imms FJ. Nitric oxide-mediated vasodilation in human pregnancy. *Am J Physiol* 1997;272(2 Pt 2):H748–52.

3. Phippard AF, Horvath JS, Glynn EM, Garner MG, Fletcher PJ, Duggin GG, et al. Circulatory adaptation to pregnancy – serial studies of haemodynamics, blood volume, renin and aldosterone in the baboon (*Papio hamadryas*). *J Hypertens* 1986;4:773–9.

4. Capeless EL, Clapp JF. Cardiovascular changes in early phase of pregnancy. *Am J Obstet Gynecol* 1989;161(6 Pt 1):1449–53.

5. Schrier RW. Pathogenesis of sodium and water retention in high-output and low-output cardiac failure, nephrotic syndrome, cirrhosis, and pregnancy (2). *N Engl J Med* 1988;319:1127–34.

6. Clapp JF 3rd, Seaward BL, Sleamaker RH, Hiser J. Maternal physiologic adaptations to early human pregnancy. *Am J Obstet Gynecol* 1988;159:1456–60.

7. Spatling L, Fallenstein F, Huch A, Huch R, Rooth G. The variability of cardiopulmonary adaptation to pregnancy at rest and during exercise. *Br J Obstet Gynaecol* 1992;99;Suppl 8:1–40.

8. Robson SC, Hunter S, Boys RJ, Dunlop W. Serial study of factors influencing changes in cardiac output during human pregnancy. *Am J Physiol* 1989;256(4 Pt 2):H1060–5.

9. Katz R, Karliner JS, Resnik R. Effects of a natural volume overload state (pregnancy) on left ventricular performance in normal human subjects. *Circulation* 1978;58(3 Pt 1):434–41.

10. Robson SC, Boys RJ, Hunter S. Doppler echocardiographic estimation of cardiac output: analysis of temporal variability. *Eur Heart J* 1988;9:313–18.

11. Mabie WC, DiSessa TG, Crocker LG, Sibai BM, Arheart KL. A longitudinal study of cardiac output in normal human pregnancy. *Am J Obstet Gynecol* 1994;170:849–56.

12. Ueland K, Hansen JM. Maternal cardiovascular dynamics. II. Posture and uterine contractions. *Am J Obstet Gynecol* 1969;103:1–7.

13. Bader RA, Bader ME, Rose DF, Braunwald E. Hemodynamics at rest and during exercise in normal pregnancy as studies by cardiac catheterization. *J Clin Invest* 1955;34:1524–36.

14. Easterling TR, Benedetti TJ, Schmucker BC, Millard SP. Maternal hemodynamics in normal and preeclamptic pregnancies: a longitudinal study. *Obstet Gynecol* 1990;76:1061–9.

15. Laird-Meeter K, van de Ley G, Bom TH, Wladimiroff JW, Roelandt J. Cardiocirculatory adjustments during pregnancy – an echocardiographic study. *Clin Cardiol* 1979;2:328–32.

16. Mashini IS, Albazzaz SJ, Fadel HE, Abdulla AM, Hadi HA, Harp R, *et al.* Serial noninvasive evaluation of cardiovascular hemodynamics during pregnancy. *Am J Obstet Gynecol* 1987;156:1208–13.

17. Robson SC, Dunlop W, Boys RJ, Hunter S. Cardiac output during labour. *Br Med J (Clin Res Ed)* 1987;295:1169–72.

18. Davies P, Francis RI, Docker MF, Watt JM, Crawford JS. Analysis of impedance cardiography longitudinally applied in pregnancy. *Br J Obstet Gynaecol* 1986;93:717–20.

19. Hendricks CH, Quilligan EJ. Cardiac output during labor. *Am J Obstet Gynecol* 1956;71:953–72.

20. Brownridge P. The nature and consequences of childbirth pain. *Eur J Obstet Gynecol Reprod Biol* 1995;59 Suppl:S9–15.

21. Lees MM, Scott DB, Kerr MG, Taylor SH. The circulatory effects of recumbent postural change in late pregnancy. *Clin Sci* 1967;32:453–65.

22. Robson SC, Hunter S, Moore M, Dunlop W. Haemodynamic changes during the puerperium: a Doppler and M-mode echocardiographic study. *Br J Obstet Gynaecol* 1987;94:1028–39.

23. MacGillivray I, Rose GA, Rowe B. Blood pressure survey in pregnancy. *Clin Sci* 1969;37:395–407.

24. Steer PJ, Little MP, Kold-Jensen T, Chapple J, Elliott P. Maternal blood pressure in pregnancy, birth weight, and perinatal mortality in first births: prospective study. *BMJ* 329:1312:2004.

25. Bailey RR, Rolleston GL. Kidney length and ureteric dilatation in the puerperium. *J Obstet Gynaecol Br Commonw* 1971;78:55–61.

26. Cietak KA, Newton JR. Serial qualitative maternal nephrosonography in pregnancy. *Br J Radiol* 1985;58:399–404.

27. Davison JM, Lindheimer MD. Changes in renal haemodynamics and kidney weight during pregnancy in the unanaesthetized rat. *J Physiol* 1980;301:129–36.

28. Marchant DJ. Alterations in anatomy and function of the urinary tract during pregnancy. *Clin Obstet Gynecol* 1978;21:855–61.

29. Davison JM. Kidney function in pregnant women. *Am J Kidney Dis* 1987;9:248–52.

30. Dunlop W. Investigations into the influence of posture on renal plasma flow and glomerular filtration rate during late pregnancy. *Br J Obstet Gynaecol* 1976;83:17–23.

31. Chesley LC, Sloan DM. The effect of posture on renal function in late pregnancy. *Am J Obstet Gynecol* 1964;89:754–9.

32. Ezimokhai M, Davison JM, Philips PR, Dunlop W. Non-postural serial changes in renal function during the third trimester of normal human pregnancy. *Br J Obstet Gynaecol* 1981;88:465–71.

33. Sturgiss SN, Martin K, Whittingham A, Davison JM. Assessment of the renal circulation during pregnancy with color Doppler ultrasonography. *Am J Obstet Gynecol* 1992;167:1250–4.

34. Yura T, Takamitsu Y, Yuasa S, Miki S, Takahashi N, Bandai H, *et al.* Total and split renal function assessed by ultrasound Doppler techniques. *Nephron* 1991;58:37–41.

35. Rigsby CM, Burns PN, Weltin GG, Chen B, Bia M, Taylor KJ. Doppler signal quantitation in renal allografts: comparison in normal and rejecting transplants, with pathologic correlation. *Radiology* 1987;162(1 Pt 1):39–42.

36. Patriquin HB, O'Regan S, Robitaille P, Paltiel H. Hemolytic-uremic syndrome: intrarenal arterial Doppler patterns as a useful guide to therapy. *Radiology* 1989;172:625–8.

37. Stevens PE, Gwyther SJ, Hanson ME, Boultbee JE, Kox WJ, Phillips ME. Noninvasive monitoring of renal blood flow characteristics during acute renal failure in man. *Intensive Care Med* 1990;16:153–8.

38. Mostbeck GH, Kain R, Mallek R, Derfler K, Walter R, Havelec L, *et al.* Duplex Doppler sonography in renal parenchymal disease. Histopathologic correlation. *J Ultrasound Med* 1991;10:189–94.

39. Katz AI, Lindheimer MD. Actions of hormones on the kidney. *Annu Rev Physiol* 1977;39:97–133.

40. Conrad KP, Novak J. Emerging role of relaxin in renal and cardiovascular function. *Am J Physiol Regul Integr Comp Physiol* 2004;287:R250–61.

41. Smith M, Davison J, Conrad K, Danielson L. Renal hemodynamic effects of relaxin in humans. *Ann NY Acad Sci* 2005;1041:163–72.

42. Ramsey EM, Houston ML, Harris JW. Interactions of the trophoblast and maternal tissues in three closely related primate species. *Am J Obstet Gynecol* 1976;124:647–52.

43. Robertson WB, Warner B. The ultrastructure of the human placental bed. *J Pathol* 1974;112:203–11.

44. Robertson WB, Brosens I, Dixon HG. The pathological response of the vessels of the placental bed to hypertensive pregnancy. *J Pathol Bacteriol* 1967;93:581–92.

45. Assali NS, Douglass RA, Junior, Baird WW, Nicholson DB, Suyemoto R. Measurement of uterine blood flow and uterine metabolism. IV. Results in normal pregnancy. *Am J Obstet Gynecol* 1953;66:248–53.

46. Blechner JN, Stenger VG, Prystowsky H. Uterine blood flow in women at term. *Am J Obstet Gynecol* 1974;120:633–40.

47. Longo LD. Maternal blood volume and cardiac output during pregnancy: a hypothesis of endocrinologic control. *Am J Physiol* 1983;245(5 Pt 1):R720–9.

48. Johnson MR, Jauniaux E, Ramsay B, Jurkovic D, Meuris S. Maternal relaxin: a determinant of fetal heart rate? *Br J Obstet Gynaecol* 1994;101:1003–4.

49. Jauniaux E, Johnson MR, Jurkovic D, Ramsay B, Campbell S, Meuris S. The role of relaxin in the development of the uteroplacental circulation in early pregnancy. *Obstet Gynecol* 1994;84:338–42.

50. Chapman AB, Zamudio S, Woodmansee W, Merouani A, Osorio F, Johnson A, *et al.* Systemic and renal hemodynamic changes in the luteal phase of the menstrual cycle mimic early pregnancy. *Am J Physiol* 1997;273(5 Pt 2):F777–82.

51. Balasch J, Arroyo V, Carmona F, Llach J, Jimenez W, Pare JC, *et al.* Severe ovarian hyperstimulation syndrome: role of peripheral vasodilation. *Fertil Steril* 1991;56:1077–83.

52. Manau D, Arroyo V, Jimenez W, Fabregues F, Vanrell JA, Balasch J. Chronology of hemodynamic changes in asymptomatic *in vitro* fertilization patients and relationship with ovarian steroids and cytokines. *Fertil Steril* 2002;77:1178–83.

53. Manau D, Balasch J, Arroyo V, Jimenez W, Fabregues F, Casamitjana R, *et al.* Circulatory dysfunction in asymptomatic *in vitro* fertilization patients. Relationship with hyperestrogenemia and activity of endogenous vasodilators. *J Clin Endocrinol Metab* 1998;83:1489–93.

54. Sealey JE, Itskovitz-Eldor J, Rubattu S, James GD. August P, Thaler I, *et al.* Estradiol- and progesterone-related increases in the renin–aldosterone system: studies during ovarian stimulation and early pregnancy. *J Clin Endocrinol Metab* 1994;79:258–64.

55. Chapman AB, Abraham WT, Zamudio S, Coffin C, Merouani A, Young D, *et al.* Temporal relationships between hormonal and hemodynamic changes in early human pregnancy. *Kidney Int* 1998;54:2056–63.

56. Trudinger BJ, Giles WB. Elaboration of stem villous vessels in growth restricted pregnancies with abnormal umbilical artery Doppler waveforms. *Br J Obstet Gynaecol* 1996;103:487–9.

57. Paller MS, Gregorini G, Ferris TF. Pressor responsiveness in pseudopregnant and pregnant rats: role of maternal factors. *Am J Physiol* 1989;257(4 Pt 2):R866–71.

58. Slater AJ, Gude N, Clarke IJ, Walters WA. Haemodynamic changes and left ventricular performance during high-dose oestrogen administration to male transsexuals. *Br J Obstet Gynaecol* 1986;93:532–8.

59. Johnson MR, Abdalla H, Allman AC, Wren ME, Kirkland A, Lightman SL. Relaxin levels in ovum donation pregnancies. *Fertil Steril* 1991;56:59–61.

60. Johnson MR, Abbas AA, Allman AC, Nicolaides KH, Lightman SL. The regulation of plasma relaxin levels during human pregnancy. *J Endocrinol* 1994;142:261–5.

61. Bell RJ, Eddie LW, Lester AR, Wood EC, Johnston PD, Niall HD. Relaxin in human pregnancy serum measured with an homologous radioimmunoassay. *Obstet Gynecol* 1987;69:585–9.

62. Kakouris H, Eddie LW, Summers RJ. Cardiac effects of relaxin in rats. *Lancet* 1992;339:1076–8.

63. Weisinger RS, Burns P, Eddie LW, Wintour EM. Relaxin alters the plasma osmolality–arginine vasopressin relationship in the rat. *J Endocrinol* 1993;137:505–10.

64. Novak J, Danielson LA, Kerchner LJ, Sherwood OD, Ramirez RJ, Moalli PA. *et al.* Relaxin is essential for renal vasodilation during pregnancy in conscious rats. *J Clin Invest* 2001;107:1469–75.

65. Johnson MR, Brooks AA, Steer PJ. The role of relaxin in the pregnancy associated reduction in plasma osmolality. *Hum Reprod* 1996;11:1105–8.

66. Lei ZM, Reshef E, Rao V. The expression of human chorionic gonadotropin/luteinizing hormone receptors in human endometrial and myometrial blood vessels. *J Clin Endocrinol Metab* 1992;75:651–9.

67. Toth P, Li X, Rao CV, Lincoln SR, Sanfilippo JS, Spinnato JA 2nd, *et al* Expression of functional human chorionic gonadotropin/human luteinizing hormone receptor gene in human uterine arteries. *J Clin Endocrinol Metab* 1994;79:307–15.

68. Davison JM, Vallotton MB, Lindheimer MD. Plasma osmolality and urinary concentration and dilution during and after pregnancy: evidence that lateral recumbency inhibits maximal urinary concentrating ability. *Br J Obstet Gynaecol* 1981;88:472–9.

69. Davison JM, Shiells EA, Philips PR, Lindheimer MD. Influence of humoral and volume factors on altered osmoregulation of normal human pregnancy. *Am J Physiol* 1990;258(4 Pt 2):F900–7.

70. Holden DP, Fickling SA, Whitley GS, Nussey SS. Plasma concentrations of asymmetric dimethylarginine, a natural inhibitor of nitric oxide synthase, in normal pregnancy and preeclampsia. *Am J Obstet Gynecol* 1998;178:551–6.

71. Holden DP, Cartwright JE, Nussey SS, Whitley GS. Estrogen stimulates dimethylarginine dimethylaminohydrolase activity and the metabolism of asymmetric dimethylarginine. *Circulation* 2003;108:1575–80.

72. Cartwright JE, Holden DP, Whitley GS. Hepatocyte growth factor regulates human trophoblast motility and invasion: a role for nitric oxide. *Br J Pharmacol* 1999;128:181–9.

73. Gangula PR, Dong YL, Wimalawansa SJ, Yallampalli C. Infusion of pregnant rats with calcitonin gene-related peptide (CGRP)(8-37), a CGRP receptor antagonist, increases blood pressure and fetal mortality and decreases fetal growth. *Biol Reprod* 2002;67:624–9..

74. Gangula PR, Supowit SC, Wimalawansa SJ, Zhao H, Hallman DM, DiPette DJ, *et al.* Calcitonin gene-related peptide is a depressor in NG–nitro–L–arginine methyl ester-induced hypertension during pregnancy. *Hypertension* 1997;29(1 Pt 2):248–53.

75. Parkington HC, Coleman HA, Tare M. Prostacyclin and endothelium-dependent hyperpolarization. *Pharmacol Res* 2004;49:509–14.

76. Mullen MJ, Kharbanda RK, Cross J, Donald AE, Taylor M, Vallance P, *et al.* Heterogenous nature of flow-mediated dilatation in human conduit arteries *in vivo*: relevance to endothelial dysfunction in hypercholesterolemia. *Circ Res* 2001;88:145–51.

77. Pyke KE, Tschakovsky ME. The relationship between shear stress and flow-mediated dilatation: implications for the assessment of endothelial function. *J Physiol* 2005;568:357–69.

78. Ginsburg J, Duncan SL. Peripheral blood flow in normal pregnancy. *Cardiovasc Res* 1967;1:132–7

Chapter 4

Antenatal care of women with cardiac disease: an obstetrician's perspective

Martin Lupton

Introduction

In 1952 Dr Forest Dewey Dodrill, supported by General Motors, built the first heart bypass machine. In doing so he revolutionised cardiac surgery. His device, alongside other new cardiothoracic interventions and improved medications, has led to a large cohort of people with congenital heart disease (CHD) surviving into adult life. It is estimated that by 2010 there will be approximately 166 000 adults with CHD in the UK, of whom about 15 000 will have complex cardiac conditions. One-half of these adults will be women and many will wish to have children.

Since the 1950s, the capacity of medicine to 'do things to people' has accelerated and the philosophical framework within which medicine is practised has also undergone startling changes. The most significant change has been the ascendancy of the principle of patient autonomy and the rapid demise of medical paternalism. Obstetrics has had to confront this philosophical paradigm shift more directly than most other specialties. For example, it is no longer considered appropriate for the obstetrician alone to decide what risks it is reasonable for a woman to undertake. Her own opinion is now the key determinant of the choice that she will make. Who else other than the woman, it is argued, can know whether a 30% risk of death is a reasonable risk to accept in order to create a new life? The obstetrician's role is therefore complex. A modern obstetrician needs to be an educator, counsellor, facilitator and coordinator. Interestingly, this concept of the obstetrician resonates with the original meaning of the word 'obstetric', which is derived from the Latin word 'obstare' meaning 'to stand by or next to'.

When caring for pregnant women with cardiac conditions, the obstetrician needs to remember two things. The first is that women with heart disease can die during pregnancy if they are not properly cared for. The second is that women with heart disease can die during pregnancy even if their care is exemplary. If the mother does die, the obstetrician will be held to account for her care. It is therefore in the interests of the obstetrician as well as of the woman to make use of the best available multidisciplinary advice at all stages in her pregnancy.

It is vital for the obstetrician to be aware of the basic cardiovascular physiology of pregnancy, as these pose a major challenge to women with heart disease who become pregnant.

Haemodynamic changes in normal pregnancy

Pregnancy causes major cardiovascular changes in healthy women. However, these changes may be poorly tolerated by women with cardiac disease. These are dealt with in detail in Chapter 3 but for convenience a summary is given here. During pregnancy there is a 50% increase in cardiac output, taking place mainly over the first and second trimesters.[1] Despite this increase, blood pressure initially falls, secondary to an even greater fall in peripheral resistance, and then rises again from approximately 34 weeks of gestation. The fall in peripheral resistance drives an increase in plasma volume of 40–45% of the prepregnancy volume.[2–4] There is also a corresponding increase in pulmonary blood flow, which in normal pregnancy does not lead to an increase in pulmonary artery pressure as it is balanced by a decrease in pulmonary vascular resistance.[5] Significant structural changes to the heart during the third trimester include myocardial hypertrophy, chamber enlargement and mild multi-valvular regurgitation. During labour, cardiac output is increased by a further 10–40% above the prelabour level, with up to 500 ml of blood joining the circulation with each contraction in women with effective anaesthesia.[6] There are also significant and rapid volume shifts in the first 2 weeks postpartum.[7]

Women are also six times more likely to have a thrombosis during pregnancy, and 11 times more likely in the immediate puerperium. This is due to the activation of the coagulation cascade and is a normal physiological process. The likelihood of thrombosis is further increased in the presence of polycythaemia secondary to cyanotic heart disease. This hypercoagulable state is of particular importance in women who require anticoagulation even when they are not pregnant.

Clearly, each of these changes to the cardiovascular system has the potential to affect women with heart disease and lead to cardiac decompensation. Most obstetricians are familiar with the normal physiology of pregnancy but are less comfortable with the altered physiology induced by cardiac disease.

Recognition of the cardiac condition

Most women with CHD will already be aware of their diagnosis but this is not always the case. For example, sudden death in young athletes is most commonly the result of undiagnosed cardiac disease.[8] Given that the incidence of serious heart disease complicating pregnancy is approximately 1%,[9] all women booking for antenatal care should have a cardiac history taken. The key questions to ask are:[10]

■ Do you ever suffer from chest pain?

■ Do you have severe breathlessness?

■ Do you have prolonged or symptomatic palpitations?

■ Do you have a history of syncope?

■ Do you have any family history of heart disease or sudden death?

Once the history has been taken, the woman should be examined. Signs such as clubbing of the fingers and cyanosis should be looked for. Her blood pressure should be measured with care, and it should be recorded. (The British Hypertension Society recommends using Korotkoff sounds 1 and 5, measured to the nearest 2 mmHg, with the woman seated comfortably and with the arm cuff at the level of the atria.[11] It is important that the blood pressure be taken manually, as most automated blood pressure measuring devices are not calibrated correctly for pregnancy and can underread the true blood pressure by as much as 30 mmHg. See also Beevers *et al.*[12] and the BHS video tutorial.[13])

The woman's urine should be tested for protein, and her heart and lungs should be auscultated. If a murmur is heard the obstetrician must decide whether it is physio-logical or pathological. If the murmur is diastolic it is considered pathological until proven otherwise. If the murmur is systolic and louder than 2/6 it should be investigated. If there is persistent splitting of S-2 or persistent jugular venous disten-sion, further cardiac investigation is required.[9] Investigations should include an echocardiograph, an electrocardiograph and possibly a chest X-ray. If an abnormality is found, an appropriate referral should be made. If the woman is hypertensive (has a raised systolic or diastolic pressure) this should be investigated and treatment instituted along with an appropriate referral.

Where should the woman be managed?

The first Confidential Enquiry into Maternal Deaths for the period 1952–54 recom-mended that 'all patients known or suspected to be suffering from heart disease should be referred for their care in pregnancy and confinement to a hospital where they can receive the necessary supervision'.[14] Thus, if a woman has a known cardiac disorder, the obstetrician needs to decide whether it is appropriate for her to remain under local care or whether she would be best served by a referral to a maternal cardiac centre. If there is obstetric uncertainty, is always appropriate to refer the woman to a maternal cardiac centre for advice. The advice may simply be how the woman could best be managed locally.

Assessment of risk

In order to decide where a woman should be cared for, the obstetrician needs to make a risk assessment. As discussed elsewhere, 'risk stratification is best accomplished before conception'[15] but in practice this does not always happen. Siu and Colman[16] have set out four areas that should be considered in an assessment of maternal cardiac risk:

■ the underlying cardiac lesion
■ maternal functional status
■ the need for further palliative or corrective surgery
■ additional associated risk factors.

The underlying cardiac lesion

Women with cardiac disease can be divided into those with trivial conditions that are unlikely to have an effect on either her or the fetus, and those with moderate or severe lesions that might have an effect on her, her fetus, or both.

Trivial and minimal-risk cardiac lesions

Trivial or insignificant lesions include small ventricular septal defects (VSDs), repaired VSDs with normal cardiac function, and trivial valve prolapse, which affects up to 10% of young women.[17]

Cardiac lesions posing a low risk to the mother (i.e. less than 1% risk of maternal death or severe disability) include corrected tetralogy of Fallot, bioprosthetic valve replacement, patent ductus arteriosus and mitral stenosis with minimal limitation of maternal physical activity (NYHA I and II; see below and Appendix A).

The major potentially serious risk of these haemodynamically insignificant lesions is endocarditis. The American College of Obstetricians and Gynecologists (ACOG)[18] does not recommend antibiotic prophylaxis for uncomplicated vaginal delivery or caesarean section in the presence of trivial cardiovascular lesions. However, most expert opinion suggests their use for instrumental or other complex deliveries.[19] It is appropriate for women with trivial or low-risk lesions to be delivered at their local hospital.

Moderate- and major-risk cardiac lesions

In contrast to the above, women with moderate or severe lesions should be delivered in maternal cardiac centres. The ACOG has described a cardiac lesion of moderate risk as one where there is a 5–15% chance of maternal death. Moderate-risk cardiac lesions include significant mitral stenosis (NYHA III and IV), aortic stenosis, uncorrected tetralogy of Fallot, Marfan syndrome, aortic coarctation and artificial valve replacement. Major risk is described as that where there is a 25–50% chance of the mother dying. These major-risk lesions include aortic coarctation with valvular involvement, pulmonary hypertension and Eisenmenger syndrome.

NYHA classification of cardiac function

Further risk stratification can be achieved using the New York Heart Association (NYHA) system, which has four classes (Appendix A):

- class I – uncompromised (no limitation of physical activity)
- class II – slight limitation of physical activity
- class III – marked limitation of physical activity
- class IV – severely compromised.

Siu, *et al.*[15] demonstrated a correlation between maternal outcome and NYHA functional status, with those women with an NYHA class higher than II having a significantly higher chance of a poor outcome. Poor maternal functional class was also predictive of a poor fetal outcome.

Additional associated risk factors

The primary associated risk factors are related to the use of medication, particularly warfarin and angiotensin-converting enzyme (ACE) inhibitors. Both of these carry significant risk to the fetus. Warfarin in particular presents a therapeutic dilemma, predominantly in the presence of an artificial heart valve. In this situation, the woman and her obstetrician need to make a stark choice between therapeutic regimens that favour the fetus (a change to other forms of anticoagulation, such as low molecular weight heparin (LMWH) and aspirin) but carry an increased risk to the mother, and those that favour the mother (e.g. remaining on warfarin) but represent a significant risk to the fetus. This is covered in detail in Chapter 7.

What should the woman be told?

Having defined the mother's underlying cardiac lesion and established the pertinent risks associated with her lesion in pregnancy, the obstetrician is in a position to determine where the woman will receive the most appropriate management and care. Wherever this might be, the primary duty of the obstetrician in the first antenatal clinic is to explain the risks that are inherent in her choice to remain pregnant. This discussion should also include how her cardiac condition might affect her fetus.

The report[20] by the British Cardiac Society (BCS) on the needs of adolescents and adults with CHD in the UK expresses the view that poor advice before pregnancy often leads to poor choices and consequent morbidity and mortality from heart disease in pregnancy. The obstetrician thus needs to discover whether or not the woman has had prepregnancy counselling and, if she has, what has been remembered and more importantly what she has understood. If she has not had counselling, the woman needs to be properly counselled. The issues that need to be covered are set out in Table 1 in the BCS report.[20] It is important that this counselling is done by an expert, and it must include both the risk of maternal mortality and morbidity and the chance of a successful outcome for the pregnancy. It should also include the risk of the fetus inheriting CHD and issues of child care should the mother die or become too ill to manage to care for the child. The standard for this sort of counselling should be very high, both in terms of content and communication. The obstetrician needs to be sure that the woman has received the information that she needs to make a valid choice. This is particularly important when the woman has a condition such as pulmonary hypertension, a dilated aortopathy or a failing heart (systemic ventricular dysfunction), all of which carry a high risk of maternal mortality. Following counselling, the choices the woman makes are ones that she, her family and her medical team will have to manage with, whatever the outcome.

Planning antenatal care

Having established a diagnosis and counselled the woman appropriately, the next task for the obstetrician and the multidisciplinary team is to plan the antenatal care and determine how it should be delivered. The obstetrician has the role of 'care coordinator' and has overall responsibility for both the mother and her fetus. Obstetricians do not have the particular expertise of the cardiologist, the anaesthetist or the midwife, but they do have a particular understanding of both the physiological changes to the woman brought about by her pregnancy and of fetal growth and wellbeing. Obstetricians are also accustomed to making judgements involving the wellbeing of both the mother and her fetus, and helping to decide when and how a baby should be delivered.

The purpose of antenatal care is to ensure the continued wellbeing of both the mother and her fetus and to manage any deviation from the norm. Prompt intervention before major cardiac decompensation can prevent significant problems, as can the early diagnosis and management of pre-eclampsia. Scrupulous attention to detail is therefore mandatory when managing women with cardiac disease in pregnancy.

The multidisciplinary team and antenatal care

The multidisciplinary team should include a cardiologist, an anaesthetist, a paediatrician, a specialist midwife, an obstetrician and trainees. Each pregnant woman's case

Combined Obstetric and Cardiac Service (COCS)
Clinical Management Plan for Delivery

Cardiac diagnosis......................................   *Please circle agreed plan*

If admitted to LW, please inform:	Consultant obstetrician on call **Y / N** Consultant anaesthetist on call **Y / N** Cornwall Team	One of COCS team **Y / N** Professor Steer Gubby Ayida Mark Johnson Martin Lupton ....(other)
Mode of delivery	Elective LSCS	Trial of vaginal delivery
Elective LSCS *(see anaesthetic sheet for anaesthetic details)*	Prophylatic compression suture Syntocinon® (oxytocin) low-dose infusion (8–12 munits/min)	*Inform COCS team member if admitted in labour before scheduled date*
Vaginal delivery first-stage Mx *(see anaesthetic sheet for anaesthetic details)*	TEDS in labour HDU chart Prophylatic antibiotics *(cardiac regimen against endocarditis)* Medication to be continued Early epidural for analgesia Continuous EFM Additional maternal monitoring	Elective / If operative delivery .... ECG in labour Arterial BP monitoring Central venous access
Vaginal delivery second-stage Mx	Normal second stage Short second stage (then assist if not del) Elective assisted delivery only	.... minutes
Vaginal delivery third-stage Mx	Normal active Mx Syntocinon® infusion 8–12 milliunits/min	Continue .... hours
Post delivery	High-dependency unit (minimum stay) LMW heparin (duration)	....................hours ....

See overleaf for exceptional clinical situations

Affix patient ID label

*Please inform the consultant obstetrician on call if there
is departure from planned management or if clinical situations
develop in women with cardiac disease*

Examples of clinical situations	Consider the following
Spontaneous labour and recent thromboprophylaxis use, e.g. LMWH/warfarin	Inform anaesthetist ASAP D/W David Williams or Mark Johnson Options may include ……………….. ……………….. ………………..
Need for Syntocinon® augmentation in labour	Use of double-strength Syntocinon® but halve rate to reduce total volume of fluids given *(this decision needs to be taken at consultant level)*
Postpartum haemorrhage	• Inform anaesthetic consultant on call • Consider use of compression suture • Consider use of intrauterine balloon (antibiotic cover is required) • Strict input/output charts to be maintained • Consider central access or arterial monitoring • Caution should be exercised in use of usual uterotonics e.g. misoprostol/ Hemabate®(carboprost)/high-dose Syntocinon® infusion
Preterm labour	Do not use ritodrine or salbutamol Atosiban (Tractocile®) should be first-line Mx

| Useful contact details of COCS team | Professor Steer (obstetrician) bleep
Gubby Ayida (obstetrician) bleep
Mark Johnson (obstetrician/physician) bleep
Martin Lupton (obstetrician) bleep
Steve Yentis (anaesthetist) bleep
Daryl Dob (anaesthetist) bleep
Dr Kaddara (cardiologist C&W) bleep
Dr Gatzoulis (cardiologist Brompton) |

*Please seek advice from COCS member if there are concerns or if
clarification is required on clinical management*

Figure 4.1.   Cardiac planning pro forma

should be considered in detail by the whole team, early on in the pregnancy, and a careful plan made for the mother's antenatal care and delivery. The plan should be recorded and should include such basic things as the frequency of appointments, the number and frequency of investigations of the mother, and the number and frequency of investigations of the fetus. In view of the number of medical staff working in any particular unit and the fact that they will not all be familiar with cardiovascular disease in pregnancy, the record should be easy to interpret and should consider foreseeable contingencies such as labour. The record should also act as an aid to the team, reminding them to perform routine tasks, which are easy to forget, at each antenatal visit. These tasks should probably include:[21]

■ measuring the pulse rate and blood pressure

■ assessing the heart rhythm

■ auscultating the heart sounds

■ listening to the lung bases

■ checking the urine for protein

■ assessing fetal growth.

An example of an antenatal record that has been designed specifically for pregnancy is shown in Figure 4.1.

The fetus and fetal surveillance

The primary risks to the fetus are inheriting a congenital cardiac disorder, the potential for harm as a result of maternal medication, intrauterine growth restriction (IUGR), which may be secondary to compromised maternal cardiac output, and prematurity (often iatrogenic). Women with cyanotic heart disease, dilated cardiomyopathy and a reduced ejection fraction, or hypertrophic cardiomyopathy and severe restrictive physiology have fetuses that are at risk of IUGR. Significant mitral stenosis may also lead to fetal growth restriction not only because of the effect of the stenosis on cardiac output but also because medical treatment classically includes beta blockade. Similarly, the fetuses of women with coarctation of the aorta are at risk of IUGR in part because a mainstay of medical treatment is beta blockade. In the presence of good haemodynamic function, however, such as that in women with NYHA class I and II disease, fetal outcome is generally good.

All women should be offered nuchal translucency screening in early pregnancy.[22] While this screening test was developed for the assessment of the risk of Down syndrome, it has also been shown to have an association with CHD. Fetal CHD is associated with approximately a 60% chance of increased nuchal thickness.[21]. Early fetal echocardiography is also available in some centres, at between 14 and 16 weeks of gestation. This can detect severe CHD but detection of less severe disorders requires additional echocardiography when the fetus is larger and easier to image. This is generally done both at the 20 week anomaly scan and at the standard fetal echocardiogram, usually performed at between 18 and 22 weeks. The fetal echo should be performed by a trained fetal cardiologist.

Provided there are no specific risk factors for growth restriction, such as cyanotic heart disease, significant hypertension or beta blockade, the routine measurement of symphysio–fundal height for the assessment of fetal growth is probably sufficient. Where there is serious concern that the fetus might be growth restricted, serial ultrasound is indicated.

Frequency of visits and admission to hospital

The care of women with cardiac lesions during pregnancy is not cheap. This is currently a particular problem for maternity units within the UK NHS. The introduction of 'payment by results' for the provision of maternity care has impacted adversely on specialist services. Specialist care to women at high risk during their pregnancy is expensive because of the cost of repeated antenatal checks, prolonged admissions to hospital and the need for a multidisciplinary team, but this is not yet officially recognised in the funding arrangements. In parts of the USA it is now almost impossible for women with CHD to find units to care for them, except as an emergency. This is as a result of the understandable reluctance of insurance companies to foot the potentially huge bills for the antenatal care of these women, and the difficulty obstetricians have in finding practice insurance to cover the threat of litigation should the mother die or the fetus sustain damage.

Antenatal appointments need to be frequent and senior members of the multidisciplinary team should provide the antenatal care. At the Chelsea and Westminster Hospital, visits are booked every fortnight until 24 weeks of gestation and weekly thereafter. The threshold for admission should be low and it is not uncommon to admit women to the unit early on in the third trimester for both medical and organisational reasons (many women live a long way from their tertiary referral unit).

References

1.   Hunter S, Robson SC. Adaptation of the maternal heart in pregnancy. *Br Heart J* 1992;68:540–3.
2.   Whittaker PG, Macphail S, Lind T. Serial hematologic changes and pregnancy outcome. *Obstet Gynecol* 1996;88:33–9.
3.   Pritchard JA. Changes in the blood volume during pregnancy and delivery. *Anesthesiology* 1965;26:393–9.
4.   Chesley LC. Plasma and red cell volumes during pregnancy. *Am J Obstet Gynecol* 1972;112:440–50.
5.   Robson SC, Hunter S, Boys RJ, Dunlop W. Serial changes in pulmonary haemodynamics during human pregnancy: a non-invasive study using Doppler echocardiography. *Clin Sci (Lond)* 1991;80:113–17.
6.   Robson SC, Dunlop W, Boys RJ, Hunter S. Cardiac output during labour. *Br Med J (Clin Res Ed)* 1987;295:1169–72
7.   Robson SC, Hunter S, Moore M, Dunlop W. Haemodynamic changes during the puerperium: a Doppler and M-mode echocardiographic study. *Br J Obstet Gynaecol* 1987;94:1028–39.
8.   Kenny A, Shapiro LM. Sudden cardiac death in athletes. *Br Med Bull* 1992;48:534–45.
9.   McFaul PB, Dornan JC, Lamki H, Boyle D. Pregnancy complicated by maternal heart disease. A review of 519 women. *Br J Obstet Gynaecol* 1988;95:861–7.
10. Burrow G, Duffy T, Copel J, editors. *Medical Complications During Pregnancy*. 6th ed. Philadelphia: Elsevier Saunders; 2004.
11. British Hypertension Society [www.bhsoc.org/bp_monitors/BLOOD_PRESSURE_1784b.pdf].
12. Beevers G, Lip GY, O'Brien E. ABC of hypertension. Blood pressure measurement. Part I –sphygmomanometry: factors common to all techniques. *BMJ* 2001;323:805.
13. British Hypertension Society [www.abdn.ac.uk/medical/bhs/tutorial/tutorial.htm].
14. Lewis, G, editor. *Why Mothers Die 2000–2002: The Sixth Report of Confidential Enquiries into Maternal Deaths in the United Kingdom*. London: RCOG Press; 2004.

15. Siu SC, Sermer M, Colman JM, Alvarez AN, Mercier LA, Morton BC, *et al.* Cardiac Disease in Pregnancy (CARPREG) Investigators. Prospective multicenter study of pregnancy outcomes in women with heart disease. *Circulation* 2001;104:515–21.
16. Siu SC, Colman JM. Heart disease and pregnancy. *Heart* 2001;85:710–15.
17. Levy D, Savage D. Prevalence and clinical features of mitral valve prolapse. *Am Heart J* 1987;113:1281–90
18. American College of Obstetricians and Gynecologists. ACOG practice bulletin number 47, October 2003: Prophylactic Antibiotics in Labor and Delivery. *Obstet Gynecol* 2003;102:875–82.
19. Thorne SA. Pregnancy in heart disease. *Heart* 2004;90:450–6.
20. Report of the British Cardiac Society Working Party. Grown-up congenital heart (GUCH) disease: current needs and provision of service for adolescents and adults with congenital heart disease in the UK. *Heart* 2002;88 Suppl 1:11–14.
21. Steer PJ. Pregnancy and contraception. In: *Adult Congenital Heart Disease.* Gatzoulis M, Swan L, Therrien J, Pantley G, editors. London: Blackwell; 2005. p. 16–36.
22. National Collaborating Centre for Women's and Children's Health. *Antenatal Care: Routine Care for the Healthy Pregnant Woman.* NICE Clinical Guideline. London: RCOG Press; 2003 [www.nice.org.uk/page.aspx?o=CG006NICEguideline].

Chapter 5
Antenatal care of women with cardiac disease: a cardiologist's perspective

Fiona Walker

Background

Depending on the obstetric population and the profile of referral, 0.5–3.0% of women have a form of heart disease already known before, or diagnosed during, pregnancy. There is usually a favourable maternal and fetal outcome but it must be borne in mind that heart disease is now the second most common cause of maternal death after suicide, and it is more common than the most frequent direct cause of maternal death, thromboembolism. Although the maternal mortality rate from cardiac disease has more than halved over the last 50 years, it was still responsible for 44 maternal deaths between 2000 and 2002 and it is therefore recognised as an important contributor to maternal mortality statistics.[1]

In the UK, maternal mortality data are collected by the Confidential Enquiry Into Maternal and Child Health (CEMACH),[1] funded by the National Institute for Health and Clinical Excellence (NICE) and the Department of Health. There is, however, no national initiative or database that records the prevalence of maternal heart disease across the UK as a whole, and there are no national guidelines that set a standard of care for these women in pregnancy. With heart disease contributing to maternal mortality statistics in such a significant way, it is clear that maternal heart disease warrants greater awareness and recognition. There is also a pressing need for national guidelines outlining optimal care provision.

Producing such guidelines is, however, difficult. Heart disease in pregnancy represents a truly interdisciplinary subject, one which at present is consigned to the perimeter of both cardiology and obstetrics. It is clear that a model of organisation of antenatal care (ANC) needs to be defined, in light of the fact that substandard care was identified as a contributing factor in 40% of deaths from heart disease in the most recent CEMACH report (2000–2002).[1] Recurring themes included failure of communication between members of the multidisciplinary team, lack of clear policies for the management of cardiac problems, and failure of individual clinicians to diagnose cardiac problems accurately, or appreciate the severity of the cardiac condition when identified.

In this chapter, therefore, I will highlight the current pattern of maternal heart disease from a cardiology perspective and suggest recommendations for the organisation of ANC provision for these women, using my experience as a tertiary centre cardiologist, the CEMACH recommendations and data submitted from some of the larger existing specialist cardiology units. These recommendations for ANC represent what I consider 'the ideal,' and have foundations based on my personal experience of setting up such a service at University College London Hospitals (UCLH).

The spectrum of maternal heart disease: past, present and future

There has been a dramatic decline in the prevalence of rheumatic heart disease in the UK over the last 40 years. It used to be found in up to 1% of young pregnant women but it is now uncommon and confined largely to areas where there are immigrant communities. Between 1952 and 1960 rheumatic heart disease was responsible for around 250 maternal deaths, whereas more recently (2000–2002) it was responsible for none.[1] This means that some perceive heart disease in pregnancy to be a vanishing problem that involves either insignificant or obscure congenital or myocardial defects.

Congenital heart disease (CHD) in pregnancy is, however, neither insignificant nor obscure and it is now both relatively and absolutely more common in pregnancy. This has occurred because of improvements in infant cardiac surgery and paediatric cardiology care over the same period. About 85% of children born with CHD now survive to adulthood. Fifty percent of these adults will be females of reproductive age. For this patient population, 'total correction' or 'cure' of CHD is the exception not the norm. The majority of these adult survivors are palliated and have a requirement for continuing surveillance and, more often than not, require recurrent medical and/or surgical interventions over the course of their life. Many lesions surgically repaired in infancy can recur in adulthood, for example, re-coarctation of the aorta or regrowth of a sub-aortic membrane. Some patients are left with residua following their primary repair, which although haemodynamically well tolerated in childhood, lead to later problems in adulthood that ultimately necessitate 're-do' surgery, for example pulmonary regurgitation in tetralogy of Fallot. Some may have simply 'outgrown' their initial repairs and need larger conduits or valves implanted. Long-term specialist follow-up of these patients is therefore essential but, even in the current era, specialist care for these adults is limited and poorly organised. Some women are thus lost to follow-up until they become pregnant, when a sternotomy scar is revealed and alarm bells ring.

Women with CHD, therefore, represent a unique patient population reaching childbearing age, with a wide variety of cardiac lesions. They may have any combination of valvular heart disease (regurgitation/stenosis/mechanical), myocardial disease (hypertrophy/dilatation/dysfunction/single ventricle), lung problems (pulmonary hypertension (PH)/restrictive ventilatory defects/single lung), cyanosis and/or arrhythmias. The exact number of such women in the UK is unknown. Accurate prevalence data are lacking and there is no national database. CHD does, however, complicate almost 1% of live births and it is estimated that there are now around 20 000 adult survivors. In an attempt to predict the future care needs of the adult population with CHD, a study in a single UK health region reviewed all births over a 10 year period (1985–94).[2] They extrapolated their results to the UK as a whole and concluded that the annual increase in numbers of adults with congenital heart disease was estimated to be approximately 1600, with 800 patients per year requiring specialist follow-up. Adding patients unknown before age 16 years, immigrants and asylum seekers, the total number will be around 2500 per year. There is thus likely to be an increase in the number of such women requiring pregnancy care over time.

Another group of cardiac diseases seen in an increasing number in women of childbearing age are inherited disorders, including cardiomyopathies (hypertrophic/dilated/arrhythmogenic right ventricular dysplasia) and Marfan syndrome. There is now greater awareness and better diagnosis of inherited cardiomyopathies with the availability of genetic screening. This, coupled with better medical treatment and risk stratification for sudden cardiac death (SCD), has significantly improved prognosis and survival for this group. These women also pose a management challenge during pregnancy, as they may have any combination of myocardial dysfunction, left ventricular outflow tract obstruction, atrioventricular valve regurgitation and/or atrial or ventricular dysrhythmias. They will often have devices *in situ* for the treatment of arrhythmias (implantable cardiac defibrillators) and/or heart failure (biventricular pacemakers), which adds another layer of complexity to management. For women with Marfan syndrome, familial screening has improved prognosis. Those with cardiac involvement, in particular aortic root dilatation (more than 50 mm), are operated on electively to prevent acute aortic dissection. A risk, of which cardiologists seem to be less aware, is that 50% of all aortic dissections in females under 40 years of age occur in pregnancy and therefore a relative contraindication to pregnancy is a woman with Marfan syndrome and an aortic root dimension of more than 40 mm (although it should be remembered that the risk of dissection does not start suddenly after 40 mm, and dissection can (and occasionally does) occur in roots with a normal diameter).[3,4]

Other important maternal heart diseases include PH, mechanical valves and puerperal cardiomyopathy. Although women with PH are advised against pregnancy owing to the significant associated mortality (30–50%), some remain undiagnosed or unaware of this risk. Others will embark on pregnancy even in the light of this knowledge as their desire to have a child is so strong. For some survivors with CHD, the diagnosis of PH can be less clear-cut (e.g. single lung hypertension), and these factors often make risk assessment and proper counselling difficult. Similarly, women diagnosed with puerperal cardiomyopathy may have recovery of ventricular function and then wish to embark on another pregnancy. These conditions are thus still encountered, even with proper specialist input and preconceptual counselling.

One can also speculate that acquired atherosclerotic heart disease is likely to become more prevalent in women of childbearing age. Current trends in smoking habits, obesity problems and poor diets in the young have already made this disease clinically manifest in women in their 40s and the numbers will inevitably rise and age at presentation fall as the adolescent cohort of today reaches adulthood.

In addition to the changes in prevalence of maternal heart diseases outlined above, patient expectation also needs to be considered when planning ANC for these women. Over the past decade or so, people have had their expectations of healthcare provision raised. They expect modern medicine to be able to 'cure all' and consider very few health threats to be insurmountable. They demand and expect high-quality care, and want it to be provided locally. It is often a disappointment for them to realise that the specialist services they require in pregnancy are not always available on their doorstep and that complications can and do occur.

Presentation of maternal heart disease

It is worth noting from the CEMACH report that the majority of maternal cardiac deaths occurred in those with previously undiagnosed underlying heart disease. More often than not, a history of heart disease or symptoms suggestive thereof that presented during pregnancy were not appreciated or fully investigated. To address this problem, strict criteria need to be defined for the assessment of women who have either a past or family history of heart diseases such as rheumatic fever or premature sudden death or women who complain of symptoms of dyspnoea. An echocardiogram will exclude the majority of important diagnoses and there should be a low threshold for referring for investigation.

Recommendations for the hierarchy of antenatal care

A useful template for organising ANC for women with heart disease can be derived by modifying the current recommendations of the European Society of Cardiology (ESC) and others for the care of adults with CHD.[5,6] Cardiac lesions can be subdivided by lesion complexity and graded from simple to highly complex (Figure 5.1). This hierarchical model of care recommends that highly complex lesions are cared for exclusively by a specialist cardiac unit that fulfils specific criteria for a minimum standard of care provision (Figure 5.2).

This care model represents the 'ideal' or 'best care' for adults with CHD. This is not currently achieved in the UK because service provision is insufficient to meet the demands of this growing population. The specialty is in its infancy and more specialists and specialist units are needed.[7] Consequently, there are (depending on definition) about eight 'specialist' cardiology units in the UK. Most fulfil the majority of the criteria for specialist unit recognition as defined by the ESC and therefore should be able to provide a specialist antenatal service.

Level I Exclusive care in a specialist unit	**Highly complex lesions:** Repairs with conduits, Rastelli, Fontan, Marfan syndrome, Ebstein anomaly, pulmonary atresia, Eisenmenger syndrome, repaired complete transposition of great arteries (arterial switch or atrial switch), congenitally corrected transposition of great arteries, pulmonary hypertension, cyanotic congenital heart disease
Level II Shared care with a regional adult cardiology unit	**Lesions of moderate complexity:** Coarctation of the aorta (repaired/native), repaired atrioventricular septal defect, aortic stenosis, pulmonary stenosis/pulmonary regurgitation, tetralogy of Fallot, ventricular septal defect and aorta regurgitation, mechanical valves, hypertrophic cardiomyopathy, dilated cardiomyopathy
Level III Care predominantly in a general adult cardiology unit	**Simple lesions:** Repaired patent ductus arteriosus/ventricular septal defect/total anomalous pulmonary venous drainage/atrial septal defect, mild pulmonary stenosis/pulmonary regurgitation, small ventricular septal defect

Figure 5.1. Hierarchy of care for adults with congenital heart disease; these care levels provide a framework for delivery of hierarchical care between general physician, non-specialist cardiologists and specialist adult congenital heart units

1.	The unit must be located in an adult medical environment.
2.	Multidisciplinary specialty provision should be available.
3.	There must be an association with strong paediatric cardiology groups with defined care pathways for the appropriate transfer of patients to the adult service when deemed appropriate.
4.	The specialist unit should serve a population of approximately 5–10 million people and it should function within the local medical community.
5.	Local cardiologists and primary care physicians should be encouraged to establish a referral relationship with the specialist unit.
6.	Specialist units should provide timely telephone advice, informal consultation, rapid consultant referrals as well as collaboration in patient follow-up.
7.	The specialist unit should include cardiologist(s) with training in management of grown-ups with congenital heart disease in a collaborative team including cardiac surgeons, anaesthetists and intensivists.
8.	Specialist consultants should be familiar with echocardiography (including transoesophageal echocardiography) and diagnostic cardiac catheterisation and one consultant per centre should have experience in interventional catheterisation.
9.	Specialist units should have access to an electrophysiologist with expertise in arrhythmia management in congenital heart disease, pacemaker insertion, ablation and defibrillator implantation.
10.	Specialist imaging including MRI and CT should be available.
11.	The specialist unit should have close links with other specialist departments and, in particular, the provision of a joint service with obstetrics to manage high-risk pregnancies.
12.	Access to a cardiac pathologist with an interest in congenital cardiac malformations is also highly desirable.
13.	A minimum of two congenital heart surgeons (often shared with paediatric cardiology units) should be available.
14.	Anaesthetists, intensive care and surgical teams with interest in congenital heart disease is desirable.
15.	The specialist unit should have an association with a transplant centre.

Figure 5.2.   Criteria for a specialist congenital heart disease unit

The recommendations I make are based on the 'ideal world', with the assumption that specialist cardiology services are abundant and distributed evenly around the UK. It is then possible to make recommendations for ANC using a modified version of the ESC hierarchical model of care (Figure 5.3), in conjunction with an assessment of risk that incorporates the Toronto risk predictor score (Figure 5.4).[8]

To provide an ANC service for these women, specialist cardiology services and high-risk obstetric services must unite, with the involvement of the following essential personnel:

- an obstetrician with experience in high-risk obstetrics
- a cardiologist or physician experienced in managing maternal heart disease who has a knowledge of congenital heart lesions
- an anaesthetist with cardiac experience

Level I Exclusive care in a specialist unit with a multidisciplinary team	Repairs with conduits, Fontan, Marfan syndrome, Ebstein anomaly, pulmonary atresia, Eisenmenger syndrome, repaired complete transposition of great arteries (arterial switch or atrial switch), congenitally corrected transposition of great arteries, pulmonary hypertension, cyanotic congenital heart disease, native coarctation of the aorta, aortic stenosis, tetralogy of Fallot with pulmonary regurgitation (moderate), ventricular septal defect/aorta regurgitation, mechanical valves, hypertrophic cardiomyopathy, dilated cardiomyopathy Toronto score ≥ 1
Level II Shared care between a specialist cardiologist and a local obstetric team	Coarctation of the aorta (repaired), atrioventricular septal defect, aortic stenosis, pulmonary stenosis/pulmonary regurgitation (mild), tetralogy of Fallot with minimal residua, ventricular septal defect and aorta regurgitation Toronto score 0
Level III Shared care between a general adult cardiology unit and a local obstetric team	Repaired patent ductus arteriosus, mild pulmonary stenosis, small ventricular septal defect, repaired atrial septal defect Toronto score 0

Figure 5.3. Hierarchy of care for pregnant women with congenital heart disease; these care levels provide a framework for delivery of hierarchical care between specialist cardiologist, general cardiologist and obstetrician

- a neonatologist and level III neonatal intensive therapy unit (ITU) services
- a fetal–maternal medicine specialist with expertise in fetal echocardiography
- a haematologist with experience in maternal medicine
- midwives with intensive care training and experience
- clinical nurse specialists (CNS) from cardiology.

Haematology services and CNS's deserve special mention. Many women with heart disease take anticoagulation medication either to reduce their risk of thrombo-embolism or because they have a mechanical valve. Meticulous monitoring is necessary, especially for mechanical valves, irrespective of the method used. Specific maternal anticoagulation guidelines should be in place, as well as a robust system for the feedback of clotting results to both the women and medical personnel. Involvement of a CNS from cardiology, who can liaise with midwifery colleagues, is also important. Each CNS can develop nursing care pathways and provide clear guidance to nursing and midwifery staff in each of their respective specialties. In the

- Prior episode of heart failure, TIA, CVA or arrhythmia
- NYHA ≥ II or cyanosis
- Left heart obstruction (MVA < 2 cm², AVA < 1.5 cm², peak LVOTO > 30 mmHg on echo)
- Reduced LV function (EF < 40%)

0 predictors: risk of a cardiac event is 5%
1 predictor: risk of cardiac event is 27%
>1 predictor: risk of cardiac event is 75%

AVA = aortic valve area
CVA = cerebrovascular accident
EF = ejection fraction
LV = left ventricular
LVOTO = left ventricular outflow tract obstruction
MVA = mitral valve area
NYHA = New York Heart Association
TIA = transient ischaemic attack

Figure 5.4.   Toronto risk markers for maternal cardiac events

event that a mother has to deliver in the cardiac unit, this co-worker relationship across the two specialties is invaluable. The CNS can be the linchpin of the multidisciplinary team.

It is wise to have cardiac surgery and an interventional cardiologist with skills in valvuloplasty in close proximity to the specialist high-risk antenatal service. In conjunction with neonatal ITU support, these specialists provide a 'comfort zone' for managing these women.

Despite preconceptual counselling and detailed prepregnancy work-up, early delivery might be needed for maternal health reasons. Not all risks or haemodynamic insults to the cardiovascular system can be predicted or anticipated in advance of pregnancy. Obstetric complications, such as twin pregnancy, pre-eclampsia or the development of unheralded arrhythmias, may compound any haemodynamic burden and lead to clinical deterioration and decompensation, even in the setting of only moderate heart lesions. Good neonatal ITU services permit timely delivery, ensuring maternal health is prioritised, while fetal welfare is not significantly compromised.

Access to an expert interventional cardiologist and cardiac surgery is also desirable for similar reasons. Not all women will have remained under specialist follow-up and some re-present in pregnancy with severe residual lesions that need urgent treatment during pregnancy if the pregnancy is to continue safely, such as mitral or aortic valvuloplasty for severe valvular obstruction. Cardiac surgery, although rarely needed, can save life if there has been an acute catastrophic event such as mechanical valve thrombosis or aortic dissection.

Obstetric cardiac case

Name: *LS*

D.O.B.:

G2P1

EDD: *30/07/2004*

Diagnosis:
Transposition of the great vessels.
Mustard repair 1975.
LV–PA conduit for LVOTO 1984.
Replacement conduit 1993.
DDDR pacemaker for tachy–brady syndrome 1998.

Prepregnancy status:

Medications:

Clinical examination findings:

Current status @ x/40:

Past obstetric history:

Recent investigations: *TTE/ETT/MRI/Angio.*

Haemodynamic issues:

Delivery plan:

Labour and delivery:
■ *Elective CS planned for 38/40 with epidural anaesthesia (previous CS).*
■ *Endocarditis prophylaxis to be given at induction.*

Drugs to be available on labour ward:

Haemodynamic monitoring and intrapartum care:

Postpartum care and monitoring:

Discharge plan and follow-up:

Plan provided by:

Figure 5.5. Template for high-risk cardiac obstetric cases

Recommendations for organisation of antenatal care

All pregnant women with heart disease should be referred to a specialist high-risk antenatal service as defined above. They should have at least one specialist cardiology review with clinical assessment and transthoracic echo (TTE) performed. Thereafter, based on lesion complexity, the severity of any residua and perceived pregnancy risk, women can be stratified to the following care pathways:

■ level I care – exclusive care by a specialist antenatal service

■ level II care – shared care; regular specialist cardiology review and local obstetric care, with defined lines of communication between specialists

■ level III care – local care; local cardiology review and local obstetric care, with clearly defined lines of communication between all specialists.

Following each review, a report should be generated which includes diagnosis, a heart diagram, a clinical summary, the anticipated haemodynamic impact of pregnancy, and recent investigations. In the later stages of pregnancy the report should also provide guidance on delivery planning (monitoring requirements, drugs to be available on labour ward, requirements for endocarditis prophylaxis and peri/postpartum care requirements). Contact details including e-mail addresses for all specialist personnel should also be included. A copy should be given to the woman and any medical personnel involved. A template for such a report is shown in Figure 5.5.

There is flexibility in this structure of ANC provision, in that care pathways can change and be reassessed if there are any unexpected complications or if any of the care providers do not feel comfortable to continue care for any reason. An overall schema for this pattern of care is shown in Figure 5.6. Eventually, when there are more specialist units and the training curricula have incorporated maternal heart disease as standard, a high-risk ANC network can be developed within designated health sectors. District general hospital (DGH) cardiologists and obstetricians with an interest in the field might then manage the majority of even moderately complex lesions. Such networks have been a success in adult cardiology and have, for example, promoted and guided the development of coronary intervention programmes in the DGH setting.

On a practical level, there are several possible ways to organise the service. Each specialist unit should have the involvement of core physicians from obstetrics, anaesthesia, haematology, and cardiology/obstetric medicine, in addition to the CNS's from midwifery and cardiology. Antenatal clinics can either be organised such that all members of the multidisciplinary team review the woman as a group or individually. At UCLH, core members of the multidisciplinary team share a clinic area, each with adjoining rooms. Women may be seen individually by a single specialist or in a combined review. In addition to outpatient review, cases should be discussed in a joint forum, which at UCLH takes place once per month. Here the finer details of lesion-specific pathophysiology are explained and delivery planning is discussed. This case conference is attended by neonatal staff and labour ward midwives, as well as by the core personnel of the high-risk team. The focus is on delivery planning and staff education. A report relaying the content of this joint case discussion should be generated and sent to the patient and all members of the multidisciplinary team. An additional copy should be placed on the labour ward in a 'cardiac high-risk' folder, which is in view, accessible at all times and known to all. Core members of the multi-disciplinary team must be made aware when a patient is admitted.

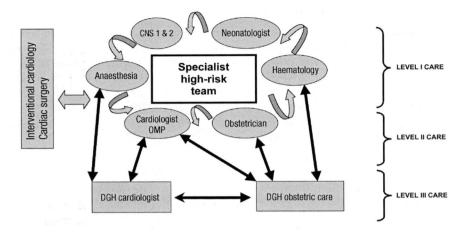

Figure 5.6. A model of antenatal care for women with heart disease; CNS = clinical nurse specialists (cardiology and midwifery); DGH = district general hospital; OMP = obstetric medical physician

The essential factors for the success and functioning of a high-risk ANC team are good communication and teamwork. All members must fulfil their individual commitments and responsibilities but communicate and function as a single unit. Good communication is the key to sharing care with local cardiology and obstetric centres but there must also be clear policies outlining the indications for re-referring back to the specialist unit.

The UCLH experience

The spectrum of heart disease seen by the service at UCLH is shown in Figures 5.7 and 5.8. This experience is not necessarily representative of that seen in other cardiac units in the UK because it is skewed by the specialist nature of cardiology services provided by The Heart Hospital (a grown-up congenital heart unit (GUCH) and an inherited cardiomyopathy service). It does, however, highlight the level of complexity that can be expected by a specialist high-risk obstetric service in the current era. Sixty-one percent of heart disease was of moderate or high complexity, as defined by the ESC guidelines. For those with inherited heart disease ($n = 20$, 11%), ten had hypertrophic cardiomyopathy, with defibrillators *in situ* in eight women. Of the 61% with moderate or complex disease, 40% continued their specialist ANC in a high-risk unit at UCLH, whereas the others were managed through local DGH services. The explanation for this is that following specialist cardiology assessment some women with moderately complex lesions were identified as having no residua or risk markers and they were therefore able to continue their obstetric care locally with intermittent specialist cardiology review.

Current limitations and interim solutions

It is currently difficult for this model of ANC to be implemented across the whole of the UK because large areas are poorly served by specialist cardiology services.

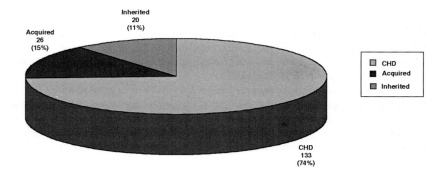

Figure 5.7.   Spectrum of maternal heart disease at UCLH, 2003–06; CHD = congenital heart disease; Acquired = rheumatic heart disease, ischaemic heart disease, puerperal cardiomyopathy, mitral valve prolapse; Inherited = hypertrophic cardiomyopathy, familial dilated cardiomyopathy, long QT syndrome, Marfan syndrome

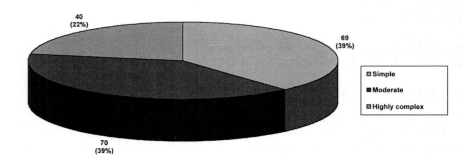

Figure 5.8.   Spectrum of heart disease at UCLH by lesion complexity, 2003–06

Although this is slowly being addressed, it does mean that women with heart disease will for the time being have to travel to receive optimum ANC. Assuming that most can be persuaded to make this journey, a single review by a specialist cardiologist will at least allow a risk assessment to be made and the haemodynamic impact of pregnancy to be predicted and anticipated. Lines of communication between the specialist and remote obstetrician can be opened, so that advice can be given from afar. For all but highly complex cases and those considered high risk, this may provide an interim solution until there are sufficient services and expertise distributed UK wide. Eventually, with sufficient services and expertise, a high-risk cardiac ANC network can be organised for each sector of the UK. This will ensure that most women with heart disease can have their ANC locally, which represents 'the ideal' for motherhood.

References

1. de Swiet M. Maternal mortality: confidential enquiries into maternal deaths in the United Kingdom. *Am J Obstet Gynecol* 2000;182:760–6.
2. Wren C, O'Sullivan JJ. Survival with congenital heart disease and need for follow up in adult life. *Heart* 2001;85:438–43.
3. Meijboom LJ, Vos FE, Timmermans J, Boers GH, Zwinderman AH, Mulder BJ. Pregnancy and aortic root growth in the Marfan syndrome: a prospective study. *Eur Heart J* 2005;26:914–20.
4. Rossiter JP, Repke JT, Morales AJ, Murphy EA, Pyeritz RE. A prospective longitudinal evaluation of pregnancy in the Marfan syndrome. *Am J Obstet Gynecol* 1995;173:1599–606.
5. Deanfield J, Thaulow E, Warnes C, Webb G, Kolbel F, Hoffman A, *et al*. Management of grown up congenital heart disease. *Eur Heart J* 2003;24:1035–84.
6. Connelly MS, Webb GD, Somerville J, Warnes CA, Perloff JK, Liberthson RR, *et al*. Canadian Consensus Conference on Adult Congenital Heart Disease 1996. *Can J Cardiol* 1998;14:395–452.
7. Report of the British Cardiac Society Working Party. Grown-up congenital heart (GUCH) disease: current needs and provision of service for adolescents and adults with congenital heart disease in the UK. *Heart* 2002;88 Suppl 1:i1–14.
8. Siu SC, Sermer M, Colman JM, Alvarez AN, Mercier LA, Morton BC, *et al*. Cardiac Disease in Pregnancy (CARPREG) Investigators. Prospective multicenter study of pregnancy outcomes in women with heart disease. *Circulation* 2001;104:515–21.

Chapter 6
Cardiac monitoring during pregnancy

Jack M Colman, Candice K Silversides, Mathew Sermer and Samuel C Siu

Fundamental to appropriate cardiac monitoring of women with heart disease during pregnancy is timely evaluation of the nature and severity of the cardiac condition and the level of risk that it poses to pregnancy. Women at intermediate and high risk require special care. Trivial and mild conditions should be re-evaluated in case they have been misdiagnosed or the condition has progressed since the last assessment. If the condition is genuinely minor, the woman can be reassured and any tendency to over-treatment counteracted.

Initial assessment

Every woman with heart disease considering pregnancy will be well served by informed preconception cardiac counselling or, if pregnancy has already begun, by a comprehensive cardiology assessment as early in pregnancy as possible. Such an assessment has the following objectives:

■ to define in detail the nature and severity of the heart condition and its impact on the woman's functional capacity

■ to ensure that the nature of the condition is well understood by the woman herself

■ to consider, if still prior to conception, whether a cardiac intervention might improve the eventual outcome of pregnancy, or may be indicated in the near future independent of pregnancy

■ to estimate the risk of an adverse maternal cardiac, obstetrical or neonatal event, using a combination of general and lesion-specific maternal cardiac risk factors, as well as classic obstetric risk factors[1]

■ to share this risk assessment with the woman and clarify her understanding and tolerance of the risks identified; there is often ambiguity in such an assessment, and this should be acknowledged

■ to be ready to deal in a sensitive fashion with the rare but important occasions when pregnancy has such high risk that advice against its attempt or continuation must be offered. It should be recognised that such advice may not only not be followed but, having been offered, may also risk alienating the woman from further specialised care. Such advice should never be provided casually without good evidence, as it may not match the mother's value system, desire for pregnancy and tolerance of risk. If a woman decides to proceed with a very high-risk pregnancy in the face of contrary advice, the decision should be respected and she should understand that the best possible care will continue to be provided.[2]

- to explore relevant issues of maternal health and life expectancy that might impact on the ability to raise and nurture a child
- to assess the likelihood of recurrence of heart disease in the offspring and, when indicated, offer clinical genetics consultation, genetic testing and other modalities for pre- and postnatal diagnosis, especially transabdominal fetal echocardiography and planned postnatal clinical and echocardiographic evaluation of the infant
- to provide recommendations from the cardiac standpoint regarding the advisability of including obstetricians that are expert in high-risk obstetrical management in the consultation process, the need for further cardiac monitoring during pregnancy, 'high risk' versus 'standard' obstetrical care, including appropriateness of local care versus management in a regional high risk centre, and the need for additional investigations or treatments
- to educate the woman regarding the sort of cardiac surveillance required during the pregnancy.

Nature and severity of the heart condition

Establishing the nature and severity of the heart condition is not a trivial task. In a woman with congenital heart disease (CHD), in particular, the history from her regarding the nature of her cardiac condition or type of repair may be incomplete or misleading. The woman often cannot provide such information from personal experience because the relevant events occurred in infancy or childhood. Parents may have misunderstood, forgotten details, or not transmitted knowledge to growing children. Surgical treatment in childhood may have led to misapprehension of 'cure' when in fact active issues remain. In women with chronic functional limitation that they have come to accept as 'normal', history alone may not properly identify the magnitude of that limitation. Furthermore, pregnancy risk cannot be assessed solely from the anatomical diagnosis. Functional status, nature and era of palliation and repair, and the presence of anatomical and electrical sequelae of prior surgery or residual abnormalities all modify the risk anticipated from the anatomical diagnosis alone.[3]

In many cases, especially in women with CHD, the cardiologist plays a crucial role at this first assessment by clarifying the meaning of eponymous diagnoses and procedures. Obstetricians and anaesthetists need and appreciate a review of the relevant anatomical and physiological issues.

Pregnancy sometimes precipitates a move from paediatric to adult medical care, and so the initial assessment may need to be expanded to deal also with issues of transition.[4]

Risk of adverse events

To fully evaluate the risk of adverse events in pregnancy one should clarify the anatomical, physiological and electrical features of the condition, define the functional status, derive a global risk score for adverse maternal cardiac events in pregnancy, consider lesion-specific risks, and also evaluate the risk of adverse obstetrical and neonatal events.

Functional status

In an early study of 482 pregnancies in women with CHD, cardiovascular morbidity was lower and live birth rate higher in mothers in NYHA functional class I (see Appendix A) compared with the others.[5] In the Canadian CARPREG study we reconfirmed the value of NYHA functional assessment, finding that maternal prepregnancy NYHA class greater than II was an independent predictor of adverse maternal cardiac events during pregnancy.[6,7]

Global risk score

In CARPREG and other studies carried out by a collaboration of Canadian investigators, maternal and fetal outcomes were analysed in 851 completed pregnancies, 252 of them in a retrospective study and subsequently another 599 in a prospective multicentre study.[6,7] In the prospective study, poor functional status (NYHA class greater than II) or cyanosis, left ventricular systolic dysfunction, left heart obstruction and history of cardiac events prior to pregnancy (arrhythmia, stroke or pulmonary oedema) were independent predictors of adverse maternal cardiac events in pregnancy.[6,7] A risk index was developed that incorporates these maternal risk factors. The risk of a cardiac event (cardiac death, stroke, pulmonary oedema or arrhythmia) during pregnancy increases with the number of predictors present at the antepartum evaluation. In a woman with heart disease and a risk index of 0, the likelihood of a cardiac event during pregnancy is under 5%, whereas with a risk index of 1 it rises to about 25% and with a risk index greater than 1 the likelihood is 75%.[7]

Lesion-specific risks

In addition to the risk defined by consideration of global and general factors, lesion-specific risks must be considered when information is available. Such lesion-specific risk data are needed to refine and supplement the global assessment for two reasons. Firstly, unique aspects of the woman's condition seen only in their specific lesion can be taken into account. Secondly, some high-risk lesions known from other studies to be important were under-represented in the population from which the global risk score was derived and as a consequence their impact is not reflected in a global score. For example, specific data are available on risks in Eisenmenger syndrome and pulmonary hypertension,[8] other cyanotic heart disease,[9] Marfan syndrome,[10] left heart obstruction,[11–13] Mustard operation,[14,15] Fontan procedure,[16] chronic hypertension[17] and peripartum cardiomyopathy.[18]

Fetal and neonatal adverse events

Women with heart disease have an increased risk of fetal and neonatal adverse events.[6,7,19–21] In a prospective study[1] incorporating a control group of pregnant women without heart disease, we showed that the risk of neonatal complications (premature birth, small-for-gestational-age birthweight, respiratory distress syndrome, intraventricular haemorrhage, fetal or neonatal death) is higher in women with heart disease, especially in the presence of poor maternal functional class, cyanosis or left heart obstruction, and that the risk is further amplified if there are concomitant maternal non-cardiac (obstetrical and other) risk factors for fetal and neonatal complications.

Where and when should cardiac monitoring during and after pregnancy take place?

Low-risk patients

Following an initial clinical assessment, some women will be considered low risk for adverse cardiac or fetal/neonatal events. Such women generally include those with small left to right shunts, repaired lesions without residual cardiac dysfunction, isolated mitral valve prolapse without significant regurgitation, bicuspid aortic valve without stenosis, mild or moderate pulmonary stenosis, or valvular regurgitation with normal ventricular systolic function. These women can reasonably be cared for in local obstetric units. Their routine care will have been enhanced by the comprehensive initial assessment because cardiac issues will have been clarified and recommendations will have been made for management and cardiac follow-up if necessary. These recommendations will often restrict rather than amplify the extra investigation and special care provided thereafter.

Intermediate- and high-risk patients

On the other hand, women with more complex conditions, with conditions in which pregnancy outcomes are not well understood and with identified risk factors for adverse outcomes are optimally managed in multidisciplinary high-risk units. Such units should include specialised medical and perinatal care. Attendance of the pregnancy cardiologist in the antenatal clinic on a regular basis is desirable. There should be on-site access to electrocardiography (ECG) and echocardiography. Collaborative arrangements with specialists in thrombosis, medical genetics, obstetrical anaesthesia, neonatology, paediatric cardiology and social work need to be in place. The advantages of such units include:

- 'one-stop shopping', thus reducing the number of medical visits for pregnant women
- enhanced, often immediate, communication among consultants
- familiarity with issues of cardiac disease in pregnancy, allowing quick recognition of women likely to need extra attention
- ready recognition of women who will do well and need little intervention, reducing the likelihood of inappropriate advice or unnecessary investigation and treatment
- good opportunities for research and teaching to enhance future care of women with heart disease.

The need for such multidisciplinary units was highlighted in the 2000–2002 report of the UK Confidential Enquiry into Maternal and Child Health.[22]

There are no experimental data to guide the development of optimal regimes for the frequency of antenatal checks of women with heart disease during pregnancy.

In the programme in Toronto, we (cardiologists) see our patients at intervals that vary according to the severity of the mother's lesion, its stability and the need for ongoing adjustment of therapy. We find it useful to provide an initial cardiology assessment early in pregnancy (this should be during the first trimester, and as early as possible in women who have not had preconception counselling) to cover issues not addressed at the preconception visit, to establish the baseline in pregnancy, to explain our role and availability, and to initiate planning. At the minimum, the cardiologist should see each woman again towards the end of the second trimester, coincident with the expected peak in cardiac output. We schedule another cardiology review in the third trimester at about 36 weeks of gestation to screen for interval changes, to ensure that plans for labour and delivery have been developed and disseminated, to answer questions, and to refresh data. Women who are symptomatic or who are expected to become so, or whose condition is anticipated to progress, are seen more frequently. An integrated multidisciplinary clinic facilitates frequent assessments since the woman can easily be seen by the cardiologist at the time of each obstetrical antenatal visit if necessary, without requiring extra trips, time and effort.

Monitoring in hospital

Cardiology review after admission for delivery may occur only postpartum. This should not normally be a disadvantage because the previously prepared plans will provide adequate guidance to the duty staff such that only the exceptional patient will require urgent involvement of the not-on-duty consultant cardiologist. Women at high risk and/or those undergoing induction for cardiac reasons do sometimes need in-hospital reassessment prior to or during labour. This is provided by the primary consultant if possible, but otherwise by on-call colleagues who have a detailed management plan, including contingency plans, available.

Women at very or extremely high risk, such as those with pulmonary hypertension, Eisenmenger syndrome, other cyanotic heart disease, Marfan syndrome with expanding aortic root, decompensated heart failure or symptomatic left-sided obstructive valve disease, may need early and extended in-hospital surveillance and management antepartum and also postpartum.

Postpartum follow-up

We provide a postpartum cardiac review at the time of the obstetric postpartum check, typically at 6 weeks after birth. At this time we ensure there is a plan for continuing follow-up of the cardiac condition after pregnancy and we discuss whether there is a need for postnatal paediatric cardiological assessment of the infant, which may be indicated in particular for the infant born to a mother with CHD, because of the increased possibility of finding previously unrecognised CHD in the infant.

Not much is known about the long-term effects of pregnancy on maternal cardiac status but there is evidence in normal women that pregnancy-related physiological changes will have resolved by 6 months postpartum.[23] Another cardiac assessment at or shortly after that point may thus be useful to refresh baseline, ensure appropriate continuing follow-up of the non-pregnant new mother and document any differences from her status prior to the index pregnancy.

Methods of cardiac monitoring during pregnancy

History, physical examination, ECG and echocardiography are the mainstays of the clinical cardiac assessment, supplemented by additional investigations when indicated.

History and physical examination

Symptoms and signs in uncomplicated pregnancy mimic those that occur because of cardiac disease. The cardiac consultant needs to clarify the true nature of these symptoms and signs, recognising their significance as markers of pathology in some cases, and in others providing reassurance to the mother that what is being experienced or seen is normal and expected. For example, cardinal cardiac symptoms such as dyspnoea, tachypnoea, fatigue, decreased exercise capacity, dizziness, palpitations and even syncope may be experienced during a normal pregnancy. Normal findings on physical examination during pregnancy that overlap typical manifestations of cardiac disease include mild elevation of jugular venous pressure, a displaced apex, a parasternal lift, increased intensity of the first heart sound, a prominent pulmonary second heart sound, persistent expiratory splitting of the second heart sound (though not fixed splitting), a third heart sound, an early peaking systolic ejection murmur, and venous hums and mammary souffles which can be mistaken for cardiac murmurs. Leg oedema is common in pregnancy for reasons other than right heart failure.[24–26] In our maternal cardiac clinic we are frequently able to reassure the woman and the other members of the care team regarding the innocence of such symptoms and signs, whereas we less frequently must attribute them to a deteriorating clinical condition. The following need particular consideration:

- Blood pressure, although this is usually managed by the obstetricians.
- Heart rate and rhythm: *de novo* arrhythmias and exacerbations of pre-existing arrhythmias are common during pregnancy in women with cardiac disease, and detecting them is important. On the other hand, 'palpitations' as perceived by the mother are more common in pregnancy and may not be due to pathological rhythm disturbance. In such cases, the mother (and sometimes the obstetrician) needs reassurance.
- Anticoagulation: for each anticoagulated patient, the optimal form of therapy must be carefully considered. There is a need for particularly precise control and dosing requirements change as pregnancy progresses. Anticoagulation in pregnancy is often best monitored in a specialised thrombosis clinic.
- Oxygen saturation: in women with shunts, right to left shunting manifesting as hypoxaemia and perhaps cyanosis may be noted for the first time or may increase during pregnancy. The normal physiological pregnancy-related fall in peripheral vascular resistance is the most important reason for this although other pathophysiological factors may play a role.[27]
- Choice of drugs: the teratogenic and fetopathic effects of cardiac drugs need to be considered and alternate therapies found when necessary. The risks and benefits of modification of drug therapy have to be addressed in terms of the health and safety of the mother and of the fetus; the needs of the two do not always coincide. Such issues arise with many drugs but are particularly problematic for coumarin anticoagulants, heparins, angiotensin-converting enzyme (ACE) inhibitors and angiotensin-receptor blockers, amiodarone and some other antiarrhythmics. Drug dosing and frequency may need adjustment

in pregnancy because of changes in the volume of distribution of many drugs, increases in glomerular filtration rate enhancing drug excretion, and changes in hepatic metabolism affecting drug processing by the liver.[28,29]

■ Plans for endocarditis prophylaxis at the time of delivery.

Electrocardiography

An ECG is invariably obtained at the baseline assessment and may be repeated to clarify symptoms or signs and serially as a screening test in women with more severe forms of heart disease. Normal changes in pregnancy must be recognised to avoid confusion with pathological processes. Sinus tachycardia is common: the average heart rate in a pregnant woman increases by about 20 beats per minute, with the rate peaking early in the third trimester. In the early postpartum period there is a transient physiological sinus bradycardia, which is occasionally profound. The frontal plane QRS axis shifts, usually to the left. Non-specific ST-T repolarisation abnormalities are common. Isolated atrial and ventricular extrasystoles are often seen in normal women during pregnancy.[30]

Echocardiography

Echocardiography is uniquely useful in pregnancy because of its safety, its ubiquitous availability, its relatively low cost and its ability to be repeated serially to follow progress. We obtain an echocardiogram at first assessment in early pregnancy unless a very recent study is available. We generally repeat the echocardiogram at the assessment late in the second trimester (26–28 weeks gestational age) to assess the impact of the interval increase in cardiac work, which is at that time near its peak, although the incremental value of such a repeat study has not yet been fully established. Similarly, it may be useful to repeat the echocardiogram after 6 months postpartum in women in whom there is concern about lesion progression, as changes noted at that point can no longer be explained by persistent physiological effects of the recent pregnancy itself.[23] There are indications for more frequent repetition of echocardiography during and following pregnancy, especially in Marfan syndrome, where serial studies every 4–6 weeks until 6 months postpartum are indicated to follow the size of the aortic root;[10] in pulmonary hypertension to screen for a rising pulmonary artery systolic pressure; and in women with a history of previous peripartum cardiomyopathy to screen for subclinical deterioration in left ventricular function. In addition, echocardiography should generally be part of a cardiac assessment performed because of new or progressive symptoms that may be of cardiac origin, whether maternal cardiac disease was previously recognised or not. Of particular interest in the echocardiographic evaluation are:

■ systemic ventricular function

■ stenosis of valves or outflow tracts, especially in the systemic circulation

■ assessment of mechanical heart valves

■ level and progression of pulmonary pressure, as estimated from the pulmonary ventricular systolic pressure reduced by any gradient across the pulmonary ventricular outflow tract

■ size of the aortic root and changes during pregnancy, relevant in women with Marfan syndrome and other ascending aortopathies

■ the echocardiographic changes in normal pregnancies that must be recognised and not mistaken for new pathology; these include modest increase in size of all cardiac chambers, new or increased regurgitation across mitral and tricuspid and occasionally pulmonary valves, and small pericardial effusions.[31]

Magnetic resonance imaging

In some women additional diagnostic modalities are needed. The most important of these in CHD is cardiac magnetic resonance imaging (MRI). Because of unresolved issues of safety in pregnant women, MRI should be done during preconception assessment. However, if such information is not available and the woman is already pregnant, and especially if alternative diagnostic tests carry the well-established risks of ionising radiation, MRI can be considered. Fetal risks of MRI include the effect of heat, the effect of noise (which can be attenuated for the mother by headphones or earplugs but not for the fetus), and the possible impact on embryonic and fetal development and growth of the static magnetic field and the superimposed induced electromagnetic gradients. However, these risks to the fetus have not been well characterised and their magnitude is not known.[32] MRI should be used during pregnancy only when clearly needed, preferably after the first trimester, with attention given to minimising time in the coil, using lower magnetic energy when possible, and preferably not using gadolinium contrast.[32] In spite of the known and unknown risks, MRI may be superior to cardiac catheterisation or computed tomography (CT) because it avoids ionising radiation and often yields diagnostic information of extremely high quality. However, more studies of safety for the fetus are needed.

Exercise testing

The role of exercise testing in pregnancy assessment of women with cardiac disease is unclear. There is evidence for the safety of moderate and even high-intensity exercise and of exercise testing in normal fit women during pregnancy,[33] but there are no data on safety or the meaning of results of testing during pregnancy in women with cardiac disease. Preconception exercise testing, especially cardiopulmonary testing using a metabolic cart to clarify exercise capacity, can be helpful in women with chronic forms of heart disease in whom functional capacity evaluated by history alone may be misleading. Nonetheless, data regarding the degree of reduction in exercise capacity that defines excessive risk in pregnancy are not available.

Ambulatory electrocardiographic monitoring

Holter monitoring and long-term external loop or event recording can be used to clarify the symptom of palpitations, which is common during pregnancy and is often due simply to awareness of pregnancy-mediated sinus tachycardia or forceful sinus beats. Since both supraventricular and ventricular arrhythmias are also more common in pregnancy in women both with a pre-existing history of arrhythmia and *de novo*,[34] it is helpful to make a specific diagnosis of the mechanism of the symptom of palpitations by Holter monitoring unless a sinus mechanism can be deduced with confidence from the history.

X-ray and nuclear medicine procedures

Procedures using ionising radiation, such as diagnostic radiography, CT, cardiac catheterisation and nuclear imaging, are usually avoided during pregnancy but should be considered, especially after the first trimester when organogenesis is complete, if the information to be obtained is critical to management and cannot be obtained in other ways. Information on radiation risks to the fetus is available.[35] No congenital abnormality has been identified in fetuses exposed to less than 100 mGy, and the vast majority of the tests that might be contemplated expose the fetus to ionising radiation well below this threshold. Steps can be taken to minimise fetal radiation dose through modification of technique (e.g. coronary angiography by the radial artery route) and shielding of the maternal abdomen (and therefore fetus). Because of radiation scattering, however, shielding is not completely effective.

Collaboration, management plans and conferences

Starting with the initial preconception or early pregnancy assessment, incorporating the subsequent clarification of diagnosis and maternal risk status, and taking into account the clinical course of the pregnancy, the cardiologist, the obstetrician or perinatologist, the anaesthetist, the neonatologist and others, as part of a multidisciplinary team, should develop a written management plan for labour, delivery and postpartum care. The elements of such a plan include:

- explanation of cardiovascular anatomy and pathophysiology in language that can be understood by competent colleagues not highly trained in cardiology; this is especially relevant for women with CHD, where a schematic diagram of the woman's cardiac anatomy is often helpful for the entire healthcare team
- recommendations for general, cardiac, obstetric, anaesthetic and paediatric management at labour and delivery
- contingency plans defining all probable and also any anticipated rare but serious adverse events that might occur, offering suggested management strategies personalised to the woman's particular condition and specific pathophysiology
- recommendations and rationale for the location, duration and nature of postpartum monitoring.

In the 24 hour per day, 365 day per year world of pregnancy management, collaborative care is the rule and the senior consultants most familiar with a particular case will not necessarily be readily available when problems arise. One of the most important roles of such consultants is thus to anticipate such circumstances and to leave adequate guidance for colleagues, developed in advance electively and thoughtfully after consultation and consensus. To facilitate the development of such plans, women with complex conditions often benefit from organised patient management conferences where all involved personnel, including obstetrics, cardiology, neonatology, anaesthesia, obstetric medicine, nursing, social work and others, meet to discuss cases. Such conferences serve multiple purposes including clarification of issues, definition of the management plan, team building and education. The 2000–2002 report on Confidential Enquiries into Maternal Deaths in the UK emphasised that 'all known information important for care must be shared among all caregivers'.[22] A comprehensive management plan and a patient management conference when appropriate are tools that facilitate such complete sharing of information and enhance the likelihood of successful pregnancy outcomes in women with heart disease.

References

1. Siu SC, Colman JM, Sorensen S, Smallhorn JF, Farine D, Amankwah KS, *et al.* Adverse neonatal and cardiac outcomes are more common in pregnant women with heart disease. *Circulation* 2002;105:2179–84.
2. Drife J, Lewis G, editors. *Why Mothers Die. Report on Confidential Enquiries into Maternal Deaths in the United Kingdom 1994–96.* London: The Stationery Office; 1998.
3. Colman JM. Non-cardiac surgery in adult congenital heart disease. In: Gatzoulis M, Daubeney P, Webb GD, editors. *Diagnosis and Management of Adult Congenital Heart Disease.* London: Churchill Livingstone; 2003. p. 99–104.
4. Foster E, Graham TP Jr, Driscoll DJ, Reid GJ, Reiss JG, Russell IA, *et al.* Proceedings of the 32nd Bethesda conference: Care of the adult with congenital heart disease. Task Force 2: special health care needs of adults with congenital heart disease. *J Am Coll Cardiol* 2001;37:1176–83.
5. Whittemore R, Hobbins J, Engle M. Pregnancy and its outcome in women with and without surgical treatment of congenital heart disease. *Am J Cardiol* 1982;50:641–51.
6. Siu SC, Sermer M, Harrison DA, Grigoriadis E, Liu G, Sorensen S, *et al.* Risk and predictors for pregnancy-related complications in women with heart disease. *Circulation* 1997;96:2789–94.
7. Siu SC, Sermer M, Colman JM, Alvarez N, Mercier L-A, Morton BC, *et al.* Prospective multicenter study of pregnancy outcomes in women with heart disease. *Circulation* 2001;104:515–21.
8. Weiss B, Zemp L, Seifert B, Hess O. Outcome of pulmonary vascular disease in pregnancy: a systematic overview from 1978 through 1996. *J Am Coll Cardiol* 1998;31:1650–7.
9. Presbitero P, Somerville J, Stone S, Aruta E, Spiegelhalter D, Rabajoli F. Pregnancy in cyanotic congenital heart disease. Outcome of mother and fetus. *Circulation* 1994;89:2673–6.
10. Rossiter J, Repke J, Morales A, Murphy E, Pyeritz R. A prospective longitudinal evaluation of pregnancy in the Marfan syndrome. *Am J Obstet Gynecol* 1995;173:1599–606.
11. Silversides CK, Colman JM, Sermer S, Siu SC. Cardiac risk in pregnant women with rheumatic mitral stenosis. *Am J Cardiol* 2003;91:1382–5.
12. Silversides CK, Colman JM, Sermer S, Farine D, Siu SC. Early and intermediate-term outcomes of pregnancy with congenital aortic stenosis. *Am J Cardiol* 2003;91:1386–9.
13. Hameed A, Karaalp IS, Tummala PP, Wani OR, Canetti M, Akhter MW, *et al.* The effect of valvular heart disease on maternal and fetal outcome of pregnancy. *J Am Coll Cardiol* 2001;37:893–9.
14. Guedes S, Mercier L-A, Leduc L, Berube L, Marcotte F, Dore A. Impact of pregnancy on the systemic right ventricle after a Mustard operation for transposition of the great arteries. *J Am Coll Cardiol* 2004;44:433–7.
15. Genoni M, Jenni R, Hoerstrup SP, Vogt P, Turina M. Pregnancy after atrial repair for transposition of the great arteries. *Heart* 1999;81:276–7.
16. Canobbio M, Mair D, van der Velde M, Koos B. Pregnancy outcomes after the Fontan repair. *J Am Coll Cardiol* 1996;28:763–7.
17. Magee LA, Ornstein MP, von Dadelszen P. Fortnightly review: management of hypertension in pregnancy. *BMJ* 1999;318:1332–6.

18. Elkayam U, Tummala PP, Rao K, Akhter MW, Karaalp IS, Wani OR, *et al.* Maternal and fetal outcomes of subsequent pregnancies in women with peripartum cardiomyopathy. *N Engl J Med* 2001;344:1567–71.

19. Shime J, Mocarski E, Hastings D, Webb G, McLaughlin P. Congenital heart disease in pregnancy: short- and long-term implications. *Am J Obstet Gynecol* 1987;156:313–22.

20. McFaul P, Dornan J, Lamki H, Boyle D. Pregnancy complicated by maternal heart disease. A review of 519 women. *Br J Obstet Gynaecol* 1988;95:861–7.

21. Avila WS, Rossi EG, Ramires JA, Grinberg M, Bortolotto MR, Zugaib M, *et al.* Pregnancy in patients with heart disease: experience with 1,000 cases. *Clin Cardiol* 2003;26:135–42.

22. Lewis G, editor. *Why Mothers Die 2000–2002: The Sixth Report of Confidential Enquiries into Maternal Deaths in the United Kingdom.* London: RCOG Press; 2004.

23. Hunter S, Robson SC. Adaptation of the maternal heart in pregnancy. *Br Heart J* 1992;68:540–3.

24. Connolly HM, Warnes CA. Pregnancy and contraception. In: Gatzoulis M, Daubeney P, Webb GD, editors. *Diagnosis and Management of Adult Congenital Heart Disease.* London: Churchill Livingstone; 2003. p. 135–44.

25. Elkayam U, Bitar F. Valvular heart disease and pregnancy. Part I. Native valves. *J Am Coll Cardiol* 2005;46:223–30.

26. vanMook WNKA, Peeters L. Severe cardiac disease in pregnancy. Part I. Hemodynamic changes and complaints during pregnancy, and general management of cardiac disease in pregnancy. *Curr Opin Crit Care* 2005;11:430–4.

27. vanMook WNKA, Peeters L. Severe cardiac disease in pregnancy. Part II. Impact of congenital and acquired cardiac diseases during pregnancy. *Curr Opin Crit Care* 2005;11:435–48.

28. Abbas AE, Lester SJ, Connolly H. Pregnancy and the cardiovascular system. *Int J Cardiol* 2005;98:179–89.

29. Reimold SC, Rutherford JD. Valvular heart disease in pregnancy. *N Engl J Med* 2003;349:52–9.

30. Gowda RM, Khan IA, Mehta NJ, Vasavada BC, Sacchi TJ. Cardiac arrhythmias in pregnancy: clinical and therapeutic considerations. *Int J Cardiol* 2003;88:129–33.

31. Campos O, Andrade JL, Bocanegra J, Ambrose JA, Carvalho AC, Harada K, *et al.* Physiologic multivalvular regurgitation during pregnancy: a longitudinal Doppler echocardiographic study. *Int J Cardiol* 1993;40:265–72.

32. DeWilde JP, Rivers AW. Price DL. A review of the current use of magnetic resonance imaging in pregnancy and safety implications for the fetus. *Prog Biophys Mol Biol* 2005;87:335–53.

33. O'Toole ML, Artol R. Clinical exercise testing during pregnancy and the post-partum period. In: Weisman IM, Zeballos RJ, editors. *Clinical Exercise Testing.* Vol. 32. London: Karger; 2002. p. 273–81.

34. Blomstrom-Lundqvist C, Scheinman MM, Aliot EM, Alpert JS, Calkins H, Camm AJ, *et al.* ACC/AHA/ESC guidelines for the management of patients with supraventricular arrhythmias. A report of the American College of Cardiology/American Heart Association Task Force and the European Society of Cardiology Committee for Practice Guidelines. *Circulation* 2003;108:1871–909.

35. Wagner LK, Lester RG, Saldana LR. *Exposure of the Pregnant Patient to Diagnostic Radiation: A Guide to Medical Management.* 2nd ed. Madison: Medical Physics Publishing; 1997.

Chapter 7

Cardiac drugs in pregnancy

Asma Khalil and Pat O'Brien

General considerations

Only 4% of developmental disorders are caused by chemical and physical agents, of which only a small proportion are due to medicinal products.[1] However, the list of known embryo/feto-toxic drugs includes several used in women with cardiac disease, including angiotensin-converting enzyme (ACE) inhibitors, phenytoin and warfarin. New drugs undergo extensive pre-market testing but the teratogenic effect of some drugs (e.g. thalidomide) is seen only in humans or other specific species. Some of the effects may thus not be evident until the drug is in general use, and these are then often brought to light by case reports or subsequent epidemiological investigations.

Potential adverse effects of drugs

The developmental toxicity of an individual drug depends on the period of pregnancy at which it has its effect. If exposure occurs in the first week after conception, i.e. pre-implantation, it may well result in early embryonic loss. The critical time for fetal organogenesis extends from 3 to 10 weeks of gestation, i.e. from 1 to 8 weeks after conception. Exposure to toxic drugs during this phase of development may result in a structural abnormality or spontaneous miscarriage. Exposure later in pregnancy can have a range of effects, including growth restriction, functional impairment of a particular organ or system, prematurity or intrauterine fetal death. This susceptibility extends into neonatal life.

Pharmacokinetics in pregnancy

Several physiological changes occur in pregnancy that may affect the blood concentration of certain drugs. Gastrointestinal motility and absorption are reduced while lung function is increased. Plasma volume and total body water increase markedly, which has a dilutional effect on some drugs, reducing their concentration. Plasma protein levels are reduced. Glomerular filtration rate rises by almost half, so that drugs which are primarily excreted unchanged by the kidneys are usually excreted more rapidly.

A few drugs that have a high molecular weight, such as heparin, do not cross the placenta. However, the placenta is effectively a lipid barrier separating the maternal and fetal circulations and, given time, most drugs of low molecular weight will cross the placenta so that maternal and fetal levels equilibrate.

Balancing of risks

The risks of embryotoxicity or feto-toxicity depend on both the duration and dose of exposure.[2-5] Prepregnancy and early pregnancy counselling needs to consider the risk–benefit analysis of prolonged exposure, i.e. throughout the pregnancy. Often, either stopping or changing the drug may be advisable. However, post-exposure counselling (after usually a relatively short exposure in early pregnancy before pregnancy is diagnosed) will require a different approach. In this situation, the short duration of exposure is often associated with a very low risk, so that termination or even additional invasive diagnostic procedures are usually not justified.[2,3,5] It should also be remembered that, in some situations, the risk to the mother and/or fetus from the underlying disease is greater than the risk associated with taking the appropriate medication. This is the case with some cardiac conditions.

When prescribing a new drug, particularly long-term medication, in women of reproductive age who have cardiac disease, the possibility of pregnancy should always be considered. By the time pregnancy is diagnosed, organogenesis is usually well under way. The woman should be asked whether she might be, or is planning to become, pregnant. If there is a risk of unplanned pregnancy, effective safe contraception should be prescribed. If pregnancy is planned or possible, medication should be chosen that is safe in pregnancy. In general, monotherapy is preferable and the lowest effective dose should be prescribed.

In the UK, expert advice can be sought from the medicines information services – contact details can be found in the *British National Formulary*.[4]

Adverse incident reporting

If any adverse fetal or maternal effect occurs in a woman taking cardiac drugs in pregnancy, in the UK it should be reported using the yellow label reporting system, whether or not this adverse effect is thought to be caused by the drug.

Breastfeeding

The benefits of breastfeeding are well established and few drugs are contraindicated during lactation (or demand that breastfeeding should be stopped).[6] The concentrations reached by most drugs in the newborn are usually well below therapeutic levels. However, prolonged exposure may lead to accumulation because of the longer half-life in the neonate and therefore caution should be exercised. Some drugs such as methyldopa have an anti-dopamine effect and may therefore lead to an increase in breast milk production.

Diuretics

In pregnancy, the diuretics of choice are the thiazides and furosemide (frusemide).

Thiazide diuretics

The thiazide diuretics include hydrochlorothiazide, chlorothiazide, indapamide and chlorthalidone. These drugs are benzthiazide derivatives that inhibit absorption of sodium and chloride in the distal renal tubule and lead to loss of potassium. They may be used in women with cardiac failure and pulmonary oedema (they are no longer used in pre-eclampsia).

They do not appear to be teratogenic. One study[7] (The Collaborative Perinatal Project) followed 233 women exposed to thiazide diuretics in the first trimester and found a slightly increased risk of malformations. However, all of these mothers had cardiac disease themselves, so the significance of these findings is unclear and further studies would be helpful. Another study[6] found no increase in birth defects among 567 pregnant women exposed to hydrochlorothiazide in the first trimester.

The thiazides cause a reduction in intravascular volume; there is thus a theoretical risk of reduced uteroplacental perfusion leading to intrauterine growth restriction (IUGR). When used long-term in pregnancy (usually for women with heart failure), the mother's electrolytes should be checked regularly. Regular ultrasound scanning is indicated to monitor for IUGR and oligohydramnios.

The neonate is also at risk of electrolyte imbalance (hyponatraemia, hypocalcaemia) if the mother had been given thiazide diuretics towards the end of pregnancy. The neonate may also suffer hypoglycaemia because of the diabetogenic effect of thiazides on the mother. Neonatal thrombocytopenia has also been reported. There have been some case reports that these drugs can inhibit uterine contractions and cause prolonged labour,[6] but this is unlikely to be of clinical significance.

Breastfeeding

Chlorothiazide is excreted in breast milk in concentrations so low that there does not seem to be any adverse effect on the neonate. Thiazides are considered compatible with breastfeeding.

Furosemide

Furosemide is a potent loop diuretic whose action wears off in 2–4 hours. Its only indications in pregnancy are cardiovascular disorders such as pulmonary oedema or heart failure; it should *not* be used for pre-eclampsia as it significantly reduces intra-vascular volume. If used long-term, this decrease in plasma volume may lead to growth restriction in the fetus, although it does not seem to significantly decrease amniotic fluid volume.[8] Furosemide does not appear to be teratogenic. In contrast to the thiazide diuretics, neonatal thrombocytopenia has not been reported with furosemide.

Breastfeeding

Although furosemide is excreted in the breast milk, no adverse neonatal effects have been reported.

Spironolactone

Spironolactone is an aldosterone antagonist that leads to potassium retention. It does not appear to be teratogenic;[6] however, experience is limited and it is thus relatively contraindicated in pregnancy. Spironolactone is known to have anti-androgenic effects and could theoretically cause feminisation of a male fetus, although this has not been reported.

Breastfeeding

The amount of spironolactone appearing in the breast milk appears to be clinically insignificant and, although data are limited, it is likely to be safe in breastfeeding.

Ethacrynic acid

Ethacrynic acid is another potent diuretic that has an effect similar to that of furosemide. One case report[9] describes ototoxicity in the baby of a woman who took ethacrynic acid and canamycin in the third trimester. However, experience with this drug in pregnancy is very limited and, for this reason, its use is not recommended in pregnancy or breastfeeding.

Amiloride

Amiloride directly influences tubular transport and is a potassium-saving diuretic. It does not appear to be teratogenic.[6] However, again data are lacking and the drug is relatively contraindicated in pregnancy. There are no reports of its use in breastfeeding women.

Mannitol

Mannitol is a potent osmotic diuretic that causes a rapid diuresis. Interstitial fluid volume falls while intravascular volume increases. Its use in pregnancy or breastfeeding has not been reported (apart from intra-amniotic injection for therapeutic termination of pregnancy).[10]

Antihypertensives

Hydralazine

Hydralazine is a vasodilator and may be used as an antihypertensive or as an afterload-reducing agent. It is well absorbed orally and is also used intravenously. The half-life is 2–8 hours; it crosses the placenta and is metabolised in the liver. In pregnancy, hydralazine is usually given parenterally in the acute management of hypertension. In this situation, it can cause symptoms similar to those of imminent eclampsia, including headache, nausea, vomiting and flushing. Experience with long-term use of hydralazine in pregnancy is limited. There is one case report[11] of a lupus-like syndrome in the mother that is thought to have resulted from hydralazine sensitivity. Data on first-trimester exposure are sparse, but currently there is no evidence of teratogenesis in humans.

When hydralazine is given intravenously, there is a significant risk of a precipitate fall in blood pressure that may lead to impaired placental perfusion and fetal heart-rate abnormalities. Intravenous administration should thus always be slow.[12]

Breastfeeding

Hydralazine is excreted in breast milk but no adverse effects in the neonate have been noted; it is probably compatible with breastfeeding.

ACE inhibitors

The ACE inhibitor class of drugs includes captopril, enalapril, lisinopril and ramipril. ACE inhibitors inhibit the conversion of angiotensin I to angiotensin II. Their use has become more widespread in recent years, but most available data on their use in pregnancy refer to captopril and enalapril. However, it is likely that the other drugs in this class have similar fetal and neonatal effects.

In contrast to exposure in the second and third trimesters, ACE inhibitors do not appear to be teratogenic in the first trimester.[6,13] Exposure in the second and third trimesters can lead to marked fetal hypotension and decreased (fetal) renal blood flow. This can lead to oligohydramnios; in some cases, there is fetal anuria and renal failure *in utero*. Severe oligohydramnios can result in pulmonary hypoplasia, limb contractures, craniofacial deformities and patent ductus arteriosus. IUGR and preterm delivery have been reported. These adverse effects persist in the neonate, with poor renal perfusion and glomerular filtration rate; there may be significant hypotension and renal failure severe enough to cause neonatal death.

Following inadvertent exposure in early pregnancy (usually in a woman who has conceived unexpectedly while still taking the drug), termination of pregnancy or invasive diagnostic procedures are not indicated, as the drug does not seem to be teratogenic at this stage of pregnancy. However, these drugs *are* contraindicated after the first trimester so the woman should be converted to another medication if possible. Where ACE inhibitors must be continued, the lowest possible dose should be used and amniotic fluid levels and fetal growth should be monitored carefully. Blood pressure and renal function should be monitored closely in the neonate.[14]

Breastfeeding

ACE inhibitors are excreted in breast milk in very low concentrations, with an average milk to plasma ratio of 0.012. No adverse effects have been observed in the neonate and these drugs are generally regarded as safe.[15]

Angiotensin II inhibitors

The angiotensin II inhibitors include losartan and valsartan. These are specific angiotensin II receptor antagonists and they thus have properties similar to those of ACE inhibitors. They are relatively recent drugs and data are still scanty. However, their mechanism of action is very similar to that of ACE inhibitors. It seems likely that the feto-toxic effects observed with ACE inhibitors in the second and third trimesters may also be associated with angiotensin II inhibitors. A case report[16] published in 2001 described anhydramnios and intrauterine fetal death, with pulmonary hypoplasia, and with facial and limb deformities typical of marked oligohydramnios. These changes were attributed to the losartan that the women had been prescribed for hypertension. These drugs are thus not recommended in pregnancy unless all other treatment avenues have been explored.

Breastfeeding

The effects of exposure in breast milk are unknown.

Antiarrhythmics

Minor arrhythmias do not need treatment but if the effectiveness of the heart as a pump becomes impaired, treatment is important. Antiarrhythmics are arranged in classes according to the effect they have on electrical conduction in the heart and the arrhythmia for which they are used.[17] As discussed below, the classes of anti-arrhythmics are 1A, 1B, 1C, 2, 3 and 4.

Class 1A antiarrhythmics

Class 1A includes disopyramide, quinidine and procainamide. The last two are used relatively commonly in pregnant women with cardiac disease and do not appear to be teratogenic.[6] In high doses, quinidine has an oxytocic effect and may cause miscarriage,[18] but this has rarely been observed in therapeutic doses and should thus not influence its choice.

Class 1B antiarrhythmics

Class 1B includes lidocaine (lignocaine), phenytoin and others. Lidocaine has no teratogenic effects. However, if maternal lidocaine toxicity occurs then some of the effects such as hyperthermia may damage the fetus.[19]

The teratogenic effects of phenytoin were first recognised back in 1964.[20] The risk of congenital abnormality associated with its use is 2–3 times greater than the background risk. Typical anomalies observed include craniofacial abnormalities, abnormalities of the distal phalanges, cardiac defects and IUGR. The typical appearance of an affected baby includes a broad nasal bridge, wide fontanelles, low-set hair and ears, cleft lip and palate and microcephaly. Neurodevelopmental delay has also been observed. Phenytoin may also lead to early haemolytic disease of the newborn, probably by depleting fetal vitamin K levels. If phenytoin must be used, maternal blood levels should be monitored and the lowest level compatible with effective treatment maintained. Consideration should be given to folic acid supplementation throughout pregnancy and extra vitamin K in the last trimester. Phenytoin appears to be safe in breastfeeding.

Class 1C antiarrhythmics

Flecainide has been used to treat fetal arrhythmias; there do not appear to be any teratogenic or feto-toxic effects in humans.[6]

Class 2 antiarrhythmics

Class 2 comprises the beta blockers, which are discussed in a separate section below.

Class 3 antiarrhythmics

Class 3 includes amiodarone, bretylium and the beta blocker sotalol. Amiodarone has been used for both maternal and fetal arrhythmias. However, it contains high levels of iodine and can lead to congenital goitre or hypothyroidism.[21] Nevertheless, most newborns do not seem to suffer any adverse long-term effects from the transient hypothyroidism.[6] Ventricular septal defects have been reported,[22] as has IUGR.

However, these effects may not be due to the amiodarone alone but may be caused by the mother's disease or other drug therapies such as beta blockers.

Because data are limited and adverse effects, particularly on the thyroid, are well documented, amiodarone should not be a first-line drug in pregnancy, either for maternal arrhythmia or for uncomplicated cases of fetal supraventricular tachycardia (SVT).

Breastfeeding

Because of its high iodine content, amiodarone could theoretically cause hypothyroidism in the nursing neonate. It is excreted in the breast milk and has a long half-life, so breastfeeding is not recommended if the mother is currently taking amiodarone or has taken it regularly within the past few months.

Sotalol has been used for both maternal and fetal arrhythmias. As with other beta blockers, it has the potential to cause IUGR and reduced placental weight. Oudijk *et al.*[23] evaluated the use of sotalol for fetal tachycardia in 21 pregnancies. They concluded that sotalol is effective in fetal atrial fibrillation, but in fetal SVT the mortality rate was high and the conversion rate low so that the risks outweighed the benefits. For maternal treatment, the risks and benefits must be weighed on an individual basis. If used, serial ultrasound scans for growth are indicated. Sotalol may also cause neonatal bradycardia or hypoglycaemia.[24]

Sotalol is concentrated in breast milk with a milk to plasma ratio of over 5. In spite of this, no adverse beta blockade effects, such as neonatal hypotension or bradycardia, have been noted. The long-term effects of exposure in breast milk are unknown.

Class 4 antiarrhythmics

Class 4 includes the calcium antagonists diltiazem and verapamil. If taken in the first trimester of pregnancy, these drugs do not appear to be teratogenic.[25,26] Data dealing with exposure at that stage are limited, however, so these drugs are not considered as first-line in early pregnancy. Having said that, exposure during the first trimester is not an indication for termination of pregnancy or invasive diagnostic procedures.

There is greater experience with calcium channel blockers in the second half of pregnancy, and they appear to be relatively safe. Two small prospective studies of calcium channel blockers, mainly nifedipine and verapamil, in pregnancy reported two birth defects of the extremities, from 100 babies.[25,27] However, the authors point out that the abnormalities may have been due to the maternal disease or other medications. In contrast, several large studies suggest that calcium channel blockers in the second and third trimesters have no significant adverse effects.[28,29] These drugs may be considered first-line for treatment of cardiac arrhythmias in the second and third trimesters in some women.[30]

Breastfeeding

Calcium channel blockers are excreted in breast milk but the infant appears to receive only a very small proportion of the mother's dose. They are considered 'probably safe' although it is recognised that data are still limited.

Nitrates

This group includes glyceryl trinitrate (GTN), isosorbide mononitrate (ISMN) and isosorbide dinitrate (ISDN). These drugs are used as coronary dilators after a myocardial infarction and for angina. They have also been used as tocolytics. Data on their use in pregnancy are limited, especially as regards the first trimester (although their use is expected to increase as the average age of women at first pregnancy increases, and as the incidence of ischaemic heart disease during pregnancy thus rises). However, they appear to be safe; occasional transient hypotension in the mother does not appear severe enough to affect placental perfusion significantly.

Breastfeeding

No data are available for nitrates in breastfeeding but the risks are likely to be low.

Electrical cardioversion

Direct current (DC) cardioversion appears to be safe and effective in pregnancy. Its use has been reported in pregnancy for the treatment of atrial fibrillation, atrial flutter and atrial tachycardia resistant to drug therapy.[18,31]

Prostacyclin

Prostacyclin has been used successfully to treat a woman with Eisenmenger syndrome in pregnancy.

Beta-adrenergic receptor blockers (beta blockers)

This class includes a long list of drugs; some of the most commonly used ones are atenolol, bisoprolol, esmolol, labetalol, metoprolol, oxprenolol, pindolol, propranolol, sotalol and timolol. They may be used an antihypertensives, in Marfan syndrome, or as antiarrhythmics. Many have both beta-1 and beta-2 activity; labetalol has both beta and alpha blocking activity. All beta blockers cross the placenta. From the evidence available to date, beta blockers do not seem to be teratogenic following exposure in the first trimester. Briggs et al.[6] reported on a case series of 105 first-trimester exposures and found that 12 infants had birth defects. However, there was no consistent pattern of malformation and other studies have failed to confirm this finding. The conclusion is that any significant teratogenic risk is unlikely.

Some studies have found an increased risk of IUGR, particularly with longer term treatment with higher doses in pregnancy. Easterling et al.[32] described IUGR following long-term use of atenolol. Butters et al.[33] reported on 33 women with chronic hypertension treated from 16 weeks of gestation with doses of atenolol up to 200 mg/day. Mean treated diastolic blood pressure was 74 mmHg (compared with 81 mmHg in controls). They reported a mean birthweight in the treated group of 2620 g compared with 3530 g in the control group. However, the underlying maternal disease could well explain this effect and other controlled studies have found no difference in the rates of IUGR between the exposed and non-exposed groups.[6,34] A Cochrane review[35] of 12 trials of beta blockers versus placebo/no treatment for mild to moderate hypertension suggested that IUGR was more common with beta blockers (RR 1.36, 95% CI 1.02–1.82). However, when the Butters trial[33] (which used large doses from an early gestation) was excluded, the relative risk fell to 1.30 and failed to achieve statistical significance (95% CI 0.97–1.74). More recently, von Dadelszen et al.[36] conducted a meta-analysis of antihypertensives for mild to moderate hypertension in pregnancy. They found that the increased risk of IUGR was proportional to the treatment-induced fall in mean arterial pressure. They concluded that this effect was not specific to beta blockers but that hypertension over-treated with any antihypertensive could impair placental perfusion and lead to IUGR. IUGR could also theoretically be mediated through the lowering of blood sugar by beta receptor blockade. However, postnatal growth and development does not seem to be affected.[37]

In summary, the risk of IUGR associated with the use of beta blockers in pregnancy seems to be small, particularly when large doses are avoided and their use is confined to the third trimester. When used, however, caution should be exercised and hypertension not over-treated. Fetal growth should be monitored with serial growth scans.

If beta blockers are used up to the time of delivery, there is a theoretical risk of neonatal bradycardia, hypotension and hypoglycaemia owing to the beta blocking effect.[38] However, in practice such adverse effects seem rare. It has been suggested that beta blockers should be stopped 24–48 hours before delivery to minimise the risk of neonatal symptoms. Because these symptoms are so mild and usually resolve quickly with no long-term adverse effects, this does not seem to be necessary. Nevertheless, neonatologists should be warned of the possibility of neonatal effects.

In theory, beta blockers could oppose the effects of beta agonists being used for tocolysis; in practice, however, this does not seem to occur.

Data on the use in pregnancy of many of the newer beta blockers are scarce. It thus seems sensible that the beta blockers that have been around for a long time, such as labetalol, atenolol and metoprolol, should be the drugs of choice when a beta blocker is required. If, however, one of the newer beta blockers is taken inadvertently in early pregnancy, the risk of teratogenesis seems low and termination of pregnancy or invasive diagnostic procedures are not justified.

Digoxin

Digoxin is one of the drugs commonly used in the treatment of women with cardiac disorders. It has been used successfully for the control of atrial flutter and fibrillation and as an inotrope. No toxic fetal effects or congenital anomalies have been reported following its use in therapeutic doses in pregnancy. Digoxin freely crosses the placenta and cord levels were found to be 50–80% of maternal levels.[39] However, myocardial sensitivity seems to be less in the fetus than in the adult.[40] Digoxin has also been shown to be effective in treating *in utero* fetal SVT.[41–43]

Monitoring of digoxin levels during pregnancy is advisable as maternal toxicity may be fatal to the fetus, and also because digoxin clearance by the kidney is increased as pregnancy advances and so the dose may need to be increased.

Breatfeeding

Digoxin appears to be safe during breastfeeding.[44]

Anticoagulants

Heparin

The molecular weight of unfractionated heparins (UHs) ranges from 4000 to 30 000 Da, with a mean of 15 000 Da. Because of this high molecular weight and their negative charge, they do not cross the placental barrier. Low molecular weight heparins (LMWH's) such as enoxaparin, dalteparin and tinzaparin have molecular weights between 4000 and 6000 Da; like UHs, LMWHs cannot cross the placenta.

Long-term UH use can cause bone demineralisation and osteoporosis; it is likely that LMWHs have the same effect.[45] This is a consideration in pregnancy and lactation, both of which can also cause osteopenia.

Breastfeeding

Neither UHs nor LMWHs are detectable in breast milk, presumably because of their high molecular weights. Furthermore, heparins are broken down in the gut, so enteral absorption is minimal.

Warfarin

Warfarin and other coumarins are vitamin K antagonists which impair synthesis of the vitamin K-dependent coagulation factors (II, VII, IX, X) in the liver. Taken orally, they are well absorbed from the gut.

Coumarins readily cross the placenta and can harm the fetus. They are embryotoxic, particularly between eight and eleven weeks of gestation, typically causing 'coumarin' (or 'warfarin') embryopathy. This is a characteristic pattern of malformations that includes nasal hypoplasia and stippled epiphyses (chondrodysplasia punctata). It does not seem to occur if the drug is stopped before 8 weeks of gestation. Exposure in later pregnancy, typically in the second trimester, may lead to IUGR, central nervous system (CNS) abnormalities and mental disability. CNS abnormalities are thought to be due to repeated small intracerebral haemorrhages and may include optic atrophy and blindness, agenesis of the corpus callosum, cerebellar atrophy or microcephaly. In fact, these sequelae, which occur in only 3% of exposed fetuses,[46] may be more serious than coumarin embryopathy. A third concern is the risk of fetal intracerebral haemorrhage at the time of delivery, if the mother is still taking oral anticoagulants.

Breastfeeding

Over 95% of warfarin is protein-bound so only minimal amounts reach breast milk. Mothers can be reassured that, in contrast to pregnancy, warfarin during lactation carries no risk to the newborn. Phenindione, on the other hand, is only 70% protein-bound and therapeutic levels have been reported in the neonate. It is contraindicated in breastfeeding.

Clopidogrel

Clopidogrel is an antiplatelet drug licensed for the reduction of atherosclerotic events (such as myocardial infarction, stroke and vascular death) in patients with a history of symptomatic ischaemic disease. Based on the relatively low molecular weight of the inactive parent drug (420 Da), it seems likely that at least some crosses the placenta (and also reaches breast milk). However, studies in rats using doses up to 78 times the recommended human adult daily dose (based on body surface area) reported no feto-toxicity.[47] There is only one case report on the use of clopidogrel throughout pregnancy,[48] and no adverse fetal or maternal effects were noted. There are no reports describing the use of clopidogrel in breastfeeding.

In summary, data are lacking but the known maternal benefits seem to outweigh any unknown fetal risks. If a woman's condition requires clopidogrel, it should not be withheld because of pregnancy.

Drugs commonly used in pregnancy: effects on women with cardiac disease

Oxytocin

Animal studies[49] have shown that oxytocin causes a reduction in heart rate that is dose specific. However, oxytocin has a direct relaxant effect on vascular smooth muscle[50,51] that can cause hypotension, and a reflex tachycardia is common. For this reason, rapid intravenous bolus doses should be avoided, particularly in women with cardiac disease.

Oxytocin also has a weak anti-diuretic hormone effect. The use of large doses (for example in the induction or termination of pregnancy or the management of postpartum haemorrhage), particularly when combined with large infusion volumes of electrolyte-free fluids, can lead to water intoxication, pulmonary oedema and hyponatraemia. Particular care should be exercised in women with cardiac disease.

Ergometrine

Ergometrine may cause sustained hypertension and is usually avoided in pregnant women with cardiac disease.

Misoprostol

Data on the use of misoprostol in women with cardiac disease are scarce. In fact, despite the fact that the drug is now in widespread use in obstetric and gynaecological practice, data on its cardiovascular effects are still limited.

The effects of misoprostol on the cardiovascular system have been examined in non-pregnant subjects. Brecht[52] randomised 20 healthy volunteers to receive either 400 μg of misoprostol enterally or placebo. Blood pressure did not change appreciably but there was a significant rise in heart rate (63 versus 59 beats per minute). Lower extremity blood flow (measured by venous occlusion plethysmography) decreased slightly while calculated peripheral vascular resistance showed a small (but non-significant) increase.

Misoprostol has been used extensively for cervical ripening and induction of labour. Several randomised trials have included women with hypertensive disorders of pregnancy but no adverse cardiovascular effects of the drug have been noted in this group of women.[53–57] Del Valle et al.[58] reported the use of misoprostol to induce labour in two women with severe pre-eclampsia, with no apparent adverse effects.

Ramsey et al.[59] examined the cardiovascular effects of intravaginal misoprostol 600 μg, given in mid-trimester to healthy pregnant women. There was no significant change in maternal heart rate, mean arterial blood pressure, mean cardiac index, stroke index, systemic vascular resistance index or end-diastolic volume index. Although this was a small study, it suggests that this dose of misoprostol is safe in healthy women, but these results cannot necessarily be extrapolated to women with cardiovascular disease.

In conclusion, no adverse effects of misoprostol have been reported in women with cardiac disease. However, data are limited, so misoprostol should be used in pregnant women with cardiac disease only when the benefits outweigh any potential risks.

Ritodrine

Ritodrine is a beta agonist used in the management of preterm labour. It causes a tachycardia and may also lead to pulmonary oedema, particularly when large volumes of intravenous fluids are administered. Fatal pulmonary oedema has been reported. Ritodrine may also interact with other drugs such as beta blockers and potassium-depleting diuretics; ritodrine has been shown to decrease plasma potassium levels. Clearly, ritodrine carries significant risks for women with cardiac disease and is probably best avoided; atosiban is preferable. If ritodrine must be used, the minimum effective dose should be used, and heart rate, fluid balance and electrolyte balance should be closely monitored and a regular check made for signs of pulmonary oedema.

Atosiban

Atosiban is a selective oxytocin receptor antagonist used in the management of preterm labour. It has been on the market only since 2000 so human pregnancy data are relatively few. Animal studies in baboons in the third trimester,[60] and isolated rat perfused hearts,[61] suggest that it has little or no effect on maternal heart rate, contractility or blood pressure. It may therefore be the tocolytic of choice in women with cardiac disease. Although atosiban crosses the placenta relatively freely, it does not seem to have any adverse effects on the fetus.[60]

References

1. Schardein JL. *Chemically-induced Birth Defects*, 4th ed. New York: Marcel Dekker; 2000.
2. Nelson K, Holmes LB. Malformations due to presumed spontaneous mutations in newborn infants. *N Engl J Med* 1989;320:19–23.
3. Wilson JD. Embryotoxicity of drugs to man. In: Wilson JD, Frazer FC, editors. *Handbook of Teratology, Vol. 1*. New York: Plenum Press; 1977. p. 309–55.
4. Joint Formulary Committee. *British National Formulary*. London: British Medical Association and Royal Pharmaceutical Society of Great Britain; 2005.
5. Heinonen OP, Slone D, Shapiro S, *Birth Defects and Drugs in Pregnancy*. Littleton, MA: Publishing Sciences Group; 1997.
6. Briggs GG, Freeman RK, Yaffe SJ. *Drugs in Pregnancy and Lactation*. 5th ed. Baltimore: Williams and Wilkins; 1998.
7. Heinonen OP, Slone D, Shapiro S. *Birth Defects and Drugs in Pregnancy*. Littleton, MA: Publishing Sciences Group; 1977. p. 371–3.
8. Votta RA, Parada OH, Windgrad RH, Alvarez OH, Tomassinni TL, Patoria A. Furosemide action on the creatinine concentration of amniotic fluid. *Am J Obstet Gynecol* 1975;123:621–4.
9. Jones HC. Intrauterine ototoxicity: a case report and review of literature. *J Natl Med Assoc* 1973;65:201–3.

10. Kraft IL, Mus BD. Hypertonic solutions to induce abortions. *Br Med J* 1971;2:49.

11. Yemini M, Shoham Z, Dgani R, Lancet M, Mogilner BM, Nissim F, *et al.* Lupus-like syndrome in a mother and newborn following administration of hydrazaline: a case report. *Eur J Obstet Gynecol Reprod Biol* 1989;30:193–7.

12. Spinnato JA, Sibai BM, Anderson GD. Fetal distress after hydralazine therapy for severe pregnancy-induced hypertension. *South Med J* 1986;79:559–62.

13. Tomlinson AJ, Campbell J, Walker JJ, Morgan C. Malignant primary hypertension in pregnancy treated with lisinopril. *Ann Pharmacother* 2000;34:180–2.

14. Brent RL, Beckman DA. Angiotensin-converting enzyme inhibitors, an embryopathic class of drugs with unique properties: information for clinical teratology counselors. *Teratology* 1991;43:543–6.

15. Committee on Drugs, American Academy of Pediatrics. The transfer of drugs and other chemicals into human milk. *Pediatrics* 2001;108:776–89.

16. Saji H, Yamanaka M, Hagiwara A, Ijira R. Losartan and fetal toxic effects. *Lancet* 2001;357:363.

17. Jogler JA, Page RL. Treatment of cardiac arrhythmias during pregnancy. *Drug Saf* 1999;20:85–94.

18. Rotmensch HH, Rotmensch S, Elkayam U. Management of cardiac arrhythmias during pregnancy: current concepts. *Drugs* 1987;33:623–33.

19. Macaulay JH, Bond K, Steer PJ. Epidural analgesia in labor and fetal hyperthermia. *Obstet Gynecol* 1992;80:665–9.

20. Janz D, Fuchs V. Are anti-epileptic drugs powerful when given during pregnancy? *German Med Monogr* 1964;9:20–3.

21. Grosso S, Berardi R, Cioni M, Morgese G. Transient neonatal hypothyroidism after gestational exposure to amiodarone: a follow-up of two cases. *J Endocrinol Invest* 1998;21:699–702.

22. Ovadia M, Breto M, Hoyer GL, Marcus FI. Human experience with amiodarone in the embryonic period. *Am J Cardiol* 1994;73:316–17.

23. Oudijk MA, Michon MM, Kleinman CS, Kapusta L, Stoutenbeek P, Visser GH, *et al.* Sotalol in the treatment of fetal dysrhythmias. *Circulation* 2000;101:2721–6.

24. Magee LA, Nulman I, Rovet JF, Koren G. Neurodevelopment after *in utero* amiodarone exposure. *Neurotoxicol Teratol* 1999;21:261–5.

25. Magee LA, Schick B, Donnenfeld AE, Sage SR, Conover B, Cook L, *et al.* The safety of calcium channel blockers in human pregnancy: a prospective, multicenter core study. *Am J Obstet Gynecol* 1996;174:823–8.

26. Czeizel AE, Rockenbauer M, Population-based case–controlled study of teratogenic potential of corticosteroids. *Teratology* 1997;56:335–40.

27. Sorensen HT, Steffensen FH, Olesen C, Nielsen GL, Pedersen L, Olsen J. Pregnancy outcome in women exposed to calcium channel blockers. *Reprod Toxicol* 1998;12:383–4.

28. Marlettini MG, Crippa S, Morselli-Labate AN, Orlandi C. Randomized comparison of calcium antagonists and beta-blockers in the treatment of pregnancy-induced hypertension. *Curr Ther Res* 1990;48:684–92.

29. Orlandi C, Marlettini MG, Cassani A. Treatment of hypertension during pregnancy with the calcium antagonist verapamil. *Curr Ther Res* 1986;39:884–93.

30. Houtzager BA, Hogendoorn SM, Papatsonis DN, Samsom JF, van Geijn HP, Bleker OP, *et al.* Long-term follow up of children exposed *in utero* to nifedipine or ritodrine for the management of preterm labour. *BJOG* 2006;113:324–31.

31. Brown CEL, Wendel GD. Cardiac arrhythmias during pregnancy. *Clin Obstet Gynecol* 1989;32:89–102.

32. Easterling TR, Brateng D, Schmucker B, Brown Z, Millard SP. The prevention of pre-eclampsia; a randomized trial of atenolol in hyperdynamic patients before onset of hypertension. *Obstet Gynecol* 1999;93:725–33.

33. Butters L, Kennedy S, Rubin PC. Atenolol in essential hypertension during pregnancy. *Br Med J* 1990;301:587–9.

34. Lydakis C, Lip GY, Beavers M, Beavers DG. Atenolol and fetal growth in pregnancies complicated by hypertension. *Am J Hypertens* 1999;12:541–7.

35. Magee LA, Duley L. Oral beta-blockers for mild to moderate hypertension during pregnancy. *Cochrane Database Syst Rev* 2003;(3):CD002863.

36. von Dadelszen P, Ornstein MP, Bull SB, Logan AG, Koren G, Magee LA. Fall in mean arterial pressure and fetal growth restriction in pregnancy hypertension: a meta-analysis. *Lancet* 2000;355:87–92.

37. Reynolds B, Butters L, Evans J, Adama T, Rubin PC. First year of life after the use of atenolol in pregnancy-associated hypertension. *Arch Dis Child* 1984;59:1061–3.

38. Rubin PC, Butters L, Kelman AW, Fitzsimons C, Reid JL. Labetalol disposition and concentration-effect relationships during pregnancy. *Br J Clin Pharmacol* 1983;15:465–70.

39. Chan V, Tse TF, Wong V. Transfer of digoxin across the placenta and into breast milk. *Br J Obstet Gynaecol* 1978;85:605–9.

40. Saarikoski S. Placental transfer and fetal uptake of 3H-digoxin in humans. *Br J Obstet Gynaecol* 1976;83:879–84.

41. Harrigan JT, Kangos JJ, Sikka A, Spisso KR, Natarajan N, Rosenfeld D, *et al.* Successful treatment of fetal congestive heart failure secondary to tachycardia. *N Engl J Med* 1981;304:1527–9.

42. Hsieh Y, Lee C, Chang C, Tsai H, Yeh L, Tsai C. Successful prenatal digoxin therapy for Ebstein's anomaly with hydrops fetalis. A case report. *J Reprod Med* 1998;43:710–12.

43. Tikanoja T, Kirkinen P, Nikolajev K, Eresmaa L, Haring P. Familial atrial fibrillation with fetal onset. *Heart* 1998;79:195–7.

44. Bennett PN, editor. *Drugs and Human Lactation.* 2nd ed. Amsterdam, Oxford: Elsevier; 1996.

45. Lindqvist PG, Dahlback B. Bleeding complications associated with low molecular weight heparin prophylaxis during pregnancy. *Thromb Haemost* 2000;84:140–1.

46. Bates SM, Ginsberg JS. Anticoagulants in pregnancy: fetal effects. *Bailliere's Clin Obstet Gynaecol* 1997;11:479–88.

47. *Product Information: Plavix.* Bristol-Myers Squibb, 2002.

48. Klinzing P, Markert UR, Liesaus K, Peiker G. Case report: successful pregnancy and delivery after myocardial infarction and essential thrombocythemia treated with clopidogrel. *Clin Exp Obstet Gynecol* 2001;28:215–16.

49. Coulson C, Thorp M, Mayer D, Cefalo R. Central hemodynamic effects of oxytocin and interaction with magnesium and pregnancy in the isolated perfused rat heart. *Am J Obstet Gynecol* 1997;177:91–3.

50. Hendricks CH, Brenner WE. Cardiovascular effects of oxytocic drugs used post partum. *Am J Obstet Gynecol* 1970;108:751–4.

51. Secher NJ, Amso P, Wallin L. Haemodynamic effects of oxytocin (syntocinon) and methyl ergometrine (methergin) on the systemic and pulmonary circulations of pregnant anaesthetized women. *Acta Obstet Gynecol Scand* 1978;57:97–107.

52. Brecht T. Effect of misoprostol on human circulation. *Prostaglandins* 1987;33:51–9.

53. Sanchez-Ramos L, Kaunitz AM, Delvalle GO, Delke I, Schroeder PA, Briones DK. Labor induction with the prostaglandin E1 methyl analogue misoprostol versus oxytocin: a randomized trial. *Obstet Gynecol* 1993;81:332–6.

54. Wing DA, Rahall A, Jones MM, Goodwin TM, Paul RH. Misoprostol: an effective agent for cervical ripening and labor induction. *Am J Obstet Gynecol* 1995;172:1811–16.

55. Wing DA, Jones MM, Rahall A, Goodwin TM, Paul RH. A comparison of misoprostol and prostaglandin E2 gel for preinduction cervical ripening and labor induction. *Am J Obstet Gynecol* 1995;172:1804–10.

56. Sanchez-Ramos L, Kaunitz AM, Wears RL, Isaac D, Gaudier FL. Misoprostol for cervical ripening and labor induction: a meta-analysis. *Obstet Gynecol* 1997;89:633–42.

57. Hofmeyr GJ, Gulmezoglu AM. Vaginal misoprostol for cervical ripening and labour induction in late pregnancy. *Cochrane Database Syst Rev* 2000;(2):CD000941. Updates in: *Cochrane Database Syst Rev* 2001;(1):CD000941, *Cochrane Database Syst Rev* 2001;(3):CD000941.

58. Delvalle GO, Sanchez-Ramos L, Jordan CW, Gaudier FL, Delke I. Use of misoprostol (prostaglandin E1 methyl analogue) to expedite delivery in severe pre-eclampsia remote from term. *J Matern Fetal Med* 1996;5:39–40.

59. Ramsey P, Hogg B, Savage K, Winkler D, Owen J. Cardiovascular effects of intravaginal misoprostol in the mid-trimester of pregnancy. *Am J Obstet Gynecol* 2000;183:1100–2.

60. Nathanielsz PW, Honnebier MB, Mecenas C, Jenkins SL, Holland ML, Demarest K. Effect of the oxytocin antagonist atosiban (1-deamino-2-D-tyr(OET)-4-thr-8-orn-vasotocin/oxytocin) on nocturanl myometrial contractions, maternal cardiovascular function, transplacental passage, and fetal oxygenation in the pregnant baboon during the last third of gestation. *Biol Reprod* 1997;57:320–4.

61. Thorp JM Jr, Mayer D, Kuller JA. Central hemodynamic effects of an oxytocin receptor antagonist (atosiban) in the isolated, perfused rat heart. *J Soc Gynecol Investig* 1999;6:186–7.

Chapter 8
Surgical and catheter intervention during pregnancy in women with heart disease

Henryk Kafka, Hideki Uemura, Michael A Gatzoulis

Introduction

Management of maternal cardiac problems associated with pregnancy involves prenatal assessment and advice regarding risks and suitability for pregnancy, assessment and intervention before pregnancy to ensure a less complicated course, and close medical management during pregnancy in order to postpone any necessary intervention until the child can be safely delivered. Nevertheless, despite these principles, practices and precautions, situations will still be encountered where an intervention during pregnancy becomes necessary.

In general, surgical and catheter interventions during pregnancy do not involve those women that have already been identified and managed before pregnancy. The women undergoing such interventions tend to be:

■ those with heart disease that has been undiagnosed

■ those with previously documented heart disease who have been lost to follow-up

■ those with an acute new problem, such as aortic dissection, acute endocarditis or myocardial infarction.

It is specifically because of thorough prepregnancy evaluation and counselling, as well as close management during pregnancy, that such interventions are rare. In a review of a population of 720 000 pregnant women in Sweden over 9 years, only 40 had undergone a cardiopulmonary operative procedure during pregnancy.[1] In a report from Brazil of 1000 women with heart disease followed through pregnancy over 10 years, 557 had rheumatic heart disease and 191 had congenital heart disease, with Chagas disease and cardiomyopathies responsible for a further 128 patients.[2] In this group of 1000 women, almost one-quarter (235) developed cardiovascular complications. Medical management alone was successful in the treatment of 161 of these women. Of the remaining 74 women, 27 died (including six of 21 women with Eisenmenger syndrome) without any cardiac interventional procedure, whereas 47 underwent some type of interventional procedure. This included cardiac surgery in

25 women, percutaneous balloon mitral valvuloplasty (PBMV) in ten, pacemaker insertion in six and coronary angioplasty in two. Cardiac surgical mortality in this group was one out of 25 (4%).

Most cardiac interventions undertaken during pregnancy involve women in developing countries. This is not only because of a higher prevalence of rheumatic heart disease, the major indication for such intervention, but also because the disorganised health network and the traditionally decreased treatment-seeking behaviour of women in such countries result in late diagnosis.[3] Even recent reports document that 35–42% of women with mitral stenosis are diagnosed for the first time when they present already pregnant.[4,5]

Even though experience with interventions during pregnancy is relatively limited, it is still important to be able to identify those who require such intervention, as well as its inherent risks and benefits. From experience with these cardiac procedures in non-pregnant patients, the relative risk and benefit profiles for the mother can be reliably estimated. However, the mother is often more concerned about the risks to the child she is carrying and counselling must be sensitive to such concerns. Although the terms 'fetal loss' or 'fetal wastage' may be used in the literature, the mother will deal with such an event as 'the death of her child' and those risks must be discussed with her before carrying out any interventional procedure.

Fetal and maternal risks of cardiopulmonary bypass

The development of cardiopulmonary bypass 50 years ago ushered in a new era of cardiac surgery that allowed for more complex procedures on increasingly complex patients.[6,7] The first documented use of cardiopulmonary bypass in pregnancy was in 1959 for a pulmonary valvotomy and atrial septal defect closure at 6 weeks of gestation.[8] The mother survived but the fetus miscarried after the procedure. This pattern of good maternal result but significant fetal loss was to repeat itself over the following four decades.[9]

Table 8.1 summarises the maternal and fetal mortality rates derived from recent systematic literature reviews and series.[2,9,10–13] Several authors have noted a trend to lower fetal mortality in the range of 10–12.5% for more recent cases but the numbers are small and no firm conclusions about decreasing fetal mortality rates can be confidently reached.[13,14] Maternal mortality rates are similar to those reported for emergency procedures in non-pregnant patients.[15]

Table 8.1. Fetal and maternal mortality rates associated with cardiopulmonary bypass procedures during pregnancy, based on recent series and systematic literature reviews

Study	Number of patients	Fetal mortality	Maternal mortality
Weiss et al.[10] (1998)	59	29%	5%
Salazar et al.[11] (2001)	15	33%	13%
de Souza et al.[12] (2001)[a]	24	33%	4%
Immer et al.[13] (2003)[b]	20	15%	5%
Arnoni et al.[9] (2003)	74	18.6%	7%
Avila et al.[2] (2003)	25	16%	4%

[a] Only open mitral commissurotomy
[b] Only aortic dissection

In general, cardiopulmonary bypass includes a number of components: hypothermia, chemical cardioplegia, haemodilution, extracorporeal circulation and oxygenation. Hypothermia was introduced to reduce myocardial and systemic oxygen demand and to increase ischaemic tolerance for the increasing complexity of surgeries.[16] Hypothermia also allowed the use of haemodilution, which reduces the need for large volumes of the blood in the circuit. The use of concomitant chemical cardioplegia permitted surgery on a non-beating flaccid heart, improving the ease and success of complex cardiac surgery.[17] Support of the rest of the circulation, as well as oxygenation, has been provided through a mechanical pump-oxygenator system that has seen significant technological advances in recent years but is still based on similar principles to those of 50 years ago.[18]

From the physiological point of view, cardiopulmonary bypass during pregnancy can be considered a form of 'controlled cardiocirculatory shock'[14] that is generally better tolerated by the mother than by the fetus. The cardiovascular changes of pregnancy result in an increase in circulating volume, an increase in cardiac output, a decrease in haematocrit and an increase in oxygen consumption. The placental blood vessels are maximally dilated. Therefore, uterine blood flow is not autoregulated and is directly proportional to maternal mean arterial pressure and inversely proportional to uterine vascular resistance. A mean arterial pressure of 70 mmHg is required for adequate placental perfusion and a higher pressure is needed during uterine contractions.[6] Furthermore, cardiopulmonary bypass brings further haemodilution, hypotension, hypothermia and non-pulsatile blood flow, as well as complement activation and the risks of particulate and air embolism.[19] This activation of complement and cytokines by the cardiopulmonary bypass circuit may even have the potential to bring about a direct deleterious effect on the placenta and fetus. Moreover, the well-established procoagulant effect of pregnancy would be expected to increase these risks further.[20] Maternal hypotension after initiation of cardiopulmonary bypass can be caused by a decrease in systemic vascular resistance due to haemodilution and release of vasoactive substances.[14,19] The use of high doses of heparin for anticoagulation during cardiopulmonary bypass and the consequent need for neutralisation with protamine can cause further difficulties in both intraoperative and postoperative haemostasis, as well as haemodynamic instability and bronchospasm related to the protamine.[21] All of these factors can result in decreased blood flow to the placenta and a reduction in oxygen supply to the fetus, with consequent fetal distress.

Uterine contractions occur frequently during cardiopulmonary bypass and are an important predictor of poor fetal outcome. They occur more frequently with increasing gestational age.[8] They may be caused by the dilutional effect of cardiopulmonary bypass on hormone levels resulting in an increased uterine excitability.[19] Uterine contractions are most common in the rewarming phase after hypothermia.[9,14] The contractions decrease placental blood flow and therefore contribute to fetal hypoxia. To reduce this deleterious effect on the fetus, it is important to monitor and control uterine contractions. Adjusting perfusion parameters may be successful. If not, the use of tocolytic agents has been recommended.[22] However, the use of these drugs (e.g. beta agonists, calcium blockers, magnesium, ritodrine, ethanol, nitroglycerine, atosiban) in any setting of preterm labour has been controversial and has been associated with cardiovascular adverse effects.[23] In a large trial, atosiban was shown to be an effective tocolytic with the fewest such adverse effects.[23,24]

The common fetal response to cardiopulmonary bypass is bradycardia. This is thought to be due to fetal hypoxia or acidosis, and may be related to maternal hypothermia. It may be transient or persistent, may show late decelerations or sinusoidal patterns, and is usually noted just after initiation of, or emergence from, cardio-pulmonary bypass.[6,22] Fetal bradycardia usually improves within 2–3 hours of the postoperative period, suggesting that it was inadequate placental perfusion that resulted in fetal hypoxia and the bradycardic response. The bradycardia has been shown to respond to measures that increase the perfusion rate and to worsen with uterine contractions that compromise placental flow.[8] Hypothermia has also been incriminated as a factor in this fetal bradycardia[25] and has been used as one of the justifications for normothermic arrest. Unfortunately, a return to normal fetal heart rate after cardiopulmonary bypass is no guarantee of a good fetal outcome.[26] Although a direct correlation between fetal heart rate and bypass flow rate has been demon-strated, with a significant and reversible decrease in fetal heart rate as flow rate is decreased, increasing the flow rate may not necessarily improve a fetal bradycardia.[27] A significant cause of fetal bradycardia is the use of high-dose opioids for maternal anaesthesia. This is reversible and transient, and should be considered if fetal brady-cardia does not respond to increasing cardiopulmonary bypass flow.[19] The potentially damaging effect of hyperkalaemic cardioplegia on the fetus has not been fully studied[14] but potassium ions can cross the placenta easily and can lead to fetal cardiac depression or even arrest.[28] Maternal hyperkalaemia must be avoided, with close monitoring of maternal potassium levels.[28,29]

A number of modifications to cardiopulmonary bypass techniques for pregnant women have been proposed.[30,31] Experimental evidence has suggested that pulsatile perfusion may help prevent placental vasoconstriction.[32] Pulsatile cardiopulmonary bypass is believed to reduce uterine contractions by releasing endothelium-derived growth factor from the vascular endothelium and to further maintain placental perfusion by preserving fetal/maternal endothelial nitric oxide synthesis and by decreasing activation of the fetal renin–angiotensin pathway.[32]

The extent of the deleterious effect on the fetus of hypothermia in cardiopulmon-ary bypass is difficult to gauge. The Pomini series[14] reported a fetal mortality of 24% with hypothermia and 0% with normothermia. Other reports have not confirmed such a strong relationship.[10,33] Experimental studies on pregnant ewes have demonstrated a number of effects of hypothermia on the fetus.[34] In all the animals, fetal temperature decreased similarly with maternal cooling. The placenta acted as a heat exchanger with a gradient of temperature during all phases of cooling. During cooling there was a direct effect on the fetal sinus node, with an average reduction in fetal heart rate of 7 beats per minute for each degree of fetal cooling. Maternal temperatures at or above 18 °C, corresponding to a fetal temperature of 25 °C or greater, were associated with fetal survival. In the fetuses that survived there was an increase in fetal heart rate with gradual rewarming. At very low temperatures, profound fetal bradycardia led to a critical reduction of cardiac output and consequently reduced feto-placental exchange with irreversible fetal acidosis and hypoxia. At 20 °C or higher, the fetus had a return to normal pH and PO_2. At 18 °C, the fetus survived but the alterations of arterial blood gases and pH were associated with a poor perinatal outcome. More profound hypothermia resulted in fetal death. Such findings have led to a variety of recom-mendations about hypothermia in cardiopulmonary bypass during pregnancy, ranging from avoidance of deep hypothermia to the use of normothermic cardiopulmonary bypass.[6,8,14,19,22,25,27,28,30,31,35–38] The so-called warm heart surgery is gaining acceptance for cardiovascular surgery in general[16,17,39] and has been used successfully in aortic valve replacement for a pregnant woman.[29]

Another modification could entail the use of a heparin-coated cardiopulmonary bypass circuit allowing reduction in the systemic heparinisation and, consequently, a reduced requirement for protamine.[21]

There have been reports of two cases where intra–aortic balloon pumping was used with cardiopulmonary bypass to improve uterine blood flow and benefit fetal haemodynamics, but its routine use in this setting remains to be determined.[40]

Of course, there are alternative techniques for cardiac surgery that do not require the use of cardiopulmonary bypass. Aortocoronary bypass surgery has been performed without cardiopulmonary bypass in pregnant women.[41,42] Closed mitral valvotomy has a long history and continues to be used in many developing countries,[43] where it has been successfully applied to pregnant women.[44,45] In developed countries, PBMV and other percutaneous techniques have obviated the need for a number of surgeries with cardiopulmonary bypass but these come with their own special risks (see the Radiation and contrast agent risks to fetus and mother section below).

The risk of cardiopulmonary bypass to a pregnant woman is similar to that of a non-pregnant patient but there is a high percentage of fetal loss as a result of cardio-pulmonary bypass. It is believed that the fetal risk can be controlled by an experienced team. When there is no alternative to an intervention, consideration should be given to delivering the woman before the intervention, if possible.[38,46] Such a decision will need to balance the risks of preterm delivery against those of fetal loss during cardiopulmonary bypass.[47,48,49]

Key points

1. Consider surgery only if the woman is deteriorating and has failed optimal medical therapy and there are no suitable percutaneous options for interventional therapy.

2. Refer the woman early to a centre with experience in intervention during pregnancy.

3. Avoid aortocaval compression by the gravid uterus by positioning the woman with the right hip elevated 15°.

4. Avoid cannulation of the femoral vein and artery, if possible. Femoral artery cannulation may result in hypoperfusion of the uterus. Venous return through a femoral vein cannula may be reduced by pressure on the inferior vena cava from the uterus.

5. Although there is no risk of fetal haemorrhage from the heparin required during cardiopulmonary bypass, heparin may increase the risk of uterine haemorrhage and must be carefully monitored. This is especially true if the fetus has been delivered by caesarean section just prior to cardiopulmonary bypass.

6. The use of high-flow, high-pressure (mean arterial pressure greater than 70 mmHg) cardiopulmonary bypass to match expected maternal cardiac output (cardiac index of 2.6–3 (l/min)/m²) is recommended.

7. Avoid deep hypothermia. Maternal temperature should not be allowed to fall below 30 °C.

8. Avoid hyperkalaemia by using cardioplegia recovery techniques and close monitoring of maternal potassium levels.

9. Continuous monitoring of uterine contraction and fetal heart rate are recommended. Intraoperative fetal echocardiography should be considered.

10. The presence of an experienced obstetric team is required for fetal monitoring and to deal with precipitous delivery or the need for caesarean section (surgical equipment for caesarean section must be readily available).

11. Consideration should be given to postponing the surgery for as long as possible to allow for fetal maturity. Delivery of the fetus prior to cardiopulmonary bypass avoids the risk of fetal loss but incurs all the risks of prematurity for the child. Careful consultation with the obstetrician and neonatologist are necessary before considering such a preterm delivery.

Radiation and contrast agent risks to fetus and mother

Percutaneous cardiac interventions during pregnancy have ranged from the relatively common PBMV,[50] to less common percutaneous coronary intervention,[51] to tricuspid valvuloplasty[52] and to implantable automatic cardioverter-defibrillator insertion.[53] These percutaneous cardiac interventions for specific lesions during pregnancy appear to be associated with a lower risk of fetal loss but they expose the mother and fetus to the risks of ionising radiation and use of contrast medium.[46] The maternal radiation risks for complications such as skin injury, cataracts, neoplasm and heritable genetic effects are likely to be similar to those for non-pregnant patients. The estimated effective dose during invasive cardiology procedures is between 1 and 20 mSv but can be as high as 45 mSv for a long and complex percutaneous coronary intervention.[54] To put this in perspective, it is important to note that the annual effective dose delivered to an individual in the USA by natural background radiation is 3–4 mSv[55] and the cosmic radiation from a US cross-country flight would result in an exposure of 0.1 mSv.[56] The major concern about the radiation risk focuses on the fetus, and the extent of that risk depends on the radiation dose and the gestational age at the time of exposure. Recent reviews and guidelines have helped to put the issue of fetal risks from radiation exposure into perspective.[55,57,58]

Much of the data on radiation safety and long-term consequences have involved the follow-up monitoring of non-X-ray exposure, such as in the survivors of the atomic bombings in Japan.[56] Any discussion of radiation risks requires some understanding of the measurement of radiation dose and its nomenclature. There have been recent changes in the nomenclature and these changes have made it more difficult for some to understand the units of measurement and their significance. There are a number of radiation measurement parameters and the most clinically valuable ones are summarised in Table 8.2. The older units are also included to allow for comparison with previously quoted standards and reports.[57,59] It should be noted that for X-rays, gamma rays and electrons there is really no difference between absorbed dose and equivalent dose, i.e. 1 mGy = 1 mSv. This is not true for neutrons and alpha particles but these radiation types are not relevant to an understanding of X-ray exposure. For the clinical purposes of this discussion, there is no practical difference between measurements in mGy and those in mSv. To further complicate the situation, monitoring systems will frequently measure the patient dose as the dose area product (DAP), which is calculated as the skin entrance dose multiplied by the area of the X-ray field and is usually reported as Gy cm². The risk to the patient is best expressed by the effective dose. The relationship of effective dose to DAP is complex and beyond the scope of this discussion. Published conversion coefficients range from 0.13 to 0.23 mSv per Gy cm², depending on the type of interventional procedure.[54,60]

Table 8.2. Clinically useful radiation dose units; adapted with permission from Hirshfeld et al.[55]

Quantity	Units of measurement	What it is	What it measures	Why it is useful	Conversion between old and new units
Absorbed dose	gray (Gy) or milligray (mGy) [rad or millirad (mrad)]	The amount of energy locally deposited in tissue per unit mass of tissue	Measures concentration of energy deposition in tissue	Assesses the potential biological risk to that specific tissue	1 rad = 10 mGy
Equivalent dose	sievert (Sv) or millisievert (mSv) [rem or millirem (mrem)]	A dose quantity that factors in the relative biological damage caused by different types of radiation	Provides a relative dose that accounts for increased biological damage from some types of radiation	This is the most common unit used to measure radiation risk to specific tissues for radiation protection of personnel	1 rem = 10 mSv
Effective dose	sievert (Sv) or millisievert (mSv) [rem or millirem (mrem)]	An attributed whole-body dose that produces the same whole-person stochastic risk as an absorbed dose to a limited portion of the body	Converts any localised absorbed or equivalent dose to a whole-body risk factor	Permits comparison of risks among several exposed individuals, even though the doses might be delivered to different sets of organs in these individuals	1 rem = 10 mSv

Ionising radiation exposure to the fetus can manifest its deleterious effects in three main ways:

■ cell death and teratogenesis
■ carcinogenesis
■ genetic effects or mutations in germ cells, for which there are no long-term data.

Exposure to high-dose radiation (1000–2000 mGy) in pregnant animals results in teratogenic effects in all those exposed. If such high-dose exposure occurs in the pre-implantation period, it tends to cause fetal death rather than congenital anomalies.[59] Based on data from atomic bomb survivors, the most common fetal effects of high-dose radiation are growth restriction, microcephaly and mental impairment.[57] During the time of active organogenesis (up to 42 days), radiation exposure may cause severe structural abnormalities. A dose of 2000 mGy will produce abnormalities in all cases, while a dose of 100 mGy will cause only a 1% increase in congenital anomalies.[59,61] The greatest risk of central nervous system (CNS) effects occurs at 8–15 weeks of gestation. In fact, there appears to be no proven CNS risk at greater than 25 weeks.[57] During the susceptible period, the risk of severe mental impairment in exposed fetuses is dose related, with no increased risk at doses of less than 200 mGy but rising to approximately 40% at 1000 mGy and 60% at 1500 mGy.[57] It can be stated that the fetal risks of malformation, growth restriction, resorption or miscarriage are not increased with radiation doses of less than 50 mGy.[55,57]

Since the dose–effect data from the Japanese atomic bomb studies of cancer incidence appear to be linear for exposures above 100 mSv, the agencies that formulate radiation protection policy have assumed a linear no-threshold model for cancer radiation risk. This means that the quantitative risks of low-level radiation are extrapolated linearly from the high-dose data all the way back to zero dose. Although the risk of very low-dose radiation remains unproved, standard practice continues with the use of this no-threshold assumption.[56] Therefore, unlike the radiation effects for malformation or growth restriction, there is not, by definition, a radiation dose threshold level below which one can state there is no increased risk of carcinogenesis.[55,56,57,62] The risk for childhood cancers, principally leukaemias, from *in utero* exposure is estimated at about 0.06% per 10 mSv, which is an increase of 1.5- to 2-fold over the natural incidence.[55,57] However, the longer term adult risk of developing cancer is unknown and believed to be greater since solid cancers are about seven times more prevalent than induced leukaemias and occur much later.[55] One can consider that such risks to the fetus would be at least as great as they are for newborn exposure to radiation. The lifetime cancer mortality risk for newborn males has been estimated to be about 0.13% per 10 mSv and to be higher (0.16%) for females because of their greater breast and thyroid sensitivity.[55,62,63]

The risk for induction of hereditary effects has been estimated at one excess case per million for every 0.1 mGy absorbed dose to the gonads.[55,64] Although this relation-ship has been used to predict heritable abnormalities in the offspring of irradiated fetuses,[64] it probably only applies to actively reproductive patients.[55] Controlling the dose to the fetus (see below) will also control the dose to the maternal ovaries. However, in cases where gonadal dose may have exceeded 100 mGy, the woman should be advised to wait 6 months before attempting conception.[55]

The harmful doses referred to above are those received by the fetus, and the relationship between the dose to the mother and the dose received by the fetus must be understood. The uterus receives only the radiation scattered from the irradiated area. This represents just a small fraction of the total dose delivered, typically less than 2%.[55] Generally speaking, interventional procedures above the diaphragm are unlikely to deliver dangerous doses to the fetus. During the most susceptible early stage, the fetus is very small and far away from the diaphragm. A study of estimated fetal dose during typical cardiac electrophysiological ablation reported doses of 0.1–0.2 mGy in the first trimester, 0.3 mGy in the second trimester and 0.55 mGy in the third trimester.[64] Based on current understanding, doses of this magnitude will not pose significant risks to the fetus or measurably increase the risk of childhood cancers. The excess lifetime risk of fatal cancer would not exceed 50 cases per million fetuses exposed to such a dose level.

Nevertheless, everything must still be done to minimise fetal exposure to ionising radiation. The first step is to ensure that there is no medical alternative to the procedure being contemplated and that there is no imaging alternative to the X-rays.[57] Cardiac catheterisation has been carried out under echocardiographic guidance alone.[65] More recently, transoesophageal echocardiography has been used in combination with fluoroscopy to reduce the amount of radiation exposure during PBMV and percutaneous balloon aortic valvuloplasty (PBAV) in pregnancy[66-69] and this has been used as the exclusive imaging technique for some cases of PBMV.[70] Transoesophageal echocardiography has also been used as the only imaging technique in pacemaker[71] and implantable cardioverter-defibrillator insertions in pregnant women[53] and to close an atrial septal communication during pregnancy.[72] Magnetic resonance imaging (MRI) has been used in pregnancy for the diagnosis of maternal and fetal lesions and is generally considered to be safe for the fetus.[73,74] Recent developments suggest that the use of MRI-guided cardiovascular interventions will increase,[75-77] which would also reduce any concerns regarding the safety of contrast agents.[57,78]

Contrary to popular belief and practice, external shielding of the pelvis and abdomen of the mother during procedures involving the head or chest is of limited protective value to the fetus.[55,64] The radiation dose absorbed by the fetus without external shielding has been found to be only 3% higher for all stages of gestation.[64] Most fetal exposure is caused by internally scattered radiation from the directly exposed structures. Previously described principles of limiting radiation to all cardiac patients must also be applied in these cases: minimising beam-on time, the use of pulsed fluoroscopy, optimal beam collimation, optimal positioning, and using the least magnification possible.[55,58,79,80] There are also other manoeuvres that may help reduce fetal radiation dose. Since the dose to the small first-trimester fetus is strongly related to fetal position, imaging the mother with her bladder empty will result in the smallest absorbed fetal dose.[64] A transradial approach for coronary intervention during pregnancy has been described and hypothesised to reduce fetal radiation exposure.[81]

Animal studies have shown no evidence of teratogenic effects from iodinated radio-contrast agents but there is a potential risk of fetal hypothyroidism for procedures performed when the fetal thyroid becomes active (after 25 weeks of gestation).[57] However, these risks have been shown to be minimal.[59] Of course, consideration must still be given to the potential for adverse effects (renal dysfunction, anaphylaxis) in the mother.

Key points

1. The mother should be counselled that there are radiation risks to the fetus but that a dose of less than 50 mGy has not been associated with any increase in fetal anomalies or pregnancy loss, and that the risk of abnormality at this

dose level is negligible in comparison with the other risks of pregnancy, and certainly negligible in comparison with the risks of not undertaking the intervention. Most interventional cardiac procedures would produce a total exposure to the woman of significantly less than 50 mGy (usually 1–10 mGy), and a dose to the fetus of only 1–2% of that total dose. Such a dose would not be expected to materially increase the baby's risk of childhood cancers. It will be necessary to help the mother keep these risks in perspective and not let the fear of fetal anomalies divert the appropriate planned management and its benefits.

2. It should be ensured that there are no other therapeutic manoeuvres or imaging techniques that can be utilised rather than an X-ray-guided intervention.

3. There are techniques for monitoring and minimising radiation exposure during every cardiac intervention and these should be used.

Valvular heart disease

Valvular heart disease, both acquired and congenital, is the most common indication for cardiac intervention during pregnancy. General issues in valvular heart disease in pregnancy are dealt with in Chapters 11, 13 and 19 and in extensive recent reviews.[46,82–84] This discussion will focus on the indications for, and the management of, cardiac intervention for valvular lesions in pregnant women.

Mitral valve stenosis

The greatest number of cardiac interventions in pregnancy involve mitral stenosis. Most of the experience has been in developing countries with higher incidences of rheumatic heart disease.[3] Worldwide, mitral stenosis is the most common symptomatic valvular abnormality seen in pregnancy.[46] The pregnancy-associated rise in circulating volume and heart rate results in a corresponding increase in the pressure gradient across the narrowed mitral valve, which can result in heart failure and pulmonary oedema. Additionally, the rise in atrial pressure may give rise to atrial arrhythmias, with increased heart rate and/or loss of atrial contraction, further exacerbating the unfavourable haemodynamics and worsening the heart failure. Recent reports confirm the high incidence (65%) of arrhythmias and heart failure in pregnant women with severe mitral stenosis, as well as an increased risk of fetal mortality and morbidity.[3,84,85] Despite these high rates of maternal complications with severe mitral stenosis, there were no reported maternal deaths in three recent series.[3,84,85] However, fetal morbidity was related to severity of mitral stenosis with a 33–44% rate of prematurity and a 33% incidence of intrauterine growth restriction.

Women with severe mitral stenosis who wish to become pregnant need to be counselled on the risks of the pregnancy to them and to the child, and to be offered therapeutic choices. Percutaneous balloon mitral valvuloplasty prior to pregnancy has been used successfully to minimise pregnancy-associated clinical deterioration in such women and to reduce the requirement for medication (with its attendant fetal risks) or cardiac intervention during the pregnancy.[46] If the presence of severe calcification or associated mitral regurgitation make the woman an unsuitable candidate for PBMV, mitral valve replacement can be considered. Despite the maternal and fetal risks in pregnant women who have had mitral valve replacement prior to pregnancy,[82,86,87] the series by Bhatla *et al.*[3] demonstrated that only 3% of those who had had valve replacement surgery deteriorated into New York Heart Association (NYHA) functional class III/IV (see Appendix A) compared with 26% of those who had had either valvotomy or no prior intervention. Furthermore, there were fewer intrauterine growth-restricted and low birthweight infants born to mothers with prosthetic valves. However, such an approach does raise the issue of whether tissue valves (needing a further replacement in 10–15 years) or metal valves (raising the problems of anticoagulation in pregnancy) should be used (see Chapter 11).

The surgical approach to mitral stenosis in developed countries focuses on open mitral valvuloplasty and mitral valve replacement, both of which require the use of cardiopulmonary bypass with its attendant risks to the fetus (see above). De Souza *et al.*[12] reported on 24 pregnant women who underwent open mitral valvuloplasty for refractory severe heart failure due to mitral stenosis. There was one maternal death but six fetal and two neonatal deaths. In another report of 73 women undergoing mitral valve replacement or open mitral valvuloplasty there was one maternal death and ten fetal deaths.[8]

Closed mitral valvotomy surgery has been performed for more than six decades and is often the preferred approach to severe mitral stenosis for patients in developing countries.[43,88] A review of 1134 patients in Turkey undergoing closed mitral valvotomy revealed an in-hospital mortality rate of 0.4% and a postoperative embolisation incidence of 0.5%.[43] Because there is no need for cardiopulmonary bypass, closed mitral valvotomy may have some advantages in pregnant women. In fact, Spencer[89] has suggested that since open mitral valvuloplasty improves haemodynamics significantly more than closed mitral valvotomy, the only role for closed mitral valvotomy might be in pregnancy in an effort to avoid cardiopulmonary bypass. Audits of closed mitral valvotomy in pregnancy in developing countries have reported no maternal mortality and fetal mortality rates of 0–12%.[44,45,90,91] However, there is a significant likelihood of re-stenosis and the need for repeat surgery. Furthermore, the closed procedure can be used only for isolated mitral stenosis, with no left atrial thrombus, no heavy calcification and reasonably preserved valvular/subvalvular apparatus.[59,90,91] In developed countries, closed mitral valvotomy has been abandoned in favour of open mitral commissurotomy and mitral valve replacement because of better haemo-dynamics and long-term results with these procedures.[89] Therefore, in these countries, cardiac surgeons are no longer being trained in the technique of closed mitral valvotomy and it cannot be considered a realistic option in that context.

Percutaneous balloon mitral valvuloplasty has been practised for more than 20 years with excellent results.[92,93] In a recent series of 2773 patients, there was a technical failure rate of 1.2% and an in-hospital death rate of 0.4%. The most common adverse events included severe mitral regurgitation in 4.1%, arterial embolism in 0.4% and tamponade in 0.2%. Good results (mitral valve area greater than 1.5 cm^2 and no regurgitation more severe than grade 2 out of 4) were obtained in 90% of patients, with only 4.7% of them having to undergo mitral surgery within the first month after the percutaneous procedure.[94] Percutaneous balloon mitral valvuloplasty has been increasingly used in pregnancy for women in NYHA class III/IV refractory to medical therapy and the experience of its use in pregnancy has been equally positive. The technique using the Inoue balloon has been well described (Figure 8.1).[95,96] Well over 400 cases in which PBMV was used to treat medically refractory symptomatic mitral stenosis in pregnancy have been described and Table 8.3 summarises some recent reports.[4,12,50,67,69,97–100] Symptomatic, haemodynamic and echocardiographic improvement is seen in the vast majority of women. The excellent results achieved are likely related to the underlying

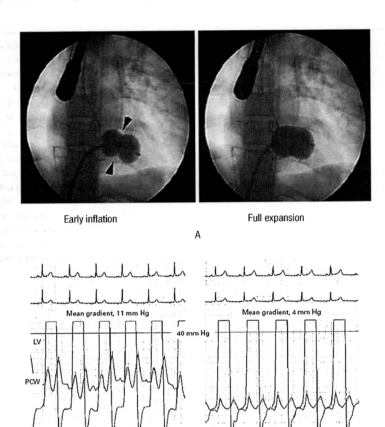

Early inflation   Full expansion

A

Mean gradient, 11 mm Hg

40 mm Hg

LV

PCW

Mean gradient, 4 mm Hg

Before valvuloplasty   After valvuloplasty

B

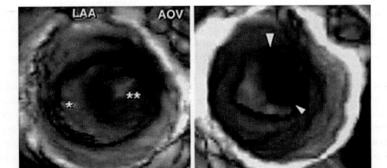

Before valvuloplasty   After valvuloplasty

C

Figure 8.1. The percutaneous balloon mitral valvuloplasty (PBMV) procedure in a pregnant 27-year-old woman newly diagnosed with heart failure and mitral stenosis; the procedure was performed while the woman was under general anaesthesia; transoesophageal echocardiographic guidance was used for inter-atrial septal puncture; a 30 mm Inoue balloon was passed through the stenotic mitral valve, its distal end was inflated (arrowheads in panel A, left), and under traction the whole balloon was expanded (panel A, right); the mean pressure gradient measured by catheter fell from 11 mmHg to 4 mmHg (panel B, LV = left ventricular pressure, PCW = pulmonary capillary wedge pressure); the transoesophageal probe was used to construct a three-dimensional image of the mitral valve before and after the procedure; a view during diastole from the left atrium before valvuloplasty (panel C, left) showed commissural fusion, with limited opening of the valve (the single asterisk denotes the posterior mitral leaflet, the double asterisk the anterior mitral leaflet, LAA = left atrial appendage, AOV = aortic valve); after dilatation (panel C, right), the anterior commissure was wide open (top arrowhead), whereas the posterior commissure was still partially fused (bottom arrowhead); the posterior leaflet was fixed; the area of the mitral valve increased from 1.1 cm² to 2.3 cm²; there was grade 1 mitral regurgitation after the procedure; reproduced with permission from Delabays and Goy[95]

Table 8.3. Recent reports of percutaneous balloon mitral valvuloplasty (PBMV) in a total of 341 pregnancies, with a haemodynamic/echocardiographic success rate of 97%, a maternal mortality of 0.3% and a reported fetal/neonatal death rate of 3%

Study	n	Success rate	Maternal deaths	Fetal/ neonatal deaths	Notes
Khaledi[67] (2004)	18	18/18	0	0/18	
Nercolini et al.[50] (2002)	44	42/44	0	3/37[a]	
Mishra et al.[4] (2001)	85	80/85	0	0/85	One episode of tamponade
Fawzy et al.[97] (2001)	23	23/23	0	1/23	
De Souza et al.[12] (2001)	21	20/21	0	1/21	
Sivadasanpillai et al.[69] (2005)	36	35/36	0	2/36	
Mangione et al.[98] (2000)	30	30/30	0	2/23[a]	
Gupta et al.[99] (1998)	40	39/40	1/40	1/23[a]	11 patients had therapeutic termination before 18 weeks
Ben Farhat et al.[100] (1997)	44	44/44	0	0/44	

[a] Not all patients returned to the centre for delivery and the fetal/neonatal status for every case is not known

valvular pathology. The valves in these young mothers are unlikely to be heavily calcified or to have significant subvalvular thickening. Commissural fusion is the major pathology and this makes them good candidates for PBMV.[101] Maternal mortality has been very low (less than 0.3%), as has the fetal/neonatal mortality (3%).

Balloon inflation has been reported to cause a transient decrease in maternal blood pressure and fetal heart rate with a return to baseline levels within a few seconds of balloon deflation.[101] The woman is recumbent for the procedure and pressure from the uterus may result in maternal hypotension and may hinder the passage of catheters.[59] The rate of reported complications has been low but maternal complications do include cardiac tamponade, residual atrial septal defect, excessive blood loss, venous thrombosis, transient atrial fibrillation, deterioration in degree of mitral regurgitation and systemic embolisation.[93] Furthermore, PBMV has precipitated uterine contractions and resulted in premature labour.[46,102] Tocolytics may be used for premature labour precipitated by the procedure. As noted above, tocolytic agents may have significant cardiovascular effects and must be used with caution.[23] Atosiban has the lowest frequency of cardiovascular adverse effects and is probably the tocolytic of choice in women with cardiac problems.

The other concern remains the radiation risk. In some series, therapeutic terminations of pregnancy were offered to women who had PBMV before 18 weeks of gestation.[99] However, early follow-up reports of children born after the procedure found no evidence of abnormal growth or development, although these studies included fewer than 70 children and follow-up of less than 8 years.[69,97,98,103] Mishra et al.[4] reviewed fluoroscopy exposure times from several series and reported that 95% of the procedures had less than 16 minutes of fluoroscopy time and that the average fluoroscopy time for their own group of 85 women was 3.6 ± 3.2 minutes. Such exposure times would not be expected to materially affect fetal risk. Even so, all measures should be taken to limit radiation risks to the fetus, including use of the Inoue balloon which requires less procedural time[46,104] and the increased use of transoesophageal echocardiography to reduce fluoroscopy time.[66-70] Because of the increased sensitivity to radiation effects in early pregnancy, PBMV should be avoided in the first trimester if possible. Fortunately, the haemodynamic changes of pregnancy are such that most women with mitral stenosis do not deteriorate clinically until the second or third trimester.[105]

A recent editorial[104] stated that PBMV by the Inoue balloon technique is the ideal treatment of significant symptomatic mitral stenosis in pregnant women. Although to date there have been no direct comparative studies of PBMV and mitral valve surgery in pregnancy (and such a future study is unlikely), cumulative descriptive reports have shown a lower maternal and fetal/neonatal mortality rate and an acceptable rate of complications with the percutaneous approach.[4,12,50,67,69,97-100] However, there are the unknown risks of future problems from radiation exposure, and the risks of precipitating premature labour. Therefore, this procedure must be limited to those symptomatic women for whom medical therapy has not been successful. Percutaneous balloon mitral valvuloplasty is no substitute for expert management during pregnancy, labour and delivery. The procedure cannot be performed in women with more than moderate mitral regurgitation, left atrial thrombus, marked calcification or absence of commissural fusion.[93,106] If such women with severe mitral stenosis cannot be controlled medically[84] they will need careful assessment for mitral valve surgery, keeping in mind the higher fetal loss associated with the cardiopulmonary bypass necessary for such surgery.

Aortic valve stenosis

Severe aortic valve stenosis has traditionally been considered a contraindication to pregnancy, with a reported maternal death rate of 17% as well as concerns about clinical deterioration leading to premature delivery and fetal morbidity.[46,85,105] However, recent reports suggest a more optimistic outcome for this group of women.[83,85] Of 49 pregnancies reviewed by Silversides et al.,[83] 16 involved moderate aortic stenosis and 29 had severe aortic stenosis. There were no cardiac complications in the women with mild or moderate aortic stenosis, but three of the 29 women with severe aortic stenosis did develop complications, including pulmonary oedema in two women and recurrent atrial arrhythmias and angina in the third. Of these three women, one required percutaneous aortic valvuloplasty during pregnancy whereas the other two could be managed medically through the rest of the pregnancy and subsequently underwent surgical repair postpartum. There were no maternal deaths. Although there were five premature births and three cases of respiratory distress syndrome, there were no fetal or neonatal deaths.[83] In the group of 12 women reported by Hameed et al.,[85] one woman with severe aortic stenosis and coarctation of the aorta died 10 days postpartum in conjunction with surgery for aortic valve replacement. As in the Silversides series, there was an increased incidence of preterm delivery but there were no fetal or neonatal deaths.

This more recent experience exemplifies the current management of severe aortic stenosis in pregnant women.[83,85] Most reports consider severe aortic stenosis to be present if the aortic valve area is less than 1 cm^2 or the peak gradient is 64 mmHg or higher.[83] All attempts should be made to identify those women with severe aortic stenosis and consider valve surgery or balloon valvotomy before pregnancy. Choice of valve replacement becomes important because of the increased risks in pregnancy for women with prosthetic valves. For women with aortic stenosis, an attractive alternative to bioprosthetic or mechanical valves would be the pulmonary autograft (Ross procedure).[107] For women with severe aortic stenosis who present already pregnant, discussion needs to focus on the risks of the pregnancy for mother and child, including termination, continuing medical management and the need for intervention, either surgical or balloon valvuloplasty.[46] These women should also be advised that, even if they deliver successfully without cardiac intervention, there is a significant likelihood of the need for such intervention postpartum.[83]

Women who develop symptoms may respond to medical therapy that includes bedrest, diuretics and close monitoring, frequently in a hospital environment.[46] Failure to respond to medical management requires decisions about termination, early delivery or cardiac intervention. Cardiac intervention must be limited to women with clinical deterioration. A high gradient across the aortic valve during pregnancy is not sufficient reason for intervention.[68,108] Aortic valve surgery has been successfully carried out in pregnancy for decades but the number of reported cases has been small. Because of the small numbers, most series on cardiac surgery in pregnancy have not separately reported the mortality or morbidity results for just the women undergoing aortic surgery.[2,9,10] Two separate reviews from 1994 and 1996 reported no maternal mortality but fetal losses of 30–38% in two small groups of 18 and 15 women.[8,33] There have been no recent large series of aortic valve replacement in pregnancy but in 2003 Jahangiri et al.[31] did report replacement of the aortic valve in four women, one with congenital aortic stenosis, two with aortic regurgitation and one with mitral and aortic stenosis. All four women did very well during surgery, were extubated within 4 hours and discharged home within 8 days. Three women delivered a normal newborn baby at

38 weeks by caesarean section. The fetus in the fourth case showed evidence of hydrops a week after surgery and the pregnancy was terminated 2 weeks after surgery. Although there have been no large series of pregnant women undergoing aortic valve surgery, it is clear that the fetal mortality remains a major concern. It is precisely for this reason that balloon aortic valvotomy has been performed in pregnant women with aortic stenosis refractory to medical therapy. There have been only 11 cases of PBAV in pregnancy reported in the literature since 1988.[68,109] In all the reported cases, there has been reduction in valvular gradient and improvement in clinical situation, without fetal loss.

Unlike PBMV, PBAV in the non-pregnant adult has been considered a palliative procedure because the improvement in haemodynamics has been transient and there has been no demonstrated improvement in long-term survival. In general, its use has been relegated to the elderly with severe aortic stenosis who are not considered candidates for aortic valve replacement and it has been used as a 'bridge to surgery' for those in cardiogenic shock or for those who require urgent non-cardiac surgery.[109,110] It cannot be considered an alternative for aortic valve replacement in the adult. On the other hand, PBAV is commonly used in the neonatal and paediatric setting to postpone the need for eventual aortic valve replacement.[111,112] Complications of PBAV have included embolic phenomena, marked aortic regurgitation, haemopericardium and aortic rupture but none of these has yet been reported with PBAV during pregnancy.[59] It should not be performed in the setting of already significant aortic regurgitation or a heavily calcified valve. It carries the risk of radiation exposure to mother and fetus but the increasing use of transoesophageal echocardiography during PBAV does reduce fluoroscopy times.[68]

There have been no reported series of PBAV in pregnancy and certainly no comparative studies with aortic valve surgery. Given the rarity of the need for intervention, such future series are unlikely. Percutaneous balloon aortic valvuloplasty must be considered palliative and the woman must understand that she will require definitive aortic valve surgery in the future and that the sole purpose of the PBAV is to allow her pregnancy to continue.[59]

Pulmonary valve stenosis

Pulmonary stenosis during pregnancy is most likely due to congenital obstruction at valvular, subvalvular or supravalvular level but has also been described in the setting of a stenosis in a homograft that had been part of a previous Ross procedure.[46,113] Unlike the situation with mitral stenosis or aortic stenosis, even severe pulmonary stenosis does not appear to have an adverse effect on maternal or fetal morbidity/mortality.[59,85,114] Balloon valvuloplasty for pulmonary stenosis has been performed in non-pregnant patients but only a handful of cases of balloon valvuloplasty during pregnancy have been reported.[59] These resulted in significant improvement and no complications but experience has been limited and the procedure should be considered only for the rare woman with severe symptomatic valvular pulmonary valve stenosis.

Mitral regurgitation and aortic regurgitation

Mitral regurgitation during pregnancy may be due to mitral valve prolapse or rheumatic mitral disease. It may also occur as a consequence of valvuloplasty for mitral stenosis. Aortic regurgitation is likely to be due to bicuspid aortic valve, rheumatic disease or enlarged aortic annulus.[46] Because of the physiological decrease in systemic resistance, both these lesions are well tolerated during pregnancy. For those pregnant women with symptoms and left ventricular dysfunction, there is well-established effective medical management with diuretics, digoxin and vasodilator therapy. Although angiotensin-converting enzyme (ACE) inhibitors are contraindicated during pregnancy, nitrates and hydralazine are an effective substitute when vasodilatation is the effect required.[46] Because women with valvular regurgitation generally do well during pregnancy (see Chapter 11), and because prosthetic valves carry particular risks during pregnancy, there is no recommendation for prepregnancy prophylactic replacement of mitral or aortic valves in women with severe regurgitation but no other established indications for surgery. On the other hand, consideration may be given to mitral valve repair or to the Ross procedure in selected women before pregnancy. Intervention during pregnancy should be undertaken only for severely symptomatic women who are refractory to optimal medical therapy. If at all possible, surgery during pregnancy should be avoided because of the high risk of fetal loss. When surgery is needed it is usually because of sudden deterioration, such as in endocarditis or dissection. Some adaptations to cardiopulmonary bypass techniques may help lower the risk of fetal death[29] but, at this time, there is no percutaneous option to open-heart surgical cardiopulmonary bypass repair of mitral regurgitation or aortic regurgitation. Preliminary work on percutaneous aortic valve replacement and mitral valve repair is in much too early a stage to predict its future role in interventions during pregnancy.[110]

Prosthetic valves

The challenges in the management of pregnant women with a prosthetic valve are discussed in Chapter 11. Interventions in pregnant women with a prosthetic valve may be considered in the setting of valve thrombosis, endocarditis or degeneration in a bioprosthetic valve or homograft. Thromboembolism is common owing to pregnancy–related thrombophilia[20] as well as to problems with inadequate anticoagulation during pregnancy.[115] Prosthetic valve thrombosis poses special problems in pregnancy because of the relative contraindications to thrombolysis in pregnancy,[81,82,116] the high operative risks of surgical thrombectomy[117] and the high fetal loss in any cardiac surgery with cardiopulmonary bypass.[9,10] Despite its relative contraindications, thrombolysis has been used successfully for other indications in pregnancy[118] and should be considered first for valve thrombosis, reserving high-risk surgery for women at particularly high risk of bleeding or when thrombolysis has failed.[82] If surgery becomes necessary, it should be noted that successful reported procedures have used simple thrombectomy,[117,119] valve replacement with conventional cardiopulmonary bypass,[120,121] or a beating-heart technique for valve replacement.[29]

Endocarditis

Antibiotic prophylaxis has not generally been recommended for uncomplicated labour and delivery, even in those women with valvular heart disease, prosthetic valves or congenital lesions that predispose them to endocarditis.[36] However, recent reports have indicated a significant incidence of bacteraemia during normal labour and delivery[46] as well as a high maternal (22.1%) and fetal (14.7%) mortality associated with endocarditis during pregnancy.[122] Antibiotic prophylaxis is thus now more frequently recommended even for uncomplicated labour in particularly high-risk women.[46] There have been successful operative procedures reported for endocarditis complications during pregnancy[38] but, in the light of the high morbidity and mortality rates for mother and fetus, it has been recommended that early delivery of the fetus should be considered, if at all possible, to allow intensive medical and surgical therapy of the infection.[122]

Dissection of the aorta

Acute dissection of the aorta is a life-threatening situation. Left untreated, it has a 50% mortality in the first 48 hours.[123] Aortic dissection in women aged under 40 years is rare; however, about half the dissections in women in this age range occur during pregnancy.[124] A review[13] of pregnant women with aortic dissection reported in the literature between 1983 and 2002 identified 45 women with Stanford type A dissection (involving the ascending aorta) and 12 with Stanford type B (not involving the ascending aorta). Maternal mortality for the type A dissections was 15% and for type B it was 0%. Fetal mortality was 32% for type A and 43% for type B. The high fetal mortality rate in type B dissection occurred despite the fact that these women usually did not go to immediate surgery, and was probably because the dissection extended down into the iliac vessels and caused decreased placental flow.[13] Of the 45 women with type A dissection, 20 had either Marfan or Ehlers–Danlos syndrome, nine had hypertension and four had a bicuspid aortic valve. The average size of the aortic root at time of presentation was 4.8 ± 0.9 cm.

Changes in the structure of arteries and veins have been described in pregnancy and oestrogen receptors have been found in human aortic tissue. Hormonal changes during pregnancy lead to gradual dilatation of the aorta and of renal and placental vessels in an effort to improve perfusion during pregnancy.[13] It is believed that these hormonal effects can lead to fragmentation of the reticulin fibres. In addition, there are the increases in cardiac output and circulating volume that increase the shear stresses on these vessels.[105] These changes occur with every pregnancy but dissection occurs only rarely and under special circumstances. The aorta in Marfan and Ehlers–Danlos syndrome already has connective tissue defects. In addition, abnormal elastic properties have been described in the aortas of patients with bicuspid aortic valve and in those with repaired tetralogy of Fallot.[125] Coarctation of the aorta has also been associated with an intrinsic aortopathy, placing these individuals at risk from dissection.[126,127] In a recent series of 50 pregnant women with coarctation, there was one episode of Stanford type A dissection that resulted in death.[126]

Every effort should be made to identify women with Marfan or Ehlers–Danlos syndrome, bicuspid aortic valve, coarctation and hypertension before pregnancy, and to assess aortic root size.[127] Women with aortic root size greater than 4 cm should be considered for elective aortic root replacement before pregnancy, as this can now be done with low mortality and morbidity.[13] In pregnant women, close clinical and echocardiographic surveillance is warranted and beta blockers should be considered if the aortic root is larger than 4 cm or is enlarging during the pregnancy (keeping in mind that a small amount of physiological enlargement of the aorta can be observed during pregnancy[13]).[105,128] Hypertension and pre-eclampsia should be controlled as well as possible.[36] High-risk women can be admitted to hospital at between 28 and 32 weeks of gestation with plans for aortic root surgery shortly after delivery. Such an admission should be to a facility with a surgical, obstetric and neonatal team experienced in cardiac surgery during pregnancy. It has been recommended that, if dissection occurs before 30 weeks, emergency surgery be undertaken with the fetus *in utero*.[13,123,124] After 30 weeks, immediate caesarean section followed by the aortic surgery is preferred, keeping in mind the increased risks of bleeding from the delivery site. (Dealing with a postpartum haemorrhage at the same time as cardiac surgery is very stressful for the surgeons as well as being dangerous for the woman; a delay of 24 hours between the two procedures may be advisable if considered safe from the cardiac point of view.) There have been no serious complications reported in the literature using this type of approach.[13,38,129,130] Of course, there will be crisis situations where it will not be possible to undertake delivery prior to the aortic surgery and the fetus will be exposed to the risks of cardiopulmonary bypass.[26]

Coronary interventions

Aortocoronary bypass surgery and coronary angioplasty and stenting are by far the most common cardiac interventions in non-pregnant patients. Such interventions in pregnant women are very rare but are likely to increase in the future because of the rising incidence of myocardial ischaemia in pregnancy.[131] There have been two large reviews of myocardial infarction in pregnancy.[116,131] In 1996, Roth and Elkayam[116] reviewed 125 myocardial infarctions during pregnancy and reported a maternal mortality rate of 21% and a total fetal loss of 16/125 (13%), with ten of those being due to maternal death. Fetal loss among mothers surviving the infarction was only 6%. Ladner et al.[131] reported 151 cases of myocardial infarction associated with 5.4 million pregnancies in California over 10 years. This included 89 myocardial infarctions during pregnancy and 62 postpartum. The mortality during pregnancy from myocardial infarction was 13% but 0% postpartum. The highest risk for death was noted intrapartum where six out of 31 women (19.2%) died. The three most powerful independent predictors for myocardial infarction in pregnancy were hypertension, diabetes and advancing maternal age. All of these factors are likely to be more common in pregnancy in the future. Indeed, Ladner et al.[131] noted a definite increase in the frequency of myocardial infarction in pregnancy from one in 73 400 at the beginning of the study decade to one in 24 600 in the final year. In another series of 14 women with established coronary disease, 13 achieved full term and seven remained free of cardiovascular events throughout the pregnancy but four developed unstable angina, necessitating percutaneous coronary intervention for two women and aortocoronary bypass surgery for one.[2]

Myocardial ischaemia and infarction during pregnancy have been linked to underlying coronary disease, hereditary dyslipidaemia,[132] coronary dissection,[42] thrombotic tendencies of pregnancy,[20] emboli from prosthetic valves,[115] and paradoxical embolism across an inter-atrial communication.[133] In the Roth and Elkayam review,[116] the coronary arteries had been studied in 68 of the 125 cases, by angiography or at autopsy. Of those 68 cases, 43% were found to have coronary disease, with or without thrombus, 21% had thrombus without coronary disease, 16% had coronary dissection and 29% had no detectable coronary abnormality. Pregnancy has a well-known thrombophilic effect[20] and this may account for a number of women presenting with myocardial infarction secondary to occluding thrombus but no evidence of coronary atherosclerosis.[133,134] Coronary dissection is known to be increased in the setting of pregnancy and its cause is unclear. It probably involves hormonally mediated morphological changes in the arterial wall[135] that are likely the same factors that increase the risk of aortic dissection in pregnancy.[13,123] These women present acutely with little in the way of classic risk factors and can deteriorate rapidly.[135,136]

The current standard treatment of acute myocardial infarction calls for rapid reperfusion.[137] This may be through thrombolysis or by percutaneous coronary intervention. Acute percutaneous coronary intervention is preferred if the myocardial infarction is complicated by shock or failure or if there are contraindications to thrombolysis. Thrombolytics have been used in pregnancy for venous thrombo-embolism and acute myocardial infarction. However, thrombolytic use has been associated with an increased risk of maternal and fetal haemorrhage, and pregnancy has generally been considered a contraindication for thrombolysis.[81,116] For those reasons, where facilities exist, percutaneous coronary intervention has become preferred for treatment of myocardial infarction in pregnancy, especially for women with coronary dissection.[51,81,135,138] Percutaneous coronary intervention carries its own risks, including those of radiation and risks associated with the use of antiplatelet agents and the 2b3a inhibitors. Any percutaneous coronary intervention for acute myocardial infarction should target only the culprit lesion[137] and the procedure is expected to be relatively short, with exposure times well within the safe range.[55,64] It has recently been proposed that a radial artery access route for percutaneous coronary intervention may reduce fetal exposure further and decrease the risk of bleeding complications.[81] In non-pregnant patients, antiplatelet agents, notably aspirin and clopidogrel, are routinely used after the percutaneous coronary intervention and 2b3a agents are used during the procedure because of proven benefits to long- and short-term mortality.[136] The safety of clopidogrel and 2b3a agents in pregnancy is unknown but there are concerns about increasing the risk of fetal intracranial bleeding during vaginal delivery.[51,81] Animal studies have been reported to show no teratogenic effects of eptifibatide.[136]

Some women will have a coronary anatomy that is unsuitable for percutaneous coronary intervention, and aortocoronary bypass surgery will need to be considered.[139] As with other cardiac surgery, it is recommended that hypothermia be avoided.[140] Nevertheless, despite the use of normothermia, fetal loss can still occur.[141] There have been several cases reported of aortocoronary bypass surgery in pregnancy where the procedure was performed off-pump, without the need for cardiopulmonary bypass.[41,42] This may improve the rate of fetal loss but the numbers reported to date are too small for any firm conclusions to be drawn.

Pregnant women presenting with acute ischaemia or infarction have a mortality rate of 13–21% and may deteriorate rapidly.[116,131] Full resuscitative measures, including the use of an intra-aortic balloon pump, and extracorporeal membrane oxygenation, need to be undertaken and will frequently allow for successful percutaneous coronary intervention or aortocoronary bypass surgery.[135,140,141] Because of the inherent instability of such situations, it is also necessary to plan for delivery of the baby by caesarean section. Infant survival is related to the time interval between death of the mother and the delivery. Roth and Elkayam[116] found that delivery more than 15 minutes after maternal death resulted in a low likelihood of a surviving infant, and those that did survive almost always had some neurological defect. Conversely, all surviving infants delivered within 5 minutes of maternal death were healthy.[116]

Pregnant women presenting with an acute infarction need rapid reperfusion using the best means at hand, be that thrombolysis, percutaneous coronary intervention or aortocoronary bypass surgery. If the anatomy is suitable and the facilities are adequate, percutaneous coronary intervention is to be preferred. Ideally, such a procedure should take place at a centre with an experienced team that has expertise in catheter-based procedures in pregnancy. However, it is recognised that women frequently present in a crisis situation and there may be no opportunity for safe transfer to such a centre. With the increasing incidence of diabetes mellitus and hypertension and a definite trend to older age of pregnancy, more women with coronary crises can be expected. Therefore, risk factors need to be identified as early as possible and controlled with medication and lifestyle change.

Congenital heart disease

In contrast to the situation in developing countries where rheumatic heart disease is still prevalent, developed countries now have congenital heart disease as the most common structural heart defect in women of childbearing age.[130] Other than for congenital aortic stenosis or pulmonary valve stenosis (see the Valvular heart disease section above), there have been very few reports of interventions for congenital heart disease during pregnancy. In general, shunt lesions are well tolerated during pregnancy and there is no need for intervention. There are, in any case, no mechanical intervention options for high-risk women such as those with Eisenmenger syndrome.[105]

Atrial septal defect is probably the most common non-valvular congenital defect seen during pregnancy.[65] Atrial septal defects or ventricular septal defects, with left to right shunting, result in a volume overload circulation that is well compensated during pregnancy.[36,142] There have been some reports of atrial septal defect and ventricular septal defect closure surgery in the past[8,11,33] but a literature search found no recent reports of defect closure surgery during pregnancy, except for an atrial septal defect closure that was undertaken in the first trimester in a stable woman who was not known to be pregnant at the time.[11] She did well with surgery and went on to have a term vaginal delivery of a normal infant. There is a continuing risk of paradoxical embolisation across a shunt defect, especially in the thrombophilic state of pregnancy. As a result, some have recommend the use of low-dose aspirin after the first trimester in women with open shunts.[36] It is reasonable to use aspirin until the 35th week of pregnancy (its safety has been established by the many trials of low-dose aspirin for the prevention of pre-eclampsia). In the occasional woman with marked breathlessness, who may be sedentary, one might wish to continue anticoagulant prophylaxis, using a prophylactic dose of low molecular weight heparin, into the early peripartum period. There has been a recent report of device closure across an inter-atrial communication during pregnancy using echocardiography as the only guide, to reduce radiation risk to the fetus.[72] This was undertaken because of recurrent strokes and not because of any haemodynamic instability. There is the potential for endocarditis on ventricular septal defects[2] and endocarditis precautions are necessary, in view of the high maternal and fetal mortality associated with endocarditis during pregnancy.[122]

Tetralogy of Fallot is the most common form of cyanotic heart disease and such women have an increased risk of fetal loss.[143] Although several cases of repair of tetralogy of Fallot during pregnancy were published more than 35 years ago, no such interventions have been reported recently.[8] In a review published in 2004,[143] there were no maternal deaths, even among the unrepaired women (all of whom eventually went on to have complete repair), but a high fetal loss rate (24%). Although severe pulmonary regurgitation occurred in some women with repaired tetralogy of Fallot, resulting in progressive right ventricular dilatation, surgical intervention was postponed safely until well after delivery.

Coarctation of the aorta is generally well tolerated in pregnancy.[126] Although there is an obstructive lesion at the coarctation site, there are no recent case reports or case series describing relief during pregnancy of such obstruction, by either surgery or trans-catheter stenting. Indeed, such an intervention during pregnancy would probably carry an increased risk of aortic dissection because of hormone-induced endothelial changes and the aortopathy associated with coarctation.[126,127] Older reports of coarctation and pregnancy quoted a 9.5% maternal mortality rate[36] but in a recent series of 50 women followed through 118 pregnancies, managed at a tertiary centre, there was only one maternal death from dissection, and a 9% miscarriage rate.[126]

Optimal blood pressure control and monitoring are clearly important, as is recommended in Marfan syndrome.[127] There may be the rare woman with severe coarctation where the need for preventing proximal hypertension with drug therapy cannot be met without significant compromise of distal circulation and, consequently, of placental perfusion and fetal wellbeing. For such a woman, trans-catheter relief of coarctation with primary stenting, under echocardiographic and limited fluoroscopy screening, may be an option and should be carefully considered, but only in a tertiary setting. Endocarditis precautions are necessary in women with coarctation. A recent report documented a successful operation, without fetal loss, to repair a pseudo-aneurysm resulting from staphylococcal endarteritis at the coarctation site.[144]

Miscellaneous interventions

Cardiac arrhythmias may require device intervention. For pregnant women with important symptomatic bradycardia or atrioventricular block, it may be necessary to insert a temporary or even a permanent pacemaker. Pacemaker insertion does carry the risk of radiation exposure to the fetus but the procedure can be carried out with echocardiographic guidance alone.[71] In the event of a cardiovascular collapse related to bradycardia or atrioventricular block, the swift placement of epicardial leads and a pacemaker generator should be considered an option in experienced hands. No X-ray or echocardiographic guidance is required but rapid general anaesthesia is necessary to open the chest. Implantable cardioverter-defibrillators can have a life-saving role in non-pregnant patients and have been shown to be well tolerated through pregnancy,[145] but there can be problems with inappropriate shocks due to the increase in pulse rate secondary to pregnancy demand or development of new supraventricular tachycardia.[146] There have been reports of implantable cardioverter-defibrillator insertion during pregnancy without any fetal compromise.[53,145] The radiation risks of the procedure can be further reduced by the use of transoesophageal echocardiography for lead placement.[53] In addition to lethal arrhythmias there may be supraventricular arrhythmias that can be dealt with using cardiac electrophysiology mapping and ablation techniques, thus avoiding the deleterious effects of antiarrhythmic medication. A decision will have to be made as to whether the risk of radiation exposure can be offset by the reduced risk of having a stable mother who can avoid high dose antiarrhythmics.[64]

The thrombophilic nature of pregnancy results in an increased risk of pulmonary thromboembolism.[20] The presence of a large thrombus in leg or pelvic vessels and the wish to suspend anticoagulation at time of delivery may call for the insertion of an inferior vena caval filter. These have been used successfully in pregnancy. Since the period of risk will be short, use of a removable temporary inferior vena caval filter is preferred unless there is another cause for thrombophilia.[147,148]

Insertion of an intra-aortic balloon pump can frequently stabilise a patient in acute cardiovascular collapse to a sufficient degree to allow definitive therapy for the underlying problem. There are no series reports of the use of intra-aortic balloon pumping in pregnancy but several other reports have clearly documented successful application in this setting and there is no specific contraindication to its use in haemo-dynamically unstable pregnant women.[132,140,141] When intra-aortic balloon pumping is insufficient to rescue the woman, consideration can be given to the use of left and right ventricular assist devices.[149] The only documented cases of the use of such a device (or a biventricular assist device) during pregnancy have been in peripartum cardio-myopathy after delivery,[150] in one case to rescue a young woman who remained unstable after emergency aortocoronary bypass surgery for acute myocardial infarction.[134] She was not known to have been pregnant at the time of her collapse and there was subsequent fetal demise. Use of these devices is undertaken only in the most extreme circumstances to save the life of the mother, and fetal concerns must therefore be considered secondary.

Removal of cardiac tumours during pregnancy has been described, with reports of four myxomas and one primary sarcoma removed being without maternal or fetal death.[8,151] It should be possible to delay the excision of a benign myxoma until after delivery unless there are significant arrhythmias or embolic phenomena linked to the myxoma. The surgical risk to the fetus relates to the risks of cardiopulmonary bypass.[2,8,13]

Conclusion

There has been extensive experience and there is much expertise in the application of surgical and catheter interventions to non-pregnant patients, even in the extreme situations of haemodynamic instability. Nevertheless, it must be emphasised that the application of these techniques to pregnant women requires additional expertise and a thorough understanding of the risks to the pregnant woman and her child, as well as careful planning before the procedure to ensure that the team is prepared for all possible outcomes. The obstetric and paediatric team members must be present and be prepared to deal with fetal distress or precipitous delivery.[102] Although a centre may be experienced in complex interventions in non-pregnant patients, the interventions in pregnant women should be carried out in specialised centres with established teams for high-risk pregnancy management.[107,128]

Key points summary

1. Only women with medically refractory symptoms, and for whom catheter-based interventions are unsuitable, should be considered for cardiac surgery during pregnancy. Because of concerns about the high rates of fetal loss during cardiopulmonary bypass, consideration should be given to early delivery if at all possible. Only centres with experienced teams and expertise in cardiac surgery during pregnancy should carry out such surgery, except in situations where transfer to such a centre would entail greater risk.

2. Percutaneous techniques for valvular, coronary and arrhythmia intervention appear to carry acceptable risks to mother and fetus and significant benefit to pregnant women whose symptoms continue to be refractory to optimal medical management. The medical personnel involved need to minimise radiation risk to mother and fetus during these procedures. Only centres with experienced teams and expertise in catheter intervention during pregnancy should carry out such procedures, except in situations where transfer to such a centre would entail greater risk.

Acknowledgements

Dr Kafka is a Detweiler Fellow of the Royal College of Physicians and Surgeons of Canada, and has received funding support from Queen's University, Canada.

References

1. Mazze RI, Kallen B. Reproductive outcome after anesthesia and operation during pregnancy: A registry study of 5405 cases. *Am J Obstet Gynecol* 1989;161:1178–85.

2. Avila WS, Rossi EG, Ramires JAF, Grinberg M, Bortolotto MRL, Zugaib M, *et al.* Pregnancy in patients with heart disease: experience with 1000 cases. *Clin Cardiol* 2003;26:135–42.

3. Bhatla N, Lal S, Behera G, Kriplani A, Mittal S, Agarwal N, *et al.* Cardiac disease in pregnancy. *Int J Gynecol Obstet* 2003;82:153–9.

4. Mishra S, Narang R, Sharma M, Chopra A, Seth S, Ramamurthy S, *et al.* Percutaneous transseptal mitral commissurotomy in pregnant women with critical mitral stenosis. *Indian Heart J* 2001;53:192–6.

5. Desai DK, Adanlawo M, Naidoo DP, Moodley J, Kleinschmidt I. Mitral stenosis in pregnancy: a four-year experience at King Edward VIII Hospital, Durban, South Africa. *BJOG* 2000;107:953–8.

6. Mora CT. Pregnancy and cardiopulmonary bypass. In: Mora CT, editor. *Cardiopulmonary Bypass. Principles and Techniques of Extracorporeal Circulation.* New York: Springer-Verlag; 1995. p. 359–75.

7. Cooley DA. Early experience with cardiopulmonary bypass: reflections. *J Card Surg* 2003;18:265–7.

8. Parry AJ, Westaby S. Cardiopulmonary bypass during pregnancy. *Ann Thorac Surg* 1996;61:1865–9.

9. Arnoni RT, Arnoni AS, Bonini RCA, de Almeida AFS, Neto, CA, Dinkhuysen JJ, *et al.* Risk factors associated with cardiac surgery during pregnancy. *Ann Thorac Surg* 2003;76:1605–8.

10. Weiss BM, von Segesser LK, Alon E, Seifert B, Turina MI. Outcome of cardiovascular surgery and pregnancy: a systematic review of the period 1984–1996. *Am J Obstet Gynecol* 1998;179:1643–53.

11. Salazar E, Espinola N, Molina FJ, Reyes A, Barragan R. Heart surgery with cardiopulmonary bypass in pregnant women. *Archivos Cardiol Mexico* 2001;71:20–7.

12. de Souza JA, Martinez EE, Ambrose JA, Alves CMR, Born D, Buffolo E, *et al.* Percutaneous balloon mitral valvuloplasty in comparison with open mitral valve commissurotomy for mitral stenosis during pregnancy. *J Am Coll Cardiol* 2001;37:900–3.

13. Immer FF, Bansi AG, Immer-Bansi AS, McDougall J, Zehr KJ, Schaff HV, *et al.* Aortic dissection in pregnancy: analysis of risk factors and outcome. *Ann Thorac Surg* 2003;76:309–14.

14. Pomini F, Mercogliano D, Cavalletti C, Caruso A, Pomini P. Cardiopulmonary bypass in pregnancy. *Ann Thorac Surg* 1996;61:259–68.

15. Alpert JS, Sabik JF III, Cosgrove DM. Mitral valve disease. In: Topol EJ, editor. *Textbook of Cardiovascular Medicine.* Philadelphia: Lippincott Williams & Wilkins; 2002. p. 483–508.

16. Cook DJ. Changing temperature management for cardiopulmonary bypass. *Anesth Analg* 1999;88:1254–71.

17. Nicolini F, Beghi C, Muscari C, Agostinelli A, Budillon AM, Spaggiari I, *et al.* Myocardial protection in adult cardiac surgery: current options and future challenges. *Eur J Cardiothorac Surg* 2003;24:986–93.

18. Daly RC, Dearani JA, McGregor CGA, Mullany CJ, Orszulak TA, Puga FJ, *et al.* Fifty years of open heart surgery at the Mayo Clinic. *Mayo Clin Proc* 2005;80:636–40.

19. Mahli A, Izdes S, Coskun D. Cardiac operations during pregnancy: review of factors influencing fetal outcome. *Ann Thorac Surg* 2000;69:1622–6.

20. Brenner B. Haemostatic changes in pregnancy. *Thromb Res* 2004;114:409–14.
21. Ovrum E, Holen EA, Tangen G, Brosstad F, Abdelnoor M, Ringdal ML, et al. Completely heparinized cardiopulmonary bypass and reduced systemic heparin: clinical and hemostatic events. *Ann Thorac Surg* 1995;60:365–71.
22. Karahan N, Ozturk T, Yetkin U, Yilik L, Baloglu A, Gurbuz A. Managing severe heart failure in a pregnant patient undergoing cardiopulmonary bypass: case report and review of the literature. *J Cardiothorac Vasc Anesth* 2004;18:339–43.
23. Caritis S. Adverse effects of tocolytic therapy. *BJOG* 2005;112:74–8.
24. Worldwide Atosiban versus Beta-agonists Study Group. Effectiveness and safety of the oxytocin antagonist atosiban versus beta-adrenergic agonists in the treatment of preterm labour. *BJOG* 2001;108:133–42.
25. Goldstein I, Jakobi P, Gutterman E, Milo S. Umbilical artery flow velocity during maternal cardiopulmonary bypass. *Ann Thorac Surg* 1995;60:1116–18.
26. Mul TFM, van Herwerden LA, Cohen-Overbeek TE, Catsman-Berrevoets CE, Lotgering FK. Hypoxic-ischemic fetal insult resulting from maternal aortic root replacement, with normal fetal heart rate at term. *Am J Obstet Gynecol* 1998;179:825–7.
27. Kawkabani N, Kawas N, Baraka A, Vogel T, Mangano CM. Severe fetal bradycardia in a pregnant woman undergoing hypothermic cardiopulmonary bypass. *J Cardiothorac Vasc Anaesth* 1999;13:346–9.
28. Cohen RG, Castro LJ. Cardiac surgery during pregnancy. In: Elkayam U, Gleicher N, editors. *Cardiac Problems in Pregnancy*. 3rd ed. New York: Wiley-Liss; 1998. p. 277–83.
29. Tehrani H, Masroor S, Lombardi P, Rosenkranz E, Salerno T. Beating heart aortic valve replacement in a pregnant patient. *J Card Surg* 2004;19:57–8.
30. Tripp HF, Stiegel RM, Coyle JP. The use of pulsatile perfusion during aortic valve replacement in pregnancy. *Ann Thorac Surg* 1999;67:1169–71.
31. Jahangiri M, Clark J, Prefumo F, Pumphrey C, Ward D. Cardiac surgery during pregnancy: pulsatile or nonpulsatile perfusion? *J Thorac Cardiovasc Surg* 2003;126:894–5.
32. Vedrinne C, Tronc F, Martinot S, Robin J, Allevard AM, Vincent M, et al. Better preservation of endothelial function and decreased activation of the fetal renin–angiotensin pathway with the use of pulsatile flow during experimental fetal bypass. *J Thorac Cardiovasc Surg* 2000;120:770–7.
33. Chambers CE, Clark SL. Cardiac surgery during pregnancy. *Clin Obstet Gynecol* 1994;37:316–23.
34. Pardi G, Ferrari MM, Iorio F, Acocella F, Boero V, Berlanda N, et al. The effect of maternal hypothermic cardiopulmonary bypass on fetal lamb temperature, hemodynamics, oxygenation, and acid–base balance. *J Thorac Cardiovasc Surg* 2004;127:1728–34.
35. Baraka A, Kawkabani N, Haroun-Bizri S. Hemodynamic deterioration after cardiopulmonary bypass during pregnancy: resuscitation by postoperative emergency caesarean section. *J Cardiothorac Vasc Anesth* 2000;14:314–15.
36. Klein LL, Galan HL. Cardiac disease in pregnancy. *Obstet Gynecol Clin North Am* 2004;31:429–59.
37. Gopal K, Hudson IM, Ludmir J, Braffman MN, Ewing S, Bavaria JE, et al. Homograft aortic root replacement during pregnancy. *Ann Thorac Surg* 2002;74:243–5.
38. Westaby S, Parry AJ, Forfar JC. Reoperation for prosthetic valve endocarditis in the third trimester of pregnancy. *Ann Thorac Surg* 1992;53:263–5.
39. Guyton RA. Warm-blood cardioplegia and normothermic cardiopulmonary bypass. In: Mora CT, editor. *Cardiopulmonary Bypass. Principles and Techniques of Extracorporeal Circulation*. New York: Springer-Verlag; 1995. p. 484–92.

40. Willcox TW, Stone P, Milsom FP, Connell H. Cardiopulmonary bypass in pregnancy: possible new role for the intra-aortic balloon pump. *J Extra Corpor Technol* 2005;37:189–91.

41. Silberman S, Fink D, Berko RS, Mendzelevski B, Bitran D. Coronary artery bypass surgery during pregnancy. *Eur J Cardio-Thorac Surg* 1996;10:925–6.

42. Klutstein MW, Tzivoni D, Bitran D, Mendzelevski B, Ilan M, Almagor Y. Treatment of spontaneous coronary artery dissection: report of three cases. *Cathet Cardiovasc Diagn* 1997;40:372–6.

43. Tutun U, Ulus AT, Aksoyek AI, Hizarci M, Kaplan S, Erbas S, et al. The place of closed mitral valvotomy in the modern cardiac surgery era. *J Heart Valve Dis* 2003;12:585–91.

44. Aggarwal N, Suri V, Goyal A, Malhotra S, Manoj R, Dhaliwal RS. Closed mitral valvotomy in pregnancy and labor. *Int J Gynecol Obstet* 2005;88:118–21.

45. Abid A, Abid F, Zargouni N, Khayati A. Closed mitral valvotomy in pregnancy – a study of seven cases. *Int J Cardiol* 1990;26:319–21.

46. Elkayam U, Bitar F. Valvular heart disease and pregnancy. Part I: native valves. *J Am Coll Cardiol* 2005;46:223–30.

47. Steer P. The epidemiology of preterm labour. *BJOG* 2005;112:1–3.

48. Draper ES, Manktelow B, Field DJ, James D. Prediction of survival for preterm births by weight and gestational age: retrospective population based study. *BMJ* 1999;319:1093–7.

49. Draper ES, Manktelow B, Field DJ, James D. Tables for predicting survival for preterm births are updated. *BMJ* 2003;327:872.

50. Nercolini DC, da Rocha Loures Bueno R, Guerios EE, Tarastchuk JC, Pacheco AL, Pia de Andrade PM, et al. Percutaneous mitral balloon valvuloplasty in pregnant women with mitral stenosis. *Catheter Cardiovasc Interv* 2002;57:318–22.

51. Sebastian C, Scherlag M, Kugelmass A, Schecter E. Primary stent implantation for acute myocardial infarction during pregnancy: use of abciximab, ticlopidine and aspirin. *Cathet Cardiovasc Diagn* 1998;45:275–9.

52. Gamra H, Betbout F, Ayari M, Addad F, Jarrar M, Maatouk F, et al. Recurrent miscarriages as an indication for percutaneous tricuspid valvuloplasty during pregnancy. *Cathet Cardiovasc Diagn* 1997;40:283–6.

53. Abello M, Peinado R, Merino JL, Gnoatto M, Mateos M, Silvestre J, et al. Cardioverter defibrillator implantation in a pregnant woman guided with transesophageal echocardiography. *Pacing Clin Electrophysiol* 2003;26:1913–14.

54. Stisova V. Effective dose to patient during cardiac interventional procedures (Prague workplaces). *Radiat Prot Dosim* 2004;111:271–4.

55. Hirshfeld JW, Balter S, Brinker JA, Kern MJ, Klein LW, Lindsay BD, et al. ACCF/AHA/HRS/SCAI Clinical competence statement on physician knowledge to optimize patient safety and image quality in fluoroscopically guided invasive cardiovascular procedures. *Circulation* 2005;111:511–32.

56. Barish RJ. In-flight radiation: counseling patients about risk. *J Am Board Fam Pract* 1999;12:195–9.

57. ACOG Committee Opinion No. 299. Guidelines for diagnostic imaging during pregnancy. *Obstet Gynecol* 2004;104:647–51.

58. Bashore T. Fundamentals of x-ray imaging and radiation safety. *Catheter Cardiovasc Interv* 2001;54:126–35.

59. Presbitero P, Prever SB, Brusca A. Interventional cardiology in pregnancy. *Eur Heart J* 1996;17:182–8.

60. Neofotistou V. Review of patient dosimetry in cardiology. *Radiat Prot Dosim* 2001;94:177–82.

61. Damilakis J, Perisinakis K, Prassopoulos P, Dimovasili E, Varveris H, Gourtsoyiannis N. Conceptus radiation dose and risk from chest screen-film radiography. *Eur Radiol* 2003;13:406–12.

62. Brenner DJ, Elliston CD, Hall EJ, Berdon WE. Estimated risks of radiation-induced fatal cancer from pediatric CT. *AJR* 2001;176:289–96.

63. Huda W, Bushong SC, Hendee WR. In x-ray computed tomography, technique factors should be selected appropriate to patient size. *Med Phys* 2001;28:1543–4.

64. Damilakis J, Theocharopoulos N, Perisinakis K, Manios E, Dimitriou P, Vardas P, et al. Conceptus radiation dose and risk from cardiac catheter ablation procedures. *Circulation* 2001;104:893–7.

65. Vidaillet HJ, Skelton TN, Kisslo KB, Kisslo J, Bashore TM. Echocardiographic guidance of cardiac catheterization for atrial septal defect in pregnancy. *Am J Cardiol* 1986;58:1133–4.

66. Poirier P, Champagne J, Alain P, Martineau A, Marquis Y, Dumesnil JG, et al. Mitral balloon valvuloplasty in pregnancy: limiting radiation and procedure time by using transesophageal echocardiography. *Can J Cardiol* 1997;13:843–5.

67. Khaledi AK. Percutaneous balloon mitral valvotomy with the guide of transesophageal echocardiography during pregnancy. *Acta Med Iran* 2004;42:248–55.

68. Myerson SG, Mitchell ARJ, Ormerod OJM, Banning AP. What is the role of balloon dilatation for severe aortic stenosis during pregnancy? *J Heart Valve Dis* 2005;14:147–50.

69. Sivadasanpillai H, Srinivasan A, Sivasubramoniam S, Mahadevan KK, Kumar A, Titus T, et al. Long-term outcome of patients undergoing balloon mitral valvotomy in pregnancy. *Am J Cardiol* 2005;95:1504–6.

70. Saleh MAAW, El Fiky AA, Fahmy M, Farag N, Khashaba AA. Use of biplane transesophageal echocardiography as the only imaging technique for percutaneous balloon mitral commissurotomy. *Am J Cardiol* 1996;78:103–6.

71. Antonelli D, Bloch L, Rosenfeld T. Implantation of permanent dual chamber pacemaker in a pregnant woman by transesophageal echocardiographic guidance. *Pacing Clin Electrophysiol* 1999;22:534–5.

72. Daehnert I, Ewert P, Berger F, Lange PE. Echocardiographically guided closure of a patent foramen ovale during pregnancy after recurrent strokes. *J Interven Cardiol* 2001;14:191–2.

73. Leyendecker JR, Gorengaut V, Brown JJ. MR imaging of maternal diseases of the abdomen and pelvis during pregnancy and the immediate postpartum period. *Radiographics* 2004;24:1301–16.

74. Garel C, Brisse H, Sebag G, Elmaleh M, Oury JF, Hassan M. Magnetic resonance imaging of the fetus. *Pediatr Radiol* 1998;28:201–11.

75. Rickers C, Seethamraju RT, Jerosch-Herold M, Wilke NM. Magnetic resonance imaging guided cardiovascular interventions in congenital heart diseases. *J Interven Cardiol* 2003;16:143–7.

76. Razavi R, Hill DIG, Keevil SF, Miquel ME, Muthurangu V, Hegde S, et al. Cardiac catheterisation guided by MRI in children and adults with congenital heart disease. *Lancet* 2003;362:1877–82.

77. Raman VK, Karmarkar PV, Guttman MA, Dick AJ, Peters DC, Ozturk C, et al. Real-time magnetic resonance-guided endovascular repair of experimental abdominal aortic aneurysm in Swine. *J Am Coll Cardiol* 2005;45:2069–77.

78. Salomon LJ, Siauve N, Balvay D, Cuenod CA, Vayssettes C, Luciani A, et al. Placental perfusion MR imaging with contrast agents in a mouse model. *Radiology* 2005;235:73–80.

79. Bashore TM. Radiation safety in the cardiac catheterization laboratory. *Am Heart J* 2004;147:375–8.

80. Geijer H, Beckman KW, Andersson T, Persliden J. Radiation dose optimization in coronary angiography and percutaneous coronary intervention (PCI). II. Clinical Evaluation. *Eur Radiol* 2002;12:2813–19.

81. Sharma GL, Loubeyre C, Morice MC. Safety and feasibility of the radial approach for primary angioplasty in acute myocardial infarction during pregnancy. *J Invasive Cardiol* 2002;14:359–62.

82. Elkayam U, Bitar F. Valvular heart disease and pregnancy: part II: prosthetic valves. *J Am Coll Cardiol* 2005;46:403–10.

83. Silversides CK, Colman JM, Sermer M, Farine D, Siu SC. Early and intermediate-term outcomes of pregnancy with congenital aortic stenosis. *Am J Cardiol* 2003;91:1386–9.

84. Silversides CK, Colman JM, Sermer M, Siu S. Cardiac risk in pregnant women with rheumatic mitral stenosis. *Am J Cardiol* 2003;91:1382–5.

85. Hameed A, Karaalp IS, Tummala PP, Wani OR, Canetti M, Akhter MW, et al. The effect of valvular heart disease on maternal and fetal outcome of pregnancy. *J Am Coll Cardiol* 2001;37:893–9.

86. Hung L, Rahimtoola SH. Prosthetic heart valves and pregnancy. *Circulation* 2003;107:1240–6.

87. Reimold S, Rutherford JD. Valvular heart disease in pregnancy. *N Engl J Med* 2003;349:52–9.

88. Salerno TA, Neilson IR, Charrette EJ, Lynn RB. A 25-year experience with the closed method of treatment in 139 patients with mitral stenosis. *Ann Thorac Surg* 1981;31:300–4.

89. Spencer FC. Results in closed mitral valvotomy. *Ann Thorac Surg* 1988;45:355.

90. Stephens SJ. Changing patterns of mitral stenosis in childhood and pregnancy in Sri Lanka. *J Am Coll Cardiol* 1992;19:1276–84.

91. Subbarao KSVK, Nachiappan M, Irineu AP. Transventricular mitral commissurotomy in critical mitral stenosis during pregnancy. *Asian Cardiovasc Thorac Ann* 2004;12:233–5.

92. Mazur W, Parilak LD, Kaluza G, DeFelice C, Raizner A. Balloon valvuloplasty for mitral stenosis. *Curr Opin Cardiol* 1999;14:95.

93. Bonow RO, Carabello B, De Leon AC, Edmunds LH, Fedderly B, Freed MD, et al. ACC/AHA Guidelines for the management of patients with valvular heart disease. *J Am Coll Cardiol* 1998;32:1486–588.

94. Iung B, Nicoud-Houel A, Fondard O, Akoudad H, Haghighat T, Brochet E, et al. Temporal trends in percutaneous mitral commissurotomy over a 15-year period. *Eur Heart J* 2004;25:701–7.

95. Delabays A, Goy JJ. Percutaneous mitral valvuloplasty. *N Engl J Med* 2001;345:e4.

96. Shirodaria CC, Mitchell ARJ, Banning AP. Emergency balloon mitral valvotomy for severe mitral stenosis during pregnancy. *Heart* 2004;90:934.

97. Fawzy ME, Kinsara AJ, Stefadouros M, Hegazy H, Kattan H, Chaudhary A, et al. Long-term outcome of mitral balloon valvotomy in pregnant women. *J Heart Valve Dis* 2001;10:153–7.

98. Mangione JA, Lourenco RM, Souza dos Santos E, Shigueyuki A, Mauro MFZ, Cristovao SAB, et al. Long-term follow-up of pregnant women after percutaneous mitral valvuloplasty. *Catheter Cardiovasc Interv* 2000;50:413–17.

99. Gupta A, Lokhandwala YY, Satoskar PR, Salvi VS. Balloon mitral valvotomy in pregnancy: maternal and fetal outcomes. *J Am Coll Surg* 1998;187:409–15.

100. Ben Farhat M, Gamra H, Betbout F, Maatouk F, Jarrar M, Addad F, et al. Percutaneous balloon mitral commissurotomy during pregnancy. *Heart* 1997;77:564–7.

101. Esteves CA, Ramos AIO, Braga SLN, Harrison JK, Sousa JEMR. Effectiveness of percutaneous balloon mitral valvotomy during pregnancy. *Am J Cardiol* 1991;68:930–4.
102. Pershad A, Byrne TJ, Morgan JM, Desser KB. Precipitous labor in association with percutaneous mitral valvuloplasty: successful delivery in the catheterization laboratory. *Catheter Cardiovasc Interv* 2000;49:459–60.
103. Kinsara AJ, Ismail O, Fawzi ME. Effect of balloon mitral valvoplasty during pregnancy on childhood development. *Cardiology* 2002;97:155–8.
104. Cheng TO. Percutaneous mitral valvuloplasty by the Inoue balloon technique is the ideal procedure for treatment of significant mitral stenosis in pregnant women. *Catheter Cardiovasc Interv* 2000;57:323–4.
105. Connolly HM, Warnes CA. Pregnancy and contraception. In: Gatzoulis MA, Webb GD, Daubeney PEF, editors. *Diagnosis and Management of Adult Congenital Heart Disease.* Edinburgh: Churchill Livingstone; 2003. p. 135–44.
106. Hameed A, Akhter MW, Bitar F, Khan SA, Sarma R, Goodwin TM, et al. Left atrial thrombosis in pregnant women with mitral stenosis and sinus rhythm. *Am J Obstet Gynecol* 2005;193:501–4.
107. Siu SC, Colman JM. Heart disease and pregnancy. *Heart* 2001;85:710–15.
108. Horstkotte D, Fassbender D, Piper C. Balloon valvotomy during pregnancy. *J Heart Valve Dis* 2005;14:144–6.
109. Radford DJ, Walters DL. Balloon aortic valvotomy in pregnancy. *Aust N Z J Obstet Gynaecol* 2004;44:577–9.
110. Vahanian A, Acar C. Percutaneous valve procedures: what is the future? *Curr Opin Cardiol* 2005;20:100–6.
111. Waight DJ, Hijazi ZM. Balloon aortic valvuloplasty: triumphs again. *Catheter Cardiovasc Interv* 2000;51:173–4.
112. Tumelero RT, Duda NT, Tognon AP, Sartori I, Giongo S. Valvoplastia aortica percutanea em adolescente gestante. *Arq Bras Cardiol* 2003;82:94–7.
113. Campbell N, Rosaeg OP, Chan KL. Anaesthetic management of a parturient with pulmonary stenosis and aortic incompetence for caesarean section. *Br J Anaesth* 2003;90:241–3.
114. Hameed A, Yuodim K, Mahboob A, Goodwin TM, Wing D, Elkayam U. Effect of the severity of pulmonary stenosis on pregnancy outcome: a case control study (abstract). *Am J Obstet Gynecol* 2004;191:93.
115. Lavoie JP, Leduc L, Mercier LA. Embolic myocardial infarction in a pregnant woman with a mechanical heart valve on low molecular weight heparin. *Can J Cardiol* 2004;20:917–19.
116. Roth A, Elkayam U. Acute myocardial infarction associated with pregnancy. *Ann Intern Med* 1996;125:751–62.
117. Saw J, Thompson C, Macdonald I. Mechanical valve thrombosis during pregnancy. *Can J Cardiol* 2001;17:95–8.
118. Patel RK, Fasan O, Arya R. Thrombolysis in pregnancy. *Thromb Haemost* 2003;90:1216–17.
119. Alessandrini F, Lapenna E, Nasso G, De Bonis M, Possati GF. Successful thrombectomy for thrombosis of aortic composite valve graft in pregnancy. *Ann Thorac Surg* 2003;75:1317–18.
120. Kole SD, Jain SM, Walia A, Sharma M. Cardiopulmonary bypass in pregnancy. *Ann Thorac Surg* 1997;63:912–22.
121. Shemin RJ, Phillippe M, Dzau V. Acute thrombosis of a composite ascending aortic conduit containing a Bjork–Shiley valve during pregnancy: successful emergency cesarean section and operative repair. *Clin Cardiol* 1986;9:299–301.

122. Campuzano K, Roque H, Bolnick A, Leo MV, Campbell WA. Bacterial endocarditis complicating pregnancy: case report and systematic review of the literature. *Arch Gynecol Obstet* 2003;268:251–5.

123. Weissmann-Brenner A, Schoen R, Divon MY. Aortic dissection in pregnancy. *Obstet Gynecol* 2004;103:1110–13.

124. Ray P, Murphy GJ, Shutt LE. Recognition and management of maternal cardiac disease in pregnancy. *Br J Anaesth* 2004;93:428–39.

125. Niwa K, Siu SC, Webb GD, Gatzoulis MA. Progressive aortic root dilatation in adults late after repair of tetralogy of Fallot. *Circulation* 2002;106:1374–8.

126. Beauchesne LM, Connolly HM, Ammash NM, Warnes CA. Coarctation of the aorta: outcome of pregnancy. *J Am Coll Cardiol* 2001;38:1728–33.

127. Plunkett MD, Bond LM, Geiss DM. Staged repair of acute type 1 aortic dissection and coarctation in pregnancy. *Ann Thorac Surg* 2000;69:1945–7.

128. Siu S, Colman JM. Cardiovascular problems and pregnancy: an approach to management. *Cleveland Clin J Med* 2004;71:977–85.

129. Murphy BA, Zvara DA, Nelson LH, Kon ND, Shore-Lesserson L, Milas BL. Aprotinin use during deep hypothermic circulatory arrest for type A aortic dissection and cesarean section in a woman with preeclampsia. *J Cardiothorac Vasc Anesth* 2003;17:252–7.

130. Abbas AE, Lester SJ, Connolly H. Pregnancy and the cardiovascular system. *Int J Cardiol* 2005;98:179–89.

131. Ladner HE, Danielsen B, Gilbert WM. Acute myocardial infarction in pregnancy and the puerperium: a population-based study. *Obstet Gynecol* 2005;105:480–4.

132. Hameed AB, Tummala PP, Godwin TM, Nuno I, Wani OR, Karaalp IS, *et al.* Unstable angina during pregnancy in two patients with premature coronary atherosclerosis and aortic stenosis in association with familial hypercholesterolemia. *Am J Obstet Gynecol* 2000;182:1152–5.

133. Agostoni P, Gasparini G, Destro G. Acute myocardial infarction probably caused by paradoxical embolus in a pregnant woman. *Heart* 2004;90:1–2.

134. Etz C, Welp H, Scheld HH, Schmid C. Near fatal infection of a patient with a left ventricular assist device due to unrecognized fetal death. *Eur J Cardio-thorac Surg* 2005;27:722–3.

135. McKechnie RS, Patel D, Eitzman DT, Rajagopalan S, Murthy TH. Spontaneous coronary artery dissection in a pregnant woman. *Obstet Gynecol* 2001;98:899–902.

136. Shah P, Dzavik V, Cusimano RJ, Sermer M, Okun N, Ross J. Spontaneous dissection of the left main coronary artery. *Can J Cardiol* 2004;20:815–18.

137. Antman EM, Anbe DT, Armstrong PW, Bates ER, Green LA, Hand M, *et al.* ACC/AHA guidelines for the management of patients with ST-elevation myocardial infarction – executive summary. *J Am Coll Cardiol* 2004;44:671–719.

138. Kamran M, Suresh V, Ahluwalia A. Percutaneous transluminal coronary angioplasty (PTCA) combined with stenting for acute myocardial infarction in pregnancy. *J Obstet Gynaecol* 2004;24:701–2.

139. Majdan JF, Walinsky P, Cowchock SF, Wapner RJ, Plzak L. Coronary artery bypass surgery during pregnancy. *Am J Cardiol* 1983;52:1145–6.

140. Garry D, Leikin E, Fleisher AG, Tejani N. Acute myocardial infarction in pregnancy with subsequent medical and surgical management. *Obstet Gynecol* 1996;87:802–4.

141. Tang ATM, Cusimano RJ. Spontaneous coronary artery dissection complicating midterm pregnancy. *Ann Thorac Surg* 2004;78:e35.

142. Zuber M, Gautschi N, Oechslin E, Widmer V, Kiowski W, Jenni R. Outcome of pregnancy in women with congenital shunt lesions. *Heart* 1999;81:271–5.

143. Veldtman GR, Connolly HM, Grogan M, Ammash NM, Warnes CA. Outcomes of pregnancy in women with tetralogy of Fallot. *J Am Coll Cardiol* 2004;44:174–80.
144. Avanzas P, Garcia-Fernandez MA, Quiles J, Datino T, Moreno M. Pseudoaneurysm complicating aortic coarctation in a pregnant woman. *Int J Cardiol* 2004;97:157–8.
145. Natale A, Davidson T, Geiger MJ, Newby K. Implantable cardioverter-defibrillators and pregnancy. *Circulation* 1997;96:2808–12.
146. Olufolabi AJ, Charlton GA, Allen SA, Mettam IM, Roberts PR. Use of implantable cardioverter defibrillator and anti-arrhythmic agents in a parturient. *Br J Anaesth* 2002;89:652–5.
147. Owen RJT, Krarup KC. The successful use and removal of the Gunther tulip inferior vena caval filter in pregnancy. *Clin Radiol* 1997;52:241–3.
148. Cheung MC, Asch MR, Gandhi S, Kingdoms JCP. Temporary inferior vena caval filter use in pregnancy. *J Thromb Haemost* 2005;3:1096–7.
149. Simon MA, Kormos RL, Murali S, Nair P, Heffernan M, Gorcsan J, et al. Myocardial recovery using ventricular assist devices. Prevalence, clinical characteristics, and outcomes. *Circulation* 2005;112(9 Suppl):I32–36.
150. Colombo J, Lawal AH, Bhandari A, Hawkins JL, Atlee JL. A patient with severe peripartum cardiomyopathy and persistent ventricular fibrillation supported by a biventricular assist device. *J Cardiothorac Vasc Anaesth* 2002;16:107–13.
151. Ceresoli G, Passoni P, Benussi S, Alfieri O, Dell'antonio G, Bolognesi A. Primary cardiac sarcoma in pregnancy: a case report and review of the literature. *Am J Clin Oncol* 1999;22:460–5.

Section 3

Antenatal care fetal considerations

Chapter 9
Antenatal diagnosis of fetal cardiac defects

Helena Gardiner and Piers Daubeney

Introduction

The treatment and prognosis of congenital heart disease (CHD) has improved dramatic-ally over the last 30 years. This has resulted from better understanding of the morpho-logy of the congenitally abnormal heart, the advent of echocardiography, balloon atrial septostomy, use of prostaglandins, better intensive care and surgical techniques, and the development of cardiac catheterisation for diagnosis, intervention and electro-physiological assessment and treatment. Almost all types of CHD are now operable, many with low mortality and morbidity. The consequence is that many more children are surviving to adulthood and becoming mothers and fathers themselves. As survival has increased, it has become evident that surgical and interventional procedures are not curative but rather palliative, leading to particular long-term issues, one of which is the management of pregnancy. This chapter discusses the search for, and management of, the fetus with a structural heart malformation or with serious arrhythmia.

Fetal cardiology has reached its 25th birthday. M-mode and then real-time cross-sectional echocardiography were used to make the first prenatal diagnoses in the 1980s. Improvements in technology, including colour mapping and tissue Doppler, have further refined the ability to assess not only structural but also functional malformations and arrhythmias. However, screening for CHD remains a challenge and the constraints placed on the current system will be increased by the planned introduction of combined screening programmes that include nuchal translucency for all in 2007.

The fetal heart is fully formed from 6–8 weeks of gestation but, using current transabdominal ultrasound technology, the morphology is not easily imaged until 12–14 weeks. CHD is both important and common and still accounts for 10% of infant deaths and nearly half of all deaths from malformations.[1] Important CHD occurs in 3.5–4 per 1000 women screened in the second trimester and is identified more commonly in those with increased nuchal translucency who are screened in early pregnancy at 11–13 weeks.[2] The traditional referral criteria for detailed fetal echocardiography are shown in Table 9.1. For most women in the UK this detailed scan is performed at the same time as, or just after, the level two screening scan at 20 weeks of gestation. Low-risk groups have a risk of CHD of about 1% overall, with children of parents with CHD having a 3–5% risk, higher when the mother is affected.[3]

Table 9.1. Fetal, maternal and ultrasound findings that should prompt referral for a detailed cardiac scan

Fetal factors	Maternal factors	Ultrasound findings
■ Extracardiac anomalies ■ Aneuploidy ■ Monochorionic fetal pregnancy ■ Fetal cardiac arrhythmia	■ Family history/maternal CHD ■ Pre-existing type 1 or 2 diabetes mellitus ■ Autoimmune antibodies (connective tissue disease) ■ Teratogenic drugs (e.g. lithium)	■ Raised nuchal translucency (> 3.5 mm)[a] ■ Suspicious or 'non-diagnostic' cardiac scan ■ Two 'soft' diagnostic markers suspicious of aneuploidy[b]

[a] Fetuses with a raised nuchal translucency less than this may have a two-fold increased risk of CHD but in most centres there is insufficient capacity to offer these mothers a detailed cardiac scan
[b] Echogenic cardiac foci, short femurs, echogenic bowel, symmetrical growth restriction, choroid plexus cysts

The first comprehensive report on the efficiency of antenatal screening in the UK was produced on behalf of the British Paediatric Cardiac Association (now the British Congenital Cardiac Association) in 1999.[4] At that time, screening protocols recommended only the four-chamber view, with very few obstetric departments looking routinely at the outflow tracts. The BPCA report suggested that antenatal detection of major CHD ranged from as little as 0%, up to 71% in areas where there had been active teaching programmes. Although the average detection rate of 23.5% appears alarmingly low, the report confirmed that teaching programmes could produce a sustained improvement in the antenatal detection of CHD.

What is essential for effective screening?

Equipment

Many practical issues regarding equipment have been surmounted and most obstetric units have high-level ultrasound machines, including harmonic imaging and the appropriate range of probes essential for the cardiac examination. The heart lies horizontally in the fetal thorax and so five transverse planes through the fetal abdomen and thorax provide a series of views similar to those seen on magnetic resonance imaging (MRI), namely abdominal situs, the four-chamber view, the great arterial crossover and the three-vessel (transverse aortic and ductal arch and superior caval vein) and trachea view. At each level the cardiac structures are assessed for symmetry, the characteristic features of left- or right-sided morphology, the cardiac connections and the presence of septal defects.[5] (Figure 9.1)

Using a transabdominal approach at 18–20 weeks of gestation, these five transverse scanning planes are suitable for diagnosis and should be achievable in most pregnancies. There may be difficulties in multifetal pregnancies because of overcrowding, and the three-vessel view, which is obtained high in the fetal chest, may not always be achievable if the fetus is in a flexed position. Pulmonary veins can only be confidently examined by the concomitant use of colour flow and Doppler and are not usually included in screening. Transvaginal probes are not essential for the cardiologist, but may be a helpful adjunct for first-trimester scanning. Storage of appropriate images by video or digital techniques is helpful for training and is a medico-legal necessity for the cardiologist.

Training and audit

Progress has been made in improving the scanning skills of obstetric sonographers in the UK by using the simple 'five views' training protocol. This is also appropriate for 14 week scans and forms a practical basis for the examination. Hands-on courses are popular and helpful for sonographers and trainee obstetricians and cardiologists, and reinforce good practice.

Audit is essential to monitor the progress of a department. Knowing what has been missed is an important part of the training process. This may be difficult to achieve without additional resources to link the newborn babies with heart defects seen in the cardiac units to the findings at the anomaly scan, which is often performed in a hospital remote to this centre. Another complication is the change of surnames after delivery, but tracking through an infant's NHS number may make this easier in future.

Following a cardiac diagnosis

The causes of CHD remain an important topic for research and mouse models are providing some interesting insights. There is a significantly higher incidence of chromosomal anomalies among fetuses with prenatally diagnosed CHD (33–42%), compared with the 5% incidence of aneuploidy reported in neonatal cardiac series.[6] Therefore, if a cardiac diagnosis has been made it is good practice to repeat the anomaly scan as cardiac lesions are often associated with extracardiac malformations, and associated chromosomal lesions should also be considered. For example, an atrioventricular septal defect is commonly associated with Down syndrome, and interrupted aortic arch with 22q11 deletion.

Multidisciplinary counselling

It is best practice, but unfortunately still rather uncommon, for the cardiologist to work within the fetal medicine unit. This would provide the patient with a 'one-stop shop' approach and the opportunity for joint counselling. This is important even if an isolated cardiac defect has been identified as there are many pregnancy-related issues to discuss and both the obstetrician and cardiologist can benefit from this team approach. Where the woman herself has significant heart disease the management plan will need to be tailored to her individual health needs.

It is preferable to counsel the mother and partner or friend in a designated counselling room rather than the scanning room. The presence of a fetal cardiac liaison nurse and midwife is helpful for at least part of the session, particularly if an invasive test is offered. Before launching into a discussion about the diagnosis it is good practice to ascertain what the woman understands about potential heart abnormalities. This assesses her understanding of any information she may have received beforehand and also her background knowledge. Counselling should then proceed in a non-directive manner without letting the clinician's private beliefs interfere (even if this is difficult to achieve).[7] The normal heart should first be discussed and preferably drawn, or a printed diagram given. The abnormality should then be drawn as a comparison, or a printed diagram of the lesion given.

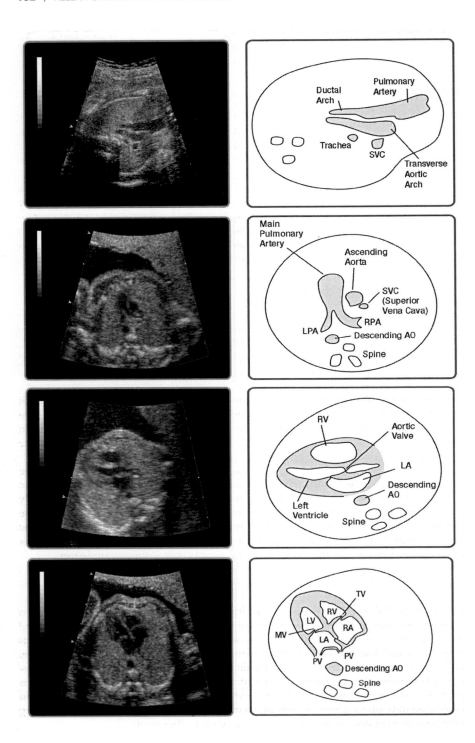

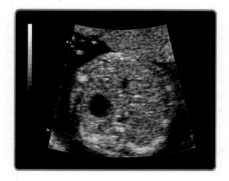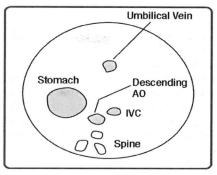

Figure 9.1. The five scanning planes taken in transverse sections through the fetal abdomen and chest that are required to examine the fetal heart; AO = aorta, IVC = inferior vena cava, LA = left atrium, LPA = left pulmonary artery, LV = left ventricle, MV = mitral valve, PV = pulmonary vein, RA = right atrium, RPA = right pulmonary artery, RV = right ventricle, SVC = superior vena cava, TV = tricuspid valve; line drawings reproduced with permission from Siemens

Parents are given a great deal of information at their first visit, much of which is entirely new to them, and it is important to guide them through the process. There is usually no time pressure for them to come to any decision, provided they are within the legal time limits for termination of pregnancy as specified by the law of the country.

Decision making may be helped by visiting the cardiac unit where surgery will be performed and by meeting various health professionals, for example a cardiac surgeon, adult congenital cardiologist and cardiac psychologist. The parents are usually guided throughout the pregnancy by the fetal cardiac liaison nurse who may be able to arrange for parents to meet other families who have had a child with similar cardiac lesion if they feel it would be helpful. Recurrence risks should be mentioned for future pregnancies, particularly where the mother herself has a cardiac lesion.

Progression of disease

Many cardiac lesions progress in severity throughout pregnancy: tetralogy of Fallot to pulmonary atresia with ventricular septal defect,[8] and pulmonary stenosis to atresia.[9] These potential changes and their likelihood should be discussed with the mother as they may entail more difficult surgical management and result in a worse outcome. Awareness of this possibility may alter a family's decision to proceed with the pregnancy. It is essential to arrange serial monitoring, particularly if the initial diagnosis is made in the early second trimester. Parents should also be made aware that certain lesions are difficult to detect in early pregnancy and that the diagnosis and counselling may be modified during the pregnancy following further scans.

Invasive testing

Counselling will usually involve the offer of an invasive test to determine karyotype and relevant specific deletions such as 22q11 deletion.[10] Most often this is an amniocentesis with a risk of miscarriage of about 1%. The timing of this procedure depends on gestational age at diagnosis and is best performed before 24 weeks to reduce the risk of preterm delivery, or it may be offered at 32 weeks if the pregnancy has reached 24 weeks by the time of diagnosis and counselling or if the parents are undecided. Some women will have had a chorionic villus sampling test in the first trimester, either because of advanced maternal age or because of an increased nuchal translucency, and in such cases the fetal karyotype is already known. A late karyotype still allows the parents to choose the outcome of the pregnancy (in the UK) if the cardiac or extracardiac condition satisfies clause E of the Termination of Pregnancy Act[11] (when the condition is sufficiently severe to result in substantial handicap (not death) to the individual). It also aids the obstetricians and neonatologists to plan the delivery and immediate perinatal care, for example to avoid caesarean section or active resuscitation in cases of trisomy 13 and 18.

In utero death

The incidence of CHD in stillbirths is ten times greater than the reported prevalence in the liveborn population, with aneuploidy accounting for this difference in most cases.[12] *In utero* death may occur secondary to fetal hydrops.[13] There are several morphological and physiological predictors, for example severe tricuspid regurgitation in Ebstein anomaly, pulmonary atresia with an intact ventricular septum[9] or an intact inter-atrial septum in transposition of the great arteries or hypoplastic left heart syndrome. It may also occur where there is a fetal arrhythmia in association with hydrops.[14] Where the mother has CHD associated with significant cyanosis or pulmonary hypertension, the fetus has a higher risk of *in utero* death, often due to placental dysfunction and growth restriction even where the fetus has a normal heart.

Management options and outcomes

Management options comprise termination of pregnancy, monitoring throughout pregnancy with an interventional approach after birth (surgical and/or catheter), monitoring with withdrawal of care after birth, and *in utero* treatment. A second opinion from another fetal cardiologist may also be of assistance, especially when the lesion is particularly unusual.

Termination of pregnancy

The logistics of a termination of pregnancy should be discussed with the family by the obstetrician involved and a midwife experienced in managing late terminations of pregnancy. For women diagnosed early (12–14 weeks of gestation) following nuchal translucency screening, surgical termination is possible, depending on local obstetric expertise.

Where the diagnosis is made later, delivery is vaginal and requires induction of labour. Guidelines exist for when feticide (usually achieved by intracardiac potassium injection after 21 weeks) is indicated and the legality of these procedures varies from country to country. A medical termination of pregnancy and a good postmortem examination assists the physicians and families in the long term, as a full diagnosis is more likely and therefore the risks of recurrence can be more confidently relayed to the family.

Serial assessment

Pulsed wave Doppler has been used since the 1970s to assess fetal wellbeing, and the introduction of the umbilical artery pulsatility index enabled protocol-driven evaluation and monitoring of fetuses with suspected growth restriction due to placental pathology. Doppler examination of ever-smaller vessels is now feasible because of improved technology and a wide variety of arteries and veins are examined routinely in the fetal medicine unit.[15] An assessment of fetal wellbeing refines fetal management and the fetal cardiologist may find serial examination of the pulmonary veins and middle cerebral artery of value in aiding patient management. This is particularly true for fetuses with simple transposition of the great arteries and hypoplastic left heart syndrome or critical aortic stenosis where restriction of the inter-atrial foramen may lead to fetal hydrops and death.

Restrictive or closed inter-atrial septum

A thickened inter-atrial septum and closure of the foramen can be detected visually and by alterations in pulse waveform of the pulmonary veins,[16] and therapeutic interventions have been performed to recreate a communication between the atria.[17] This is not only important to offload the increased systemic venous pressures of the right side, but also to optimise the pulmonary bed and reduce damage to the pulmonary veins resulting from sustained high left atrial pressures.

This should result in a change in management and, if fetal intervention is not considered appropriate, the fetus should be monitored carefully. Early delivery may be required and certainly delivery with the cardiologist available to perform an early balloon atrial septostomy or early cardiac surgery would be the most appropriate line of management.[18]

Cerebral redistribution

It has been recognised that fetuses with left heart obstruction show redistribution in the middle cerebral artery akin to that seen in growth restriction. Magnetic resonance imaging (MRI) and magnetic resonance spectroscopy have identified preoperative brain injury in newborns with simple transposition of the great arteries.[19] Protocols should ideally include serial evaluation of the fetal circulation for signs of redistribution by both the fetal medicine team and the cardiologist. Fetal MRI is helpful to detect structural brain lesions and estimate their timing, and neurologists should form part of the team to help decide on appropriate antenatal and postnatal management and investigations.[20]

Planning for delivery

Birth planning requires the input of the multidisciplinary team. The choice of where to deliver (whether in a maternity unit local to the mother's home or at the tertiary centre) depends on the maternal and fetal issues. Mothers with fetuses with duct-dependent lesions should be delivered as close to the cardiac centre as possible and obstetric care is usually transferred at 34 weeks of gestation to the tertiary centre, with a plan for induction of labour at 38–39 weeks. It is important to warn the mother that failure of induction may occur in up to one-third of nulliparous women, and caesarean section may be required. If the mother lives locally she can come to the hospital in early labour. If the mother has cardiac disease she should be managed by a team specialised in adult CHD, whether the fetus has heart disease or not.

The method of delivery is dependent on maternal factors and the presence of fetal cardiac disease does not usually affect this. Babies with CHD usually tolerate delivery well whatever route is chosen. The exception to this is where there is poor ventricular function or fetal hydrops, or when the fetal heart-rate pattern used for monitoring wellbeing may be difficult to interpret, as in cases of heart block, when elective caesarean section is preferable.

Postnatal assessment

One advantage of a fetal diagnosis is that the parents and staff have a clear idea of the management plan for an individual baby. If there is a duct-dependent lesion then admission to the neonatal unit for a period of stabilisation is indicated. A prosta-glandin infusion is commenced before transfer, which can either be to the tertiary cardiac hospital or to a paediatric ward in the hospital of delivery, depending on local facilities and preferences. The paediatric cardiac team will assess the infant and plan for surgical or catheter interventional management. Consent is required from the mother (and father if married). This may be difficult to obtain if the mother has had a caesarean section and is in a different hospital, and arrangements to deal with this problem should be discussed during the pregnancy.

If the lesion is minor then the baby can remain with its mother on the postnatal wards provided there are no immediate concerns, with routine referral to the paediatric cardiac service in due course. Common neonatal interventions and their outcomes are given in Table 9.2.

Modern surgical outcomes

Paediatric cardiac surgeons in the UK are required to report their outcomes to the Central Cardiac Audit Database (www.icservices.nhs.uk/ncasp/pages/audit_topics/chd/pcschds-old.asp). The UK surgical data thus collected report a mortality of less than 5% for the five benchmark lesions used to monitor early cardiac mortality in the UK. The medium-term outlook for most babies who have isolated CHD operated upon is good. However, where there are associated extracardiac malformations or more complex malformations (for example where a valve, chamber or great artery is hypo-plastic or missing), the outlook is more guarded. An assessment is made postnatally as to whether the child may ultimately achieve a biventricular (i.e. normal) circulation or whether they will have a functionally univentricular circulation. Once this decision is made, a surgical strategy is set to achieve that goal. The timing of procedures and their outcome for some of the more common lesions is set out in Table 9.2. Children with 'single ventricle' physiology will undergo an initial procedure to control pulmonary blood flow: too little requires a systemic to pulmonary artery (Blalock–Taussig) shunt and too much requires a pulmonary artery band. The subsequent strategy is to divert the vena cavae directly into the lungs so that blood flows passively into the pulmonary arteries. This is usually performed sequentially with a superior cavo-pulmonary anastomosis (Glenn) at about 3–12 months, followed a year or so later with a total cavo-pulmonary anastomosis (TCPC or Fontan) (see Chapter 13).

Table 9.2. Management and outcome from some of the more common types of congenital heart disease in infancy

Lesion	Age at procedure(s)	Procedure(s)	Risk
ASD	4 years	Trans-catheter device closure	Nearly zero
		Surgical repair	Nearly zero
Small VSD	–	Observation only	Zero
Large VSD	< 6 months	Surgical repair	Low
AVSD	< 4 months	Surgical repair	Low
Patent arterial duct	1 week to	Surgical in neonatal period	Low/moderate
	12 months	Trans-catheter device closure	Nearly zero
Pulmonary stenosis	any	Balloon valvuloplasty	Low
		Surgical valvotomy (more severe anatomy)	Low
Aortic stenosis	any	Balloon valvuloplasty	Low/moderate
		Surgical valvotomy/replacement	Low/moderate
Tetralogy of Fallot	< 12 months	Complete repair, may be preceded by Blalock–Taussig shunt	Low
Transposition	< 1 month	Balloon atrial septostomy	Low
		Surgical switch repair (previously Mustard/Senning	Low
Coarctation	any	Surgical repair neonatally	Low
		Balloon dilatation and stenting older children and adults	
Pulmonary atresia with intact septum	< 1 week	Trans-catheter radiofrequency perforation for good anatomy	Low to high (depending on anatomy)
		Surgical outflow reconstruction	
		Blalock–Taussig shunt for poor anatomy then as for 'single ventricle'	
Pulmonary atresia with VSD	< 1 week	Blalock–Taussig shunt	Low/moderate
		Surgical repair with homograft if good anatomy	
Common arterial trunk	< 3 months	Surgical repair with homograft	Low/moderate
DORV	variable	Too much pulmonary flow: pulmonary artery band; too little: Blalock–Taussig shunt	Low/moderate
		Surgical repair or, if more complicated anatomy, as for 'single ventricle'	
HLHS	< 3 weeks	Norwood procedure	High
		Superior cavo-pulmonary anastomosis	
		Total cavo-pulmonary anastomosis	
'Single ventricle' physiology	< 2 months	Too much pulmonary flow: pulmonary artery band; too little: Blalock–Taussig shunt	Moderate
		Superior cavo-pulmonary anastomosis	
		Total cavo-pulmonary anastomosis	
Ebstein anomaly	variable	Observation	Low to high (depending on severity)
		If severe anatomy Starnes procedure or valve repair	
Congenitally corrected transposition	variable	Repair of individual lesions (VSD, PS) or double switch procedure if warranted	Low/moderate
Isomerism	variable	Dependent on individual lesions	Moderate

Patent arterial duct included although it cannot be predicted from prenatal scanning; ages at procedure are approximate and relate to when the procedure is commonly rather than always performed; these are contemporary postnatal outcomes and encompass a wide range of individual morphologies that may worsen/improve outcomes; low risk is defined as less than 10%, moderate 10–20% and high risk as greater than 20% mortality; the outcome for fetuses at diagnosis is generally lower as it can represent a worse end of the spectrum

ASD = atrial septal defect; AVSD = atrioventricular septal defect; DORV = double outlet right ventricle; HLHS = hypoplastic left heart syndrome; PS = pulmonary stenosis; VSD = ventricular septal defect

Fetal therapy

Fetal arrhythmias

Transplacental treatment of fetal tachycardia is a well-established intervention and can be life-saving. Although there are many different drug regimens, most fetuses without hydrops do well and may be delivered at or near term with minimal morbidity.[14] Treatment strategies for heart block (due to anti-Ro or anti-La antibodies or in association with structural heart disease) have been less effective, although there have been some reports of success with systemic steroid therapy to the mother.[21,22] This is not without significant maternal morbidity, including maternal diabetes and psychosis, and fetal growth restriction, and this method of treatment is currently not widely supported.[23] New technologies such as non-invasive fetal electrocardiography (ECG) detection and magnetocardiography are becoming available to refine the diagnosis of tachyarrhythmia and heart block. These technologies may improve the monitoring of fetuses at risk, and help to determine the optimal course of treatment. It may be that screening for familial problems such as long QT syndrome proves possible in the mid-trimester fetus, but much work is required to make this a practical reality. Fetal pacing has been introduced without great success in the past decade, although more recent reports are encouraging.[24] More research is required to determine its efficacy and safety in the human fetus.

Fetal surgery and interventional catheter approaches

The rationale underlying fetal surgical and catheter procedures is to prevent extra-cardiac and secondary cardiac damage resulting from the malformation. Open fetal cardiac surgery on cardiopulmonary bypass represents a considerable challenge in fetal therapy. It is likely to be introduced for those fetuses where there is significant com-promise to normal pulmonary development, as in absent pulmonary valve syndrome (often associated with tracheobronchial compression) or Ebstein anomaly with lung hypoplasia, and to promote pulmonary artery arborisation and growth in fetuses with small central pulmonary arteries and major collateral vessels. Technical solutions to reduce the deleterious effects of the reactive placental vasculature have been found, at least in animal models, and investigators have reported a 90% survival in such models.[25]

Catheter interventions have been used to treat severe aortic and pulmonary stenosis or atresia and to open a closed or restrictive inter-atrial communication.[26,27] The underlying rationale is to promote growth of the supporting ventricle in order to achieve a two-ventricle circulation, prevent secondary damage to the myocardium and lungs, and improve the fetal circulation in cases of hydrops. There has been some initial success but larger numbers are required to assess outcome compared with natural history. However, to attempt a two-ventricle circulation repair in cases with borderline ventricular size may lead to demise, whereas a one-ventricle circulation may provide a satisfactory quality of life.

Paradoxically, antenatal surgery may be cost effective for although it certainly will use more resources initially, if it is successful and improves the pulmonary circulation and ventricular function in this group of fetuses, postoperative care is provided by and within the mother herself. This may reduce mortality and morbidity for babies who would otherwise have had long postoperative intensive care stays.

New challenges in fetal cardiology

A combined early screening with first-trimester biochemistry and a nuchal translucency measurement at 11 to 14 weeks (proposed by the UK National Screening Committee in 2004) will be widely available in 2007. Recent studies suggest that about two-thirds of cases with both CHD and an increased nuchal translucency have abnormal chromosomes.[28] Many women will choose termination of pregnancy in these circumstances. However, there is a high natural rate of demise in these fetuses anyway. Such fetuses thus do not figure in the liveborn cardiac data, and terminating pregnancies that would have been lost naturally will require considerable additional staffing resources.

Cardiac training programmes for those performing level two screening have increased the overall detection rate to 70% and more[29,30] and, when fully implemented, should remove 'postcode inequality'. To produce similar results in early pregnancy is challenging and will require further comprehensive support. Specifically, maternity units will require increased staffing and state-of-the-art equipment to provide nuchal translucency scans for all pregnancies, and cardiac scans for those with abnormal test results. Although a cardiac examination will not commonly be performed at the time of nuchal translucency measurement, as is done in some specialised centres, once an increased nuchal fold is detected the women will require diagnostic services to assess fetal chromosomes and a timely cardiac scan. Best practice indicates this should be performed at about 14 weeks of gestation to minimise wait and enable a mother to make earlier choices about the pregnancy rather than waiting for a 20 week cardiac scan. The number of pregnant women likely to require early fetal echocardiography has been calculated from existing screening programmes in the UK to be about 2%. Based on existing delivery figures, about 14 000 women would have an increased nuchal and at least those with normal karyotype (perhaps one-third) will require a 14 week scan. Support for such a service would require about six additional dedicated fetal cardiologists scanning for 20 hours a week (taking into account the repetition of cardiac scans at 20 weeks). There are about 70 paediatric cardiology consultants in the UK, fewer than half of whom perform fetal cardiac scans, and so this represents a significant expansion of the service, which is currently unrealistic in terms of available expertise and finance. Alternative strategies will thus have to be considered in order to cope with this increased demand. The most obvious solution is to improve the skills of the more senior screening sonographers and obstetricians working in fetal medicine units. It will be expensive to roll out a programme of training for these groups, but this will be necessary if appropriate support for the new screening programme is to be provided.

Fetal cardiac scanning at 14 weeks of gestation is more difficult but with practice diagnostic scans are possible in more than 85%.[31] However, effective scanning at this gestation is not possible without good-quality echocardiography equipment and hospital trusts will be required to ensure that the standard of their equipment is sufficient to cope with the demands placed on it by nuchal translucency screening, in terms of the number of extra machines required, additional sonographers employed and maintenance of quality.

Currently, fetal cardiologists perform a detailed scan on women whose fetus has a nuchal translucency equal to or above 3.5 mm. In such cases the fetus has a four-fold increased risk for CHD and this relative risk rises with increasing nuchal translucency measurements. Although it is recognised that measurements above average but below 3.5 mm are associated with some increased risk both of aneuploidy and CHD,[32,33] there are currently insufficient resources to incorporate these women into the existing system. If the skill base increases to encourage senior sonographers and obstetricians to perform early scans, all women who have had an abnormal screening scan and have normal chromosomes should ideally receive a cardiac examination at 14 weeks of gestation. Storage of appropriate images by video or digital techniques may be helpful for remote diagnosis, for example by a telelink to a local cardiac centre, if this is considered the most cost effective way of managing the increased caseload, and good precedents have been set for this both in the UK and abroad.[34,35]

Conclusions

There are many positive consequences of a screening programme. Training programmes have led to increased referrals for echocardiography because of identified ultrasound abnormality. It is likely that this will continue, resulting in increased demand for specialised fetal echocardiography. To manage this in a practical way, the traditional 'high-risk' women may be better screened in their local obstetric units and only referred if an abnormality is detected. Cardiologists will be asked to provide early 14 week cardiac scans and strategies must be set in place to cope with this before nuchal translucency screening is introduced across the UK in 2007. Although it is difficult to prove there is benefit to the fetus from an early cardiac diagnosis, and paradoxically many series report worse outcomes, fetuses with isolated CHD have survival rates similar to those reported in individuals diagnosed with CHD in postnatal life,[36] and those with duct-dependent lesions have reduced morbidity.[9,18,37]

We can use all non-invasive technologies to learn more about the fetal cardiovascular system and hopefully establish benefit. There is the potential to give babies with heart defects a better start in life and a better future, but this will require considerable cross-specialty collaboration and a team approach that is appropriately funded to meet these new challenges.

References

1.   Wren C, Richmond S, Donaldson L. Presentation of congenital heart disease in infancy: implications for routine examination. *Arch Dis Child Fetal Neonatal Ed* 1999;80:F49–53.

2.   Ghi T, Huggon IC, Zosmer N, Nicolaides KH. Incidence of major structural cardiac defects associated with increased nuchal translucency but normal karyotype. *Ultrasound Obstet Gynecol* 2001;18:610–14.

3.   Burn J, Brennan P, Little J, Holloway S, Coffey R, Somerville J, et al. Recurrence risks in offspring of adults with major heart defects: results from first cohort of British collaborative study. *Lancet* 1998;351:311–16.

4.   Bull C. Current and potential impact of fetal diagnosis on prevalence and spectrum of serious congenital heart disease at term in the UK. British Paediatric Cardiac Association. *Lancet* 1999;354:1242–7.

5.   Gardiner HM. Antenatal detection of heart defects is important and achievable. *Ultrasound* 2005;13:164–9.

6.   Wimalasundera RC, Gardiner HM. Congenital heart disease and aneuploidy. *Prenat Diagn* 2004;24:1116–22.

7.   Shinebourne EA, Carvalho JC. Ethics of fetal echocardiography. *Cardiol Young* 1996;6:261–3.

8.   Hornberger LK, Sanders SP, Sahn DJ, Rice MJ, Spevak PJ, Benacerraf BR, et al. *In utero* pulmonary artery and aortic growth and potential for progression of pulmonary

outflow tract obstruction in tetralogy of Fallot. *J Am Coll Cardiol* 1995;25:739–45.

9. Daubeney PEF, Sharland GK, Cook AC, Keeton BR, Anderson RH, Webber SA. Pulmonary atresia with intact ventricular septum: Impact of fetal echocardiography on incidence at birth and postnatal outcome. *Circulation* 1998;98:562–6.

10. Ryan AK, Goodship JA, Wilson DI, Philip N, Levy A, Seidel H, *et al.* Spectrum of clinical features associated with interstitial chromosome 22q11 deletions: a European collaborative study *J Med Genet*;34:798–804.

11. Addison PH. Abortion Act 1967. *Lancet* 1968;2:503–7.

12. Hook EB. Chromosome abnormalities and spontaneous fetal death following amniocentesis: further data and associations with maternal age. *Am J Hum Genet* 1983;35:110–16.

13. Allan L, Sharland G. Outcome of fetal congenital heart disease. In: Allan L, Hornberger LK, Sharland G, editors. *Textbook of Fetal Cardiology*. London: Greenwich Medical Media Limited; 2000. p. 417.

14. Simpson JM, Sharland GK. Fetal tachycardias: management and outcome of 127 consecutive cases. *Heart* 1998;79:576–81.

15. Harman CR, Baschat AA. Comprehensive assessment of fetal wellbeing: which Doppler tests should be performed? *Curr Opin Obstet Gynecol* 2003;15:147–57.

16. Michelfelder E, Gomez C, Border W, Gottliebson W. Franklin C. Predictive value of fetal pulmonary venous flow patterns in identifying the need for atrial septoplasty in the newborn with hypoplastic left ventricle. *Circulation* 2005;112:2974–9.

17. Marshall AC, van der Velde ME, Tworetzky W, Gomez CA, Wilkins-Haug L, Benson CB, *et al.* Creation of an atrial septal defect *in utero* for fetuses with hypoplastic left heart syndrome and intact or highly restrictive atrial septum. *Circulation* 2004;110:253–8.

18. Bonnet D, Coltri A, Butera G, Fermont L, Le Bidois J, Kachaner J, *et al.* Detection of transposition of the great arteries in fetuses reduces neonatal morbidity and mortality. *Circulation* 1999;23:99:916–18.

19. Miller SP, McQuillen PS, Vigneron DB, Glidden DV, Barkovich AJ, Ferriero DM, *et al.* Preoperative brain injury in newborns with transposition of the great arteries. *Ann Thorac Surg* 2004;77:1698–706.

20. Cowan F, Rutherford M, Groenendaal F, Eken P, Mercuri E, Bydder GM, *et al.* Origin and timing of brain lesions in term infants with neonatal encephalopathy. *Lancet* 2003;1:736–42.

21. Jaeggi ET, Fouron JC, Silverman ED, Ryan G, Smallhorn J, Hornberger LK. Transplacental fetal treatment improves the outcome of prenatally diagnosed complete atrioventricular heart block. *Circulation* 2004;110:1542–8.

22. Copel JA, Buyon JP, Kleinman CS. Successful *in utero* therapy of fetal heart block. *Am J Obstet Gynecol* 1995;173:1384–90.

23. Stanbury RM, Graham EM. Systemic corticosteroid therapy – side effects and their management. *Br J Ophthalmol* 1998;82:704–8.

24. Assad RS, Zielinsky P, Kalil R, Lima G, Aramayo A, Santos A, *et al.* New lead for *in utero* pacing for fetal congenital heart block. *J Thorac Cardiovasc Surg* 2003;126:300–2.

25. Ikai A, Riemer RK, Ramamoorthy C, Malhotra S, Cassorla L, Amir G, *et al.* Preliminary results of fetal cardiac bypass in nonhuman primates. *J Thorac Cardiovasc Surg* 2005;129:175–81.

26. Tworetzky W, Wilkins-Haug L, Jennings RW, van der Velde ME, Marshall AC, Marx GR, *et al.* Balloon dilation of severe aortic stenosis in the fetus: potential for prevention of hypoplastic left heart syndrome: candidate selection, technique, and results of successful intervention. *Circulation* 2004;110:2125–31.

27. Tulzer G, Arzt W, Franklin RC, Loughna PV, Mair R, Gardiner HM. Fetal pulmonary valvuloplasty for critical pulmonary stenosis or atresia with intact septum. *Lancet* 2002;360:1567–8.

28. Chitty LS, Kagan KO, Molina FS, Waters JJ, Nicolaides KH. Fetal nuchal translucency scan and early prenatal diagnosis of chromosomal abnormalities by rapid aneuploidy screening: observational study. *BMJ* 2006;332:452–5.

27. Carvalho JS, Mavrides E, Shinebourne EA, Campbell S, Thilaganathan B. Improving the effectiveness of routine prenatal screening for major congenital heart defects. *Heart* 2002;88:387–91.

28. McKenna C, Pasquini L, Pather J, Weston W, Wimalasundera R, Gardiner HM. Perfect prenatal detection of congenital heart disease – is it a practical possibility? *Ultrasound Obstet Gynecol* 2005;26:P03.16.

29. Simpson JM, Jones A. Accuracy and limitations of transabdominal fetal echocardiography at 12–15 weeks of gestation in a population at high risk for congenital heart disease. *BJOG* 2000;107:1492–7.

30. Makrydimas G, Sotiriadis A, Huggon IC, Simpson J, Sharland G, Carvalho JS, *et al.* Nuchal translucency and fetal cardiac effects: a pooled analysis of major fetal echocardiography centres. *Am J Obstet Gynecol* 2005;192:89–95.

31. Hyett JA, Perdu M, Sharland GK, Snijders RJM, Nicolaides KH. Using fetal nuchal translucency to screen for major congenital cardiac defects at 10–14 weeks of gestation: population based cohort study. *BMJ* 1999;318:81–5.

32. Casey F, Brown D, Craig BG, Rogers J, Mulholland HC. Diagnosis of neonatal congenital heart defects by remote consultation using a low-cost telemedicine link. *J Telemed Telecare* 1996;2:165–9.

33. Bonacina S, Draghi L, Masseroli M, Pinciroli F. Understanding telecardiology success and pitfalls by a systematic review. *Stud Health Technol Inform* 2005;116:373–8.

34. Paladini D, Russo M, Teodoro A, Pacileo G, Capozzi G, Martinelli P, *et al.* Prenatal diagnosis of congenital heart disease in the Naples area during the years 1994–1999 – the experience of a joint fetal–pediatric cardiology unit. *Prenat Diagn* 2002;22:545–52.

35. Franklin O, Burch M, Manning N, Sleeman K, Gould S, Archer N. Prenatal diagnosis of coarctation of the aorta improves survival and reduces morbidity. *Heart* 2002;87:67–9.

Chapter 10
Fetal care and surveillance in women with congenital heart disease

Christine KH Yu and TG Teoh

In the most recent Confidential Enquiry into Maternal and Child Health report (2000–02),[1] cardiac disease was identified as the second most common cause of indirect maternal death and the mortality rate from congenital heart disease (CHD) is almost the same today as it was 40 years ago. CHD is also associated with increased fetal complications such as fetal loss, intrauterine growth restriction (IUGR), premature delivery and an increased risk of fetal CHD. The two main determinants of fetal prognosis are maternal functional class and the degree of cyanosis. When the mother is in New York Heart Association (NYHA) functional class III or IV (see Appendix A), or has high-risk diseases such as severe aortic stenosis and Eisenmenger syndrome, this is associated with high maternal and fetal mortality and morbidity. Fetal monitoring should be optimised in these women. In women with cyanotic heart disease, regular assessment of fetal growth is mandatory as it often slows down and ceases before term. The use of mid-trimester uterine artery Doppler as a screening test for the prediction of uteroplacental insufficiency may be valuable in identifying fetuses at risk of IUGR and perinatal death.[2] The controversial issue of fetal monitoring during cardiac surgery in pregnancy will also be discussed below.

Maternal risk factors

Haemodynamic changes during pregnancy can exacerbate the problems associated with CHD, resulting in cardiovascular complications in the mother, which in turn may have fetal implications.[3] The outcome is influenced by functional class (NYHA classification),[4] the nature of the disease and previous cardiac surgery.

Congenital heart defects that are likely to give rise to problems include those that are complicated by pulmonary hypertension, cyanosis and severe left ventricular outflow tract obstruction. Siu et al.[5] examined the outcomes of 221 women with heart disease. Poor maternal exercise tolerance (functional class) or cyanosis, myocardial dysfunction, left heart obstruction, prior arrhythmia and prior cardiac events were predictive of maternal cardiac complications and these predictors were incorporated into a point score to estimate the probability of a cardiac complication in the mother. The rate of cardiac complications for a woman with 0, 1 and more than 1 of the above factors was 3%, 30% and 66%, respectively. Neonatal complications occurred in 17% ($n = 42$) of completed pregnancies. Neonatal events included death ($n = 2$), respiratory distress syndrome ($n = 16$), intraventricular haemorrhage ($n = 2$), premature birth ($n = 35$) and small-for-gestational-age (SGA) birthweight ($n = 14$). Poor maternal functional class or cyanosis was predictive of neonatal events.[5]

Pulmonary hypertension

Pulmonary hypertension is the most hazardous cardiac condition for a pregnant woman and can be an indication for termination of pregnancy in order to avoid maternal mortality. Severe pulmonary vascular disease, whether with (in the Eisenmenger syndrome) or without septal defects, carries a high risk, with a maternal mortality rate of 30–50%. Pulmonary hypertension is poorly tolerated in pregnancy because of the insufficient ability of the right heart to adapt to increases in cardiac output, in association with a poorly compliant pulmonary vasculature. If chronic maternal hypoxia results, this can lead to IUGR.

Severe left ventricular outflow tract obstruction

A fixed outflow tract resistance, such as aortic valvular or sub-aortic stenosis or coarctation of the aorta, may not accommodate the increased cardiac output caused by increased plasma volume. This can lead to heart failure with a rise in left ventricular and pulmonary capillary pressures, low cardiac output and pulmonary congestion.

Maternal indices

Whittemore et al.[6] showed that if the maternal haematocrit is more than 44% it is associated with birthweights below the 50th centile, and if the maternal haemoglobin is greater than 20 g/dl the live birth rate falls to 8%. If the maternal oxygen saturation falls below 85% it is predictive of poor pregnancy outcome, with a 12% live birth rate (Table 10.1).

Another series reported by Presbitero et al.[7] examined 1238 women with CHD in London and Italy. The incidence of maternal cardiovascular complications was high (32%) and included one death from endocarditis 2 months after delivery. Of 96 pregnancies, 43% resulted in a live birth, 37% ($n = 15$) of which were premature. There were 49 spontaneous miscarriages at between 6 weeks and 5 months of gestation and six stillbirths at 26–38 weeks. Mean birthweight at term was 2575 g (range 2100–3600 g). The basic maternal cardiac abnormality also influences fetal outcome. Women with single ventricles, tricuspid atresia, tetralogy of Fallot or pulmonary atresia were found to have a worse pregnancy prognosis than those with, for example, Ebstein anomaly with an atrial septal defect (ASD), corrected transposition of the great arteries, a ventricular septal defect (VSD) or pulmonary stenosis.

Cyanotic versus acyanotic heart disease

The fetal and maternal outcome in women with acyanotic heart disease is much more favourable. Chia et al.[8] examined 19 151 deliveries retrospectively with 143 cases of acyanotic heart disease. There was no significant difference in the rate of induction, use of epidurals or operative deliveries between the acyanotic heart disease group and those women without heart disease. Perinatal mortality rates were not significantly different in the two groups (15.3 per 1000 versus 14 per 1000).

Table 10.1. Live birth rates associated with various maternal oxygen saturation and haemoglobin levels; data from Whittemore *et al.*[6]

SaO$_2$ (%)	Live birth rate (%)	Hb (g/dl)	Live birth rate (%)
>90	92	<16	71
85–90	45	17–19	45
<85	12	>20	8

Conversely, cyanotic CHD is associated with reduced fertility as well as increased fetal loss. This is because cyanosis worsens owing to the increase in intracardiac right to left shunting as peripheral vascular resistance falls. For example, the right to left shunt in Eisenmenger syndrome, which occurs as a result of a fixed and high pulmonary vascular resistance, increases during pregnancy. Thromboembolic risk is increased owing to polycythaemia secondary to hypoxaemia. Maternal cyanosis is poorly tolerated by the fetus and is associated with a high incidence of fetal loss (28%), stillbirths, IUGR (30%) and preterm delivery (55%), both iatrogenic and spontaneous.[9] This is especially true if the oxygen saturation falls below 80–85%.

Sawhney *et al.*[10] compared 251 pregnancies in women with acyanotic heart disease with 24 in women with cyanotic heart disease. The incidences of miscarriage (8.3%), stillbirth (0.8%) and SGA babies (36.4%) were higher in women with cyanotic heart disease than in those with acyanotic heart disease (stillbirth 0.8%, SGA 6.9%).

Cyanotic conditions that have been surgically repaired are not associated with increased risk to either mother or fetus. Cardiac surgery improves perinatal outcome in women with cyanotic heart disease. Singh *et al.*[11] reviewed 40 pregnancies in 27 women with surgically corrected tetralogy of Fallot and reported good maternal and perinatal outcome. Whittemore *et al.*[6] observed that live births occurred in 42% of pregnancies with unrelieved cyanosis, in 72% with palliative shunts and in 78% with total surgical correction. These data were reported in 1982 and should thus be interpreted with caution, as there have been major advances in the treatment of CHD since then.

There are about 100 new Fontan repairs performed each year in the UK. This is a form of surgical palliation for patients who have only one effective ventricular chamber. It involves directly connecting the systemic venous return to the pulmonary arteries, although the precise method of doing this has varied over the last 20 years. While it is likely that fewer than half of these patients will reach reproductive age in 10–20 years' time, and half are men, they are clearly becoming a small but important group at high risk during pregnancy. Pregnancy carries additional risk owing to the increased haemodynamic burden on the Fontan connection itself and the single ventricular chamber. It is associated with a 2% risk of maternal mortality. Spontaneous miscarriage is frequent and occurs in up to 40% of pregnancies, probably owing to congestion of the intrauterine veins. Women with a successful Fontan with a small right atrium or total cavopulmonary connection and in NYHA class I or II can probably complete pregnancy and achieve a successful live birth rate of about 45%.[12]

Valvular heart disease

Regurgitant valvular disease is much better tolerated than stenosis. Mitral stenosis is associated with 10% maternal mortality, which increases to 50% in NYHA class III and IV. Fetal mortality can reach 12–31% in NYHA class III and IV. This is because a gradient develops between the left atrium and ventricle and the resultant increase in left atrial pressure can cause pulmonary oedema, a rise in pulmonary arterial and right ventricular pressures and eventually right ventricular pressures and right ventricular failure. Surgical commissurotomy and balloon mitral valvotomy have been performed for severe mitral stenosis in the second trimester of pregnancy with marked symptomatic relief and good maternal and fetal outcome. However, mitral valve surgery should be performed in selected women only.[13]

Hameed et al.[14] reported a significantly increased preterm delivery rate (23% versus 6%; $P = 0.03$) and IUGR (21% versus 0%; $P < 0.0001$) in women with valvular heart disease.

Malhotra et al.[13] carried out a retrospective comparison of the maternal and fetal pregnancy outcomes of 312 women with valvular heart disease and 321 healthy women. Women with valvular heart disease had a significantly higher incidence of surgical intervention during pregnancy (13.4%), congestive heart failure (5.1% versus 0%, $P < 0.001$) and mortality (0.64% versus 0%). There was also an increased rate of preterm delivery (48.3% versus 20.5%), reduced birthweight (2434 + 599 g versus 2653 + 542 g, $P < 0.001$) and a higher incidence of APGAR scores less than 8 (8.3% versus 4%, $P < 0.001$).

Recurrence risk

The risk of the fetus having a congenital heart defect is higher if the mother (5%) rather than the father (2%) has CHD.[15] The level of risk is dependent on the specific lesion and is higher for outflow tract lesions (Table 10.2). If the fetus is affected, the same or a related lesion is the most likely.[16] In women with an ASD, the risk of an ASD in the fetus is about 5–10%; for aortic stenosis, the risk is higher at about 18–20%. Both Marfan syndrome and hypertrophic cardiomyopathy carry an autosomal dominant inheritance pattern (50% recurrence risk).[17,18]

Table 10.2. Congenital heart disease (CHD) risk in the offspring of a parent with CHD

Congenital heart defect in a parent	Risk of CHD in offspring if one parent is affected
Intracardiac shunts	
Atrial septal defect	3–11%
Ventricular septal defect	4–22%
Patent ductus arteriosus	4–11%
Obstruction to flow	
Left-sided obstruction[a]	3–26%
Right-sided obstruction	3–22%
Complex abnormalities	
Tetralogy of Fallot	4–15%
Ebstein anomaly	Uncertain
Transposition of the great arteries	Uncertain

[a] Includes coarctation, aortic stenosis, discrete sub-aortic stenosis and supravalvular stenosis

Fetal surveillance

Early ultrasound examination is essential to confirm the gestational age. Increased fetal nuchal translucency (NT) is a common phenotypic expression of trisomy 21 and other chromosomal abnormalities[19–21] but it is also associated with fetal death and a wide range of fetal malformations, deformations, dysgeneses and genetic syndromes. There is an association between increased NT and cardiac defects in both chromosomally abnormal and normal fetuses.[22] A meta-analysis of screening studies reported that the detection rate of CHD was about 23% in chromosomally normal fetuses with an increased NT greater than 3.5 mm, and even higher at 59% in babies with chromosome abnormalities.[23]

The prevalence of major cardiac defects increases exponentially with fetal NT thickness, from 4.9 per 1000 in fetuses with an NT below the median, to 35.2, 64.4 and 126.7 per 1000 for respective NTs of 3.5–4.4 mm, 4.5–5.4 mm and 5.5 mm and above. There was no obvious difference in the distribution of NT in the various types of cardiac defect.[24] In the low-risk population, a normal NT constitutes a two-fold reduction in the risk of congenital heart defects.[22] On the other hand, women with an increased NT, especially those above the 99th centile, are at high risk for cardiac defects and therefore should not wait until 20 weeks of gestation for specialist echocardiography. With improvements in technology in ultrasound, it is possible to undertake a detailed cardiac assessment by 14 weeks.[25]

Echocardiography has been successfully applied to the prenatal assessment of fetal cardiac function and structure and in specialist centres leads to the detection and diagnosis of most cardiac abnormalities. Studies from these specialist centres report accurate diagnosis of over 90% of defects. However, the majority of such studies refer to the prenatal diagnosis of moderate to major defects in high-risk populations. An acceptable sensitivity in low-risk pregnancies is achieved by the correct examination of the four-chamber view at the routine 20 week scan, as screening studies have reported a detection rate of about 60% for major cardiac defects. Therefore, in high-risk groups such as congenital cardiac defects in one parent or in previous pregnancies, maternal diabetes or ingestion of teratogenic drugs, detailed fetal echocardiography should be carried out at specialist centres. Where there is a suspected cardiac defect, referral to a specialist centre is essential to obtain the correct diagnosis and for optimum counselling of the parents. Extracardiac anomaly and abnormal karyotype should be excluded by a fetal medicine unit, especially if the heart defect detected has a known association with chromosomal anomalies, such as an atrioventricular septal defect with trisomy 21, or common arterial trunk or interrupted aortic arch with a microdeletion of chromosome 22q11.

An early diagnosis of major CHD in the fetus allows the option of termination of pregnancy. In cases where the parents opt for the pregnancy to continue, the progression of the disease should be monitored as frequently as appropriate, usually about every 6–8 weeks. In some forms of CHD, the affected fetus will benefit from delivery in a tertiary care centre, where perinatal management can be optimised.

The assessment of fetal growth with serial ultrasound scans is essential in women with severe heart disease and cyanotic congenital heart lesions. Uterine blood flow increases to 200 ml/min by the 28th week of gestation, and reaches approximately 1200 ml/min at term. Therefore, uterine blood flow and thus perfusion of the fetus is vulnerable if the cardiac output is in any way compromised. If the overall maternal cardiac output falls, vascular resistance is altered primarily to protect the mother and particularly to maintain cerebral and coronary artery blood flow. Uterine blood flow is therefore the first to suffer and is affected by changes in perfusion pressure and uterine vascular resistance. Hence, in women with cyanotic heart disease with reduced maternal cardiac output, uterine blood flow is further reduced, and this leads to IUGR.

Uterine artery Doppler screening

Blood flow through the uteroplacental circulation can be studied non-invasively using Doppler ultrasound.[26] The impedance to flow in the uterine arteries decreases with gestation in normal pregnancies, reflecting the trophoblastic invasion of the spiral arteries and their conversion into low-resistance vessels. Impaired trophoblast invasion is one of the key features of pre-eclampsia and IUGR.[27] Previous histological findings from placental bed biopsies of women with pre-eclampsia and IUGR have shown good correlation with high resistance in uterine artery Doppler waveforms.[28] Persistence of high impedance to flow in the uterine arteries constitutes indirect evidence of abnormal placentation. This pragmatic approach of incorporating uterine artery Doppler as a screening tool in the routine antenatal setting can identify the great majority of women destined to develop serious complications of impaired placentation. This can be followed by increased surveillance and timely intervention that may improve both maternal and fetal outcomes.

One-stage screening tests in pregnant women attending for routine antenatal care at 23–24 weeks of gestation suggest that increased impedance to flow in the uterine arteries identifies about 20% of those that develop IUGR. Abnormal Doppler velocities are better at predicting severe, rather than mild, growth restriction, and the sensitivity is increased to 35%, 53%, 64% and 74% for birthweight below the tenth centile delivering before 38, 36, 34 and 32 weeks, respectively. In women with increased impedance to flow in the second trimester the likelihood ratio for the development of a growth-restricted infant is about 4, while it is about 0.8 for those with normal Doppler results. The likelihood of perinatal death in those with an abnormal Doppler result is about 2.4 times higher than the background risk.[3]

Uterine artery Doppler screening may help to stratify antenatal care by identifying the majority of pregnancies destined to develop the complications of uteroplacental insufficiency, but also by identifying a large group of women at particularly low risk of developing such complications. At St Mary's Hospital, London, women with CHD are routinely screened with uterine artery Doppler at 22–24 weeks for the prediction of IUGR.

Fetal assessment

If IUGR is confirmed, fetal wellbeing should be assessed with umbilical and fetal Doppler velocimetry as this will allow appropriate timing for delivery. Systematic reviews and meta-analyses of randomised controlled trials using umbilical artery Doppler to monitor high-risk pregnancies show a significant reduction in perinatal morbidity and mortality.[29] Pathological studies have demonstrated that abnormal placental pathology was significantly associated with abnormal umbilical artery Doppler velocimetry and these placentas had a significantly increased number of villous infarcts, cytotrophoblast proliferation and thickening of the villous trophoblastic basal membrane.[30] Clinical studies of umbilical arterial flow velocimetry waveforms in IUGR have reported progressive increase in impedance to flow until absence, and in extreme cases, reversal of end-diastolic frequencies occurs. Absent or reversed end-diastolic flow are associated with increased perinatal mortality and morbidity.[31–33] The odds ratios for perinatal mortality in pregnancies complicated by absent end-diastolic flow (AED) and reversed end-diastolic flow (RED) were 4.0 and 10.6, respectively, compared with when end-diastolic flow was present.[31] The incidences of respiratory distress syndrome and necrotising enterocolitis were not increased with AED or RED but there was an increase in neonatal cerebral haemorrhage, anaemia and hypoglycaemia.[31] In addition to increased fetal and neonatal mortality, growth restriction with AED or RED in the umbilical artery is associated with increased incidence of permanent neurological damage.[34]

Fetal arterial blood flow redistribution

In fetal hypoxaemia there is redistribution of well-oxygenated blood to vital organs such as the brain, myocardium and the adrenal glands and reduction in the perfusion of the kidneys, gastrointestinal tract and the lower extremities. This compensatory mechanism to prevent fetal damage is known the 'brain-sparing' effect. The umbilical artery (UA) pulsatility index (PI) increases and the fetal middle cerebral artery (MCA) PI decreases, and thus the UA/MCA PI ratio increases. However, compensation through cerebral vasodilatation is limited and a plateau corresponding to a nadir of PI in cerebral vessels is reached at least 2 weeks before the cerebral development of the fetus is jeopardised. Consequently, arterial vessels are unsuitable for longitudinal monitoring of growth-restricted fetuses. Cardiac and venous velocity waveforms provide more information regarding fetal wellbeing or compromise.

Fetal venous Doppler

Cerebral vasodilatation produces a decrease in left ventricle afterload, whereas increased placental and systemic resistance produce increased right ventricle afterload. Examination of the right heart and venous system show a good correlation between fetal acid–base balance and perinatal outcome. In animal studies, in severe hypoxaemia there is redistribution in the umbilical venous blood towards the ductus venosus at the expense of hepatic blood flow. In growth-restricted sheep fetuses, reversal of flow in the inferior vena cava and ductus venosus and pulsations in the umbilical vein have been observed at the end of diastole. These abnormal pulsations occur synchronously with atrial contraction and are thought to represent transmission of atrial contractions into the venous circulation. These abnormal venous waveforms are significantly associated with deterioration in acid–base status and poor perinatal outcome.[35]

The interval between first occurrence of AED and an abnormal cardiotocograph (CTG) fetal heart rate pattern, or abnormal biophysical profile (BPP), has ranged from 1–26 days.[36,37] Gestational age, the presence of hypertension and venous Doppler abnormalities (notably pulsations in the umbilical vein) are the key prognostic factors affecting this interval.[36] The optimal surveillance strategy in fetuses with AED/RED is unclear. Options include daily CTG/BPP and/or venous Doppler, with delivery when the CTG becomes pathological (decelerations with reduced variability),[36] the BPP becomes abnormal (4 or below),[38] there is reversal of Doppler velocities in the ductus venosus during atrial contraction,[39] or there are umbilical vein pulsations.[40] Under any of these circumstances, delivery needs to be expedited.

Women needing heart surgery in pregnancy

Definitive data concerning heart surgery with cardiopulmonary bypass during pregnancy are limited. Such surgery is associated with significant maternal and fetal risk and should thus only be advised in extreme cases where there is failed medical treatment. Contributing risk factors include the use of vasoactive drugs, other preoperative medication, age, nature of surgery, reoperation and functional class. Overall, functional class is the best predictor for adverse maternal outcome.[41] In a systematic review of the outcomes of 161 women undergoing cardiac surgery during pregnancy, the fetal morbidity and mortality were 9% and 30%, respectively, and the maternal morbidity and mortality were 24% and 6%, respectively.[42]

In women with significant mitral stenosis (mitral valve area less than 1.0 cm[2]) and more than NYHA class II despite aggressive medical therapy, urgent surgical intervention should be considered. Percutaneous balloon mitral valvuloplasty and closed valvotomy have been safely performed in pregnancy. However, the effect of the use of radio-opaque contrast agents on the fetus remains unknown.[43,44]

Cardiopulmonary bypass produces a non-physiological state that alters the cellular components of blood and adversely affects the coagulation factors. This results in the release of vasoactive substances from leucocytes, and complement activation.[45,46] The uteroplacental blood flow is directly proportional to the maternal mean arterial pressure and inversely proportional to the uterine vascular resistance.[45] Maternal hypotension can significantly reduce the placental perfusion and result in fetal loss.[47] Combined with non-pulsatile perfusion, uterine arteriovenous shunts, obstruction of inferior vena cava drainage, uterine artery spasm and particulate and gaseous embolism, this can lead to fetal hypoxia, bradycardia and even death.[46] In addition, hypothermia can cause fatal fetal arrhythmias. Maternal alkalosis during cardio-pulmonary bypass can shift the maternal oxyhaemoglobin dissociation curve to the left, leading to reduced fetal partial arterial oxygen pressure and oxygen content.

Effects of anaesthetic drugs on the fetus

All anaesthetic drugs administered to pregnant women will rapidly cross the placenta and be distributed to the fetus. Most of the commonly used induction agents, narcotics and muscle relaxants are safe in pregnancy. Halothane will equilibrate in fetal tissues after 60 minutes of maternal exposure and is associated with stable fetal haemodynamics and acid–base response.[48,49] However, isoflurane will produce a reduction in fetal cardiac output and redistribution of fetal circulation away from the placenta. Prolonged exposure to isoflurane can lead to hypercarbic acidosis in sheep fetuses.[50]

Fetal monitoring during surgery

Fetal heart-rate monitoring will help guide the management of maternal cardio-respiratory parameters.[51] Anaesthetic drugs can create loss of heart-rate variability by anaesthetising the brainstem centre in the fetus that modulates the intrinsic cardiac automaticity. They can thus influence the interpretation of fetal monitoring. Abrupt changes in heart rate and baseline rates outside the acceptable range of 110–160 beats per minute should prompt the anaesthetist to look for obvious causes of uteroplacental insufficiency and to implement measures to increase blood pressure and oxygen delivery to the mother.

High-pressure, high-flow cardiopulmonary bypass is recommended for the man-agement of cardiac surgery in pregnant women.[52] Successful fetal outcome has been reported using mean pump pressures above 60 mmHg and flows above 2.0 (l/min)/m[2].

Systemic cooling to temperatures below 28 °C carries a high risk of fetal cardiac arrest and demise. It is now possible to use systemic normothermia on bypass to minimise the risk of hypothermia.[53] However, despite high peak flows, normal mean arterial pressure and normothermia, fetal outcome is still dismal. This is related to the changes in fetal and uterine haemodynamics during surgery. Intraoperative fetal bradycardia is often observed after aortic clamping with a rise in umbilical artery PI and a non-pulsatile uterine artery flow noted.[54] Therefore, there may be a role for fetal heart–rate monitoring during surgery. The variables of the maternal bypass perfusion are adjusted according to the fetal heart–rate pattern observed, in order to limit the effects of bypass on the fetus as much as possible. However, if fetal monitoring is used, the best method of surveillance, either by CTG, ultrasound or Doppler assessment of umbilical and uterine arteries, remains controversial.

In cases where there is fetal or maternal compromise, caesarean delivery while on cardiac bypass has been reported. However, the decision for immediate delivery is dependent on the gestational age and viability of the fetus. Neonatal mortality is 90% at 25 weeks of gestation and decreases to about 15% by week 30.[55] Premature labour presents the greatest risk to the fetus in the perioperative period. The benefits of postponing surgery until the second trimester to allow adequate fetal lung maturation should be balanced against the potential hazards to the mother.

Summary

Women with CHD are a high-risk group and are more likely to experience fetal complications such as fetal demise, IUGR, premature delivery and fetal CHD. Increased fetal surveillance, comprising serial growth scans, is mandatory in these women. The use of Doppler ultrasound is helpful in fetal monitoring and there may be a role for using uterine artery Doppler in screening for IUGR. Umbilical and middle cerebral artery Doppler assessment and CTG can optimise the management of growth-restricted fetuses. The role of cardiac and venous velocity waveforms is evolving and should further enhance fetal surveillance.

References

1. Lewis G, editor. *Why Mothers Die 2000–2002: The Sixth Report of Confidential Enquiries into Maternal Deaths in the United Kingdom.* London: RCOG Press; 2004. p. 137–150.
2. Papageorghiou AT, Yu CKH, Bindra R, Pandis G, Nicolaides KN. Multicentre screening for pre-eclampsia and fetal growth restriction by transvaginal uterine artery Doppler at 23 weeks of gestation. *Ultrasound Obstet Gynecol* 2001;18:441–9.
3. Clark SL. Cardiac disease in pregnancy. *Obstet Gynecol Clin North Am* 1991;18:237–56.
4. Clark SL. Labor and delivery in the patient with structural cardiac disease. *Clin Perinatol* 1986;13:695–703.
5. Siu SC, Sermer M, Harrison DA, Grigoriadis E, Liu G, Sorensen S, *et al.* Risk and predictors for pregnancy-related complications in women with heart disease. *Circulation* 1997;96:2789–94.
6. Whittemore R, Hobbins JC, Engle MA. Pregnancy and its outcome in women with and without surgical treatment of congenital heart disease. *Am J Cardiol* 1982;50:641–51.
7. Presbitero P, Somerville J, Stone S, Aruta E, Spiegelhalter D, Rabajoli F. Pregnancy in cyanotic congenital heart disease. Outcome of mother and fetus. *Circulation* 1994;89:2673–6.

8. Chia P, Raman S, Tham SW. The pregnancy outcome of acyanotic heart disease. *J Obstet Gynaecol Res* 1998;24:267–73.

9. Gleicher N, Midwall J, Hochberger D, Jaffin H. Eisenmenger's syndrome and pregnancy. *Obstet Gynecol Surv* 1979;34:721–41.

10. Sawhney H, Suri V, Vasishta K, Gupta N, Devi K, Grover A. Pregnancy and congenital heart disease – maternal and fetal outcome. *Aust N Z J Obstet Gynaecol* 1998;38:266–71.

11. Singh H, Bolton PJ, Oakley CM. Pregnancy after surgical correction of tetralogy of Fallot. *Br Med J* 1982;285:168–70.

12. Canobbio MM, Mair DD, van der Velde M, Koos BJ. Pregnancy outcomes after the Fontan repair. *J Am Coll Cardiol* 1996;28:763–7.

13. Malhotra M, Sharma JB, Tripathii R, Arora P, Arora R. Maternal and fetal outcome in valvular heart disease. *Int J Gynaecol Obstet* 2004;84:11–16.

14. Hameed AH, Karaalp IS, Tummala PP, Wani OR, Canetti M, Akhter MW, et al. The effect of valvular heart disease on maternal and fetal outcome of pregnancy. *J Am Coll Cardiol* 2001;37:893–9.

15. Burn J, Brennan P, Little J, Holloway S, Coffey R, Somerville J, et al. Recurrence risks in offspring of adults with major heart defects: results from first cohort of British collaborative study. *Lancet* 1998;351:311–16.

16. Allan LD, Crawford DC, Chita SK, Anderson RH, Tynan MJ. Familial recurrence of congenital heart disease in a prospective series of mothers referred for fetal echocardiography. *Am J Cardiol* 1986;58:334–7.

17. Mitchell SC, Korones SB, Berendes HW. Congenital heart disease in 56,109 births. Incidence and natural history. *Circulation* 1971;43:323–32.

18. Nora JJ, Nora AH. The evolution of specific genetic and environmental counseling in congenital heart diseases. *Circulation* 1978;57:205–13.

19. Hyett J, Moscoso G, Nicolaides K. Abnormalities of the heart and great arteries in first trimester chromosomally abnormal fetuses. *Am J Med Genet* 1997;69:207–16.

20. Moyano D, Huggon IC, Allan LD. Fetal echocardiography in trisomy 18. *Arch Dis Child Fetal Neonatal Ed* 2005;90:F520–2.

21. Surerus E, Huggon IC, Allan LD. Turner's syndrome in fetal life. *Ultrasound Obstet Gynecol* 2003;22:264–7.

22. Hyett J, Perdu M, Sharland G, Snijders R, Nicolaides KH. Using fetal nuchal translucency to screen for major congenital cardiac defects at 10–14 weeks of gestation: population based cohort study. *BMJ* 1999;318:70–1.

23. Makrydimas G, Sotiriadis A, Huggon IC, Simpson J, Sharland G, Carvalho JS, et al. Nuchal translucency and fetal cardiac defects: a pooled analysis of major fetal echocardiography centers. *Am J Obstet Gynecol* 2005;192:89–95.

24. Atzei A, Gajewska K, Huggon IC, Allan L, Nicolaides KH. Relationship between nuchal translucency thickness and prevalence of major cardiac defects in fetuses with normal karyotype. *Ultrasound Obstet Gynecol* 2005;26:154–7.

25. Huggon IC, Ghi T, Cook AC, Zosmer N, Allan LD, Nicolaides KH. Fetal cardiac abnormalities identified prior to 14 weeks' gestation. *Ultrasound Obstet Gynecol* 2002;20:22–9.

26. Papageorghiou AT, Yu CK, Nicolaides KH. The role of uterine artery Doppler in predicting adverse pregnancy outcome. *Best Pract Res Clin Obstet Gynaecol* 2004:1–14.

27. Carbillon L, Challier JC, Alouini S, Uzan M, Uzan S. Uteroplacental circulation development: Doppler assessment and clinical importance. *Placenta* 2001;22:795–9.

28. Sagol S, Ozkinay E, Oztekin K, Ozdemir N. The comparison of uterine artery Doppler velocimetry with the histopathology of the placental bed. *Aust N Z J Obstet Gynaecol* 1999;39:324–9.

29. Alfirevic Z, Neilson JP. Doppler ultrasonography in high-risk pregnancies: systematic review with meta-analysis. *Am J Obstet Gynecol* 1995;172:1379–87.

30. Madazli R, Somunkiran A, Calay Z, Ilvan S, Aksu MF. Histomorphology of the placenta and the placental bed of growth restricted foetuses and correlation with the Doppler velocimetries of the uterine and umbilical arteries. *Placenta* 2003;24:510–16.

31. Karsdorp VH, van Vugt JM, Van Geijn HP, Kostense PJ, Arduini D, Montenegro N, *et al.* Clinical significance of absent or reversed end diastolic velocity waveforms in umbilical artery. *Lancet* 1994;344:1664–8.

32. Pattinson RC, Norman K, Odendaal HJ. The role of Doppler velocimetry in the management of high-risk pregnancies. *Br J Obstet Gynaecol* 1994;101:114–20.

33. Todros T, Ronco G, Fianchino O, Rosso S, Gabrielli S, Valsecchi L, *et al.* Accuracy of the umbilical arteries Doppler flow velocity waveforms in detecting adverse perinatal outcomes in a high-risk population. *Acta Obstet Gynecol Scand* 1996;75:113–19.

34. Valcamonico A, Danti L, Frusca T, Soregaroli M, Zucca S, Abrami F, *et al.* Absent end-diastolic velocity in umbilical artery: risk of neonatal morbidity and brain damage. *Am J Obstet Gynecol* 1994;170:796–801.

35. Baschat AA, Gembruch U, Reiss I, Gortner L, Weiner CP, Harman CR. Relationship between arterial and venous Doppler and perinatal outcome in fetal growth restriction. *Ultrasound Obstet Gynecol* 2000;16:407–13.

36. Arduini D, Rizzo G. Romanini C. The development of abnormal heart rate patterns after absent end-diastolic velocity in umbilical artery: analysis of risk factors. *Am J Obstet Gynecol* 1993;168:43–50.

37. Forouzan I. Absence of end-diastolic flow velocity in the umbilical artery: a review. *Obstet Gynecol Surv* 1995;50:219–27.

38. Divon MY, Girz BA, Lieblich R, Langer O. Clinical management of the fetus with markedly diminished umbilical artery end-diastolic flow. *Am J Obstet Gynecol* 1989;161:1523–7.

39. Hecher K, Hackeloer B-J. Cardiotocogram compared to Doppler investigation of the fetal circulation in the premature growth-retarded fetus: longitudinal observations. *Ultrasound Obstet Gynecol* 1997;9:152–61.

40. Gudmundsson S, Tulzer G, Huhta JC, Marsal K. Venous Doppler in the fetus with absent end diastolic flow in the umbilical artery. *Ultrasound Obstet Gynecol* 1996;7:262–7.

41. Pomini F, Merccogliano D, Cavaletti C, Caruso A, Pomini P. Cardiopulmonary bypass in pregnancy. *Ann Thorac Surg* 1996;61:259–68.

42. Weiss BM, Von Segesser LK, Alon E, Seifert B, Turina MI. Outcome of cardiovascular surgery and pregnancy: a systematic review of the period 1984–1996. *Am J Obstet Gynecol* 1998;179:1643–53.

43. Goon MS, Raman S, Sinnathuray TA. Closed mitral valvotomy in pregnancy – a Malaysian experience. *Aust N Z J Obstet Gynaecol* 1987;27:173–7.

44. Kalra GS, Arora R, Khan JA, Nigam M, Khalillulah M. Percutaneous mitral commissurotomy for severe mitral stenosis during pregnancy. *Cathet Cardiovasc Diagn* 1994;33:28–30.

45. Mahli A, Izdes S, Coskun D. Cardiac operations during pregnancy: review of factors influencing fetal outcome. *Ann Thorac Surg* 2000;69:1622–6.

46. Strickland RA, Oliver WC, Chantigian RC. Anesthesia, cardiopulmonary bypass and the pregnant patient. *Mayo Clin Proc* 1991;66:411–29.

47. Jahangiri M, Clark J, Prefumo F, Pumphrey C, Ward D. Cardiac surgery during pregnancy: pulsatile or nonpulsatile perfusion? *J Thorac Cardiovasc Surg* 2003;126:894–5.

48. Biehl DR, Tweed WA, Cote J, Wade JG, Sitar D. Effect of halothane on cardiac output

and regional flow in the fetal lamb *in utero*. *Anesth Analg* 1983;62:489–92.

49. Cheek DB, Hughes SC, Dailey PA, Field DR, Pytka S, Rosen MA, *et al*. Effect of halothane on regional cerebral blood flow and cerebral metabolic oxygen consumption in the fetal lamb *in utero*. *Anesthesiology* 1987;67:361–6.

50. Biehl DR, Yarnell R, Wade JG, Sitar D. The uptake of isoflurane by the foetal lamb *in utero*: effect on regional blood flow. *Can Anaesth Soc J* 1983;30:581–6.

51. Liu PL, Warren TM, Ostheimer GW, Weiss JB, Liu LM. Foetal monitoring in parturients undergoing surgery unrelated to pregnancy. *Can Anaesth Soc J* 1985;32:525–32.

52. Conroy JM, Bailey MK, Hollon MF, Cooke JE, Baker JD 3rd. Anesthesia for open heart surgery in the pregnant patient. *South Med J* 1989;82:492–5.

53. Salerno TA, Houck JP, Barrozo CA, Panos A, Christakis GT, Abel JG, *et al*. Retrograde continuous warm blood cardioplegia: a new concept in myocardial protection. *Ann Thorac Surg* 1991;51:245–9.

54. Khandelwal M, Rasanen J, Ludormirski A, Addonizio P, Reece EA. Evaluation of fetal and uterine hemodynamics during maternal cardiopulmonary bypass. *Obstet Gynecol* 1996;88:667–71.

55. Draper ES, Manktelow B, Field DJ, James D. Prediction of survival for preterm births by weight and gestational age: retrospective population based study. *BMJ* 1999;319:1093–7.

Section 4

Antenatal care specific maternal conditions

Chapter 11
Prosthetic heart valves

Carole A Warnes

Introduction

Pregnancy for a woman with a prosthetic heart valve poses risks for both the mother and the fetus. As such, it has been appropriately described as a 'double jeopardy' situation.[1] The selection of the most appropriate prosthetic valve for a woman who might become pregnant requires careful review and a detailed discussion of the relative risks with the woman, preferably before she becomes pregnant. A key issue is that bioprostheses (tissue valves) are, in general, much less thrombogenic than mechanical prostheses and, if the mother is in sinus rhythm, warfarin can be avoided. Pregnancy in the presence of a tissue prosthesis is associated with a much lower risk of maternal/fetal complications, but structural valve degeneration inevitably occurs and the woman requires reoperation, with all the attendant risks, at some point later.

Mechanical prostheses are much more problematic during pregnancy and mothers are especially vulnerable to valve thrombosis and thromboembolism. Considerable controversy still exists about the most appropriate anticoagulant management during each of the three trimesters in order to avoid these life-threatening complications. No consensus exists as to the ideal anticoagulant strategy and no large prospective series are available to provide evidence-based data. Whichever anticoagulant modality is chosen, there is the potential for increased risk of valve thrombosis and thrombo-embolism (especially with heparin) and the potential for miscarriage, placental bleeding or fetal embryopathy with the use of warfarin. Each type of prosthesis thus has a relative risk–benefit ratio in pregnancy, and these issues will be reviewed in detail along with proposed management strategies.

Tissue prostheses

The most commonly used bioprostheses (heterografts) are usually porcine (pig) valves. For patients in sinus rhythm, anticoagulation is not required, although some are prescribed aspirin either in a full adult dose (325–500 mg) or a dose of 75–81 mg (UK–USA standard preparations). For women who have a normally functioning tissue prosthesis, normal ventricular function and no significant pulmonary hypertension, a pregnancy is often uncomplicated. Tissue valves, however, have a finite lifespan and develop structural valve degeneration. In general, mitral prostheses degenerate at a faster rate than aortic prostheses.[2,3] In addition, the rate of structural valve deterioration is considerably faster in younger patients (under 40 years of age) than for older patients.[4,5] As a result, a repeat valve replacement is inevitable, on average about a decade after the first operation. The mortality risks of a reoperation vary considerably among different centres: in the author's institution the risk is less than 1%, but in other institutions it may be significantly higher. Earlier reports suggest a risk between 3.8% and 8.8%.[6,7] Moreover, while recent data in high-volume cardiac centres reveal a lower reoperative mortality than earlier reports, the surgical results of the individual institution should be considered when counselling women of childbearing age about which type of valve replacement is preferable.[8] In each case, the risks and benefits need to be carefully balanced, and it also should be recognised that if a mother dies at reoperation the baby will be left without a biological mother.[9]

Some authors have reported that pregnancy accelerates structural valve degeneration, perhaps via an effect on calcium turnover.[10-13] Badduke et al.[6] reviewed 87 women with bioprostheses: the need for reoperation for structural valve degeneration after 10 years was 59% for women having had pregnancies versus 19% for those who did not. In women who had a pregnancy, the mean interval from operation to reoperation was only 72.1 months. A retrospective European study[10] reported that 17 (35%) of 49 bioprostheses deteriorated significantly in function during pregnancy or shortly after it.

Other reports, however, have failed to confirm the suggestion of accelerated valve degeneration during pregnancy.[14,15] Jamieson et al.[7] evaluated the long-term performance of bioprostheses in women under 35 years of age to determine whether pregnancy influenced structural valve deterioration. Between 1972 and 1992, 237 women received 255 tissue prostheses. Of the total operations, 53 were performed in women who subsequently had a pregnancy and 202 in women who were never subsequently pregnant. The mean interval from implantation to reoperation for the whole group was 99.6 months. The freedom from structural valve deterioration at ten and 15 years for the non-pregnant group was 54% and 18%, respectively, and for the pregnant group 45% and the 34%, respectively (P = not significant). In a retrospective review of 232 New Zealand women followed for 1499 patient-years, North et al.[3] also found that pregnancy did not influence structural valve deterioration, with a relative risk of 0.96. Avila et al.[14] compared 48 women with tissue prostheses who had a pregnancy with a control group of 37 women who did not and reported a similar rate of valve degeneration at 5 years (27% versus 30%). Thus, while some reports suggest acceleration of valve degeneration by pregnancy, several large series suggest that pregnancy does not significantly influence the incidence of structural valve disease. This has also been the author's experience at the Mayo Clinic. The issue thus remains unresolved, although some authors have suggested that the appearance of accelerated valve degeneration in association with pregnancy might simply reflect the well-established deterioration of tissue valves in younger patients.[8] In my experience, most women during the childbearing years elect to have a tissue prosthesis, with the knowledge that approximately half of them will need a valve replacement at 10 years. A mechanical prosthesis is then selected at the time of reoperation.

Mechanical prosthetic heart valves

Pregnancy induces a hypercoagulable state and is therefore associated with an increased risk of valve thrombosis and thromboembolism in women; this is especially important with mechanical prosthetic heart valves that are already at risk of clotting. During pregnancy, there is an increased concentration of clotting factors, decreased fibrinolysis and increased platelet adhesiveness. Anticoagulation management is thus critical, and one should not extrapolate the same therapies used for women with mechanical prostheses having non-cardiac surgery to those in the pregnant state. Appropriate anticoagulation, however, is challenging because anticoagulation with warfarin can be associated with important fetal adverse effects, while anticoagulation with heparin is probably less effective and therefore associated with important fetal and maternal complications.

In many series, valve thromboses and thromboembolic events occur in approximately 10% of cases and are often fatal.[10,16–18] It should also be noted that some women are at an even higher risk of valve thrombosis, particularly those with mitral tilting disc valves and those with older-generation valves such as the Bjork–Shiley and Starr–Edwards valves.

Unfractionated heparin

Heparin is a large molecule and does not cross the placenta to affect the fetus. It has a relatively short circulating half-life, however, and is given either subcutaneously or intravenously. The use of heparin can be associated with osteoporosis[19] and an immune IgG-mediated thrombocytopenia.[20] It has frequently been the anticoagulant of choice, particularly in the first trimester, for women with mechanical prostheses in an effort to avoid the potential complications of fetal embryopathy due to warfarin. The laboratory control of anticoagulation, however, is challenging and there is a wide variability in the sensitivity of activated partial thromboplastin time (APTT) reagents for monitoring the dosage and considerable variability in response to standard dosing. In addition, the APTT may vary by as much as 50% in response to the same continuous intravenous dose of heparin with a higher anticoagulant effect at night-time. This diurnal variation may relate to a circadian rhythm in the pharmacokinetics of heparin or more likely a spontaneous circadian variation in coagulation also seen in normals.[21]

During pregnancy the APTT response to heparin is often attenuated because of the increased levels of factor VIII and fibrinogen.[22] It is thus imperative that heparin should be given at an adequate intensity, with frequent measurements of trough and peak levels. Contemporary APTT reagents are more sensitive to the anticoagulant effect of heparin and an APTT ratio of 1.5 is likely to be inadequate.[23] The APTT ratio should be at least 2, which correlates with an antifactor Xa level of more than 0.55 IU/ml in approximately 90% of women.[24] Because of the variability in the laboratory sensitivities for monitoring heparin, APTT alone may be insufficient and anti-Xa assays periodically may be more useful in guiding therapy. If this is done, it is recommended that the anti-Xa level be maintained between 0.35 and 0.7.[23] It may be that sub-optimal target APTT ratios account for some of the treatment failures reported in the literature.

In the author's experience, unfractionated heparin is difficult to manage via the subcutaneous route because of wide peaks and troughs, and a period of hospitalisation is usually necessary to achieve a stable dosage regimen. Sometimes, rather than twice daily dosing, it must be given three times a day to maintain a more stable APTT level. Intravenous administration is often preferable, particularly in high-risk cases.

The results of heparin use during pregnancy have suggested that it may not be the best anticoagulant from the perspective of the mother. Salazar et al.[18] used subcutaneous heparin during 40 pregnancies in 37 women. Unfractionated heparin was administered from the sixth to the end of the 12th week and in the last 2 weeks of gestation. It was given every 8 hours in the first 36 cases and every 6 hours in the last four cases, and the dose adjusted to maintain the APTT at 1.5–2.5 times the control level. Warfarin was used at all other times during the pregnancies. The incidence of miscarriage was 37.5% and there was one neonatal death (2.5%) due to cerebral haemorrhage. No warfarin embryopathy was noted in any of the 16 liveborn infants studied by a geneticist. There were two cases of fatal massive thrombosis of mitral tilting disc prostheses during the period of heparin therapy in the first trimester. One woman had been receiving 9500 iu of subcutaneous heparin every 8 hours since the end of week four, and the other had been receiving 6500 iu every 6 hours. Both women had followed their heparin treatment, and monitoring of the APTT had shown ranges of 55–95 seconds with a control of 30–35 seconds. The authors concluded that subcutaneous heparin with doses adjusted to keep the APTT from 1.5 to 2.5 times the control value, did not provide adequate prophylaxis against thromboembolism in these women. Whether a more aggressive protocol to keep the APTT at least twice the control value with periodic monitoring of anti-Xa levels would afford a better outcome remains to be determined; the use of low molecular weight heparin may also allow better control.

The retrospective European study by Sbarouni et al.[10] reviewed 133 women with mechanical valves having 151 pregnancies. These women were managed through pregnancy utilising three anticoagulant strategies. The first used subcutaneous unfractionated heparin throughout pregnancy. The second used subcutaneous unfractionated heparin in the first trimester and warfarin thereafter until 2–4 weeks prior to delivery when intravenous heparin was administered prior to delivery. The third regimen involved the use of warfarin throughout pregnancy. Of these 151 pregnancies, 73% produced a healthy baby, but there were 13 valve thromboses (four fatal), eight embolic events (two fatal) and seven episodes of bleeding. Most of these complications occurred with heparin therapy. Notably, the complications were almost all in those women with mitral prostheses (12 of 13 valves), and the one woman with an aortic valve thrombosis had refused to use any anticoagulant. The author's recommendation, therefore, was that since heparin was a poor anticoagulant, warfarin was the safer choice and should be maintained throughout pregnancy. Importantly, however, this study was retrospective, different centres were involved, and the adequacy of anticoagulation was not reported in every case where a thrombotic complication was observed. It is possible that an inadequate target therapeutic range may explain the reported failure.[25]

Chan et al.[26] also performed a meta-analysis from 1966 to 1997 looking at 976 women with 1234 pregnancies, comparing the same three management strategies described in the previous paragraph. The risks of miscarriage and fetal loss for those on warfarin throughout pregnancy were 25% and 34%, respectively, and (perhaps surprisingly from a theoretical point of view, as heparin does not cross the placenta) the use of heparin in the first trimester yielded similar results with a miscarriage rate of 25% and a fetal loss rate of 27% (Table 11.1). They reported that the use of warfarin throughout pregnancy was associated with embryopathy in 6.4% of live births but that if heparin were substituted at or prior to 6 weeks of gestation and continued until 12 weeks the risk of embryopathy was eliminated (Table 11.2). The overall risks of fetal loss (miscarriage, stillbirth and neonatal death) were similar in women treated with oral anticoagulants (warfarin) throughout compared with women treated with heparin in the first trimester.

The maternal mortality in this whole series was 2.9% and major bleeding events occurred in 2.5% of all pregnancies, most commonly at the time of delivery. The maternal risk, however, was quite different among the various anticoagulant strategies,

Table 11.1. Frequency of fetal complications reported with various anticoagulant strategies; the warfarin regimen involved warfarin throughout pregnancy with or without heparin prior to delivery; the heparin/warfarin regimen used heparin in the first trimester then warfarin throughout pregnancy with or without heparin prior to delivery; the heparin regimen used heparin throughout pregnancy; those on no anticoagulants included the use of antiplatelet agents alone; modified with permission from Chan *et al., Arch Intern Med* 2000:160:191–6, copyright©2000, American Medical Association, all rights reserved.[26]

Regimen	Miscarriage	Fetal anomalies	Fetal loss
Warfarin	196/792 (25%)	35/549 (6%)	266/792 (34%)
Heparin/warfarin	57/230 (25%)	6/174 (3%)	61/230 (27%)
Heparin	5/21 (24%)	0/17 (0%)	9/21 (43%)
No anticoagulants	10/102 (10%)	3/92 (3%)	20/102 (20%)

and the regimen associated with the lowest maternal risk of valve thrombosis was the use of oral anticoagulants throughout pregnancy, with a risk of 3.9% (Table 11.3). While the use of heparin between six and 12 weeks of gestation eliminated the risk of fetal embryopathy, the maternal risk increased considerably and this regimen was associated with an increased risk of valve thrombosis, at 9.2% (Table 11.3). It thus appears that the window between six and 12 weeks is pivotal since the continued exposure to warfarin resulted in an increase in the risk of fetal loss by more than 50%. The apparent advantages of reduced fetal loss and embryopathy gained from the use of heparin, however, appeared to be counterbalanced by an increase in maternal complications and an increased risk of thromboembolism.

These findings were confirmed by Meschengieser *et al.*[17] in a study of 92 pregnancies in 59 women. They reported that miscarriage or fetal losses were similar in women exposed to oral anticoagulants in the first trimester (15/61 (25%) compared with those who received adjusted subcutaneous heparin (6/31 (19%) ($P = 0.5717$). Embolic events, however, were more common in women receiving heparin. The authors concluded that heparin did not offer a clear advantage over oral anticoagulants in the pregnancy outcome.

Table 11.2. Fetal outcomes of early anticoagulant strategies in the first trimester, comparing the results of discontinuing warfarin in the first 6 weeks and substituting heparin, versus those who continued on warfarin beyond 6 weeks into the more vulnerable period before heparin was substituted; modified with permission from Chan *et al., Arch Intern Med* 2000:160:191–6, copyright©2000, American Medical Association, all rights reserved.[26]

Early anticoagulant strategy	Miscarriage	Fetal anomalies	Fetal loss
Regimen 2: heparin < 6 weeks	19/129 (15%)	0/108 (0%)	21/129 (16%)
Heparin > 6 weeks	19/56 (34%)	4/36 (11%)	20/56 (36%)

Table 11.3. Frequency of maternal complications reported with the various anticoagulation regimens described in Table 11.1; modified with permission from Chan *et al., Arch Intern Med* 2000:160:191–6, copyright©2000, American Medical Association, all rights reserved.[26]

Regimen	Thromboembolic complications	Death
Warfarin	31/788 (4%)	10/561 (2%)
Heparin/warfarin	21/229 (9%)	7/167 (4%)
Heparin	7/21 (33%)	3/20 (15%)
No anticoagulants	26/107 (24%)	5/106 (5%)

These studies highlight the dilemma that caregivers face when managing pregnant women with mechanical heart valves. While the risk and severity of warfarin embryopathy may not be as high as previously reported, the continued use of warfarin until close to term can result in a high risk of fetal loss. The use of warfarin throughout pregnancy, however, confers the greatest protection to the mother against valve thrombosis and death. Substituting heparin in the first trimester as early as possible avoids fetal embryopathy but exposes the woman to a period of increased risk of thrombosis.[26]

Subcutaneous heparin can cause a persistent anticoagulant effect at the time of delivery, although the mechanism for this prolonged effect is unclear.[23] This can complicate its use prior to labour. In one small study,[27] an anticoagulant effect persisted for up to 28 hours after the last injection of subcutaneous heparin, resulting in deliveries that were complicated by a prolonged APTT. This would suggest that intravenous heparin use, which can be started and stopped instantly, might be preferable prior to delivery.

Warfarin

The use of warfarin, particularly between the sixth and twelfth week of pregnancy, is associated with an embryopathy (warfarin embryopathy). The manifestations of warfarin embryopathy can vary widely and range from minor stippling of the epiphyses on X-ray (chondrodysplasia punctata)[28] and/or nasal hypoplasia to serious central nervous system abnormalities and optic atrophy.[28,29] Stippling of the epiphyses occurs during early childhood and disappears with age. The incidence of embryopathy in reported series also varies widely, from zero to more than 20%.[9,10,12,30–33] This has been the subject of considerable debate in the literature, and the incidence of warfarin embryopathy varies by the degree of scrutiny the baby receives (whether examined by a primary care physician or a geneticist) and whether the miscarried babies are examined for features of embryopathy. Concern has also been expressed that there may be long-term effects of warfarin exposure with minor neurological dysfunction and low intelligence quotients.[34] Other complications of warfarin administration may also occur, including a higher frequency of miscarriages and fetal loss.[26]

More recently, it has been suggested that the risk of fetal embryopathy is related to the dose of warfarin used and that it occurs mostly in women taking a daily dose over 5 mg.[31] In a relatively small series of 58 pregnancies, women whose warfarin doses were more than 5 mg had 22 fetal complications, whereas those taking a dose of 5 mg or less, had only five fetal complications ($P = 0.0001$).[31] These complications included four miscarriages and one woman with fetal growth restriction. None of the babies born to mothers taking warfarin in a dose of 5 mg or less had evidence of embryopathy. In the higher dose group, two fetuses miscarried in the sixth month of pregnancy, showing typical features of warfarin embryopathy. In these women the doses of warfarin were 6.5 and 7.5 mg.[31] The authors noted a relatively high miscarriage rate in this overall series, most commonly in the first 3 months of pregnancy, but argued that it was similar to the miscarriage rate reported in other series of women treated with subcutaneous heparin in the first trimester.[18,33] The authors suggested, therefore, that there was no advantage in the use of heparin during the first trimester to prevent fetal loss.

While this dose-related response to warfarin is not reported in all series, it merits serious consideration and might permit a risk stratification approach for women who have high-risk prostheses. These would include those with mitral tilting disc valves who might be at a greater risk of valve thrombosis, particularly those in atrial fibrillation or those with a prior thromboembolic event. If the potential mother is taking a low dose of warfarin, therefore, the possibility of continuing oral anticoagulants throughout the pregnancy to reduce the risk of valve thrombosis should be carefully discussed with the mother at the time of preconception counselling. This also has medico-legal implications since, in North America, warfarin is sold on the basis that it is contraindicated in pregnancy, so the prospective mother must be well informed about the potential risks and benefits of each anticoagulant approach, and must agree to its use on this basis, if the practitioner is to avoid being sued.

Warfarin should certainly be discontinued at around 35 weeks of gestation prior to anticipated labour, and heparin should be substituted at that point. The fetus is effectively 'overdosed' on warfarin because of its immature liver enzyme systems and low levels of vitamin K-dependent clotting factors.[35] Warfarin takes some days to be eliminated from the fetus, and as such, these babies are at increased risk of intracranial haemorrhage and should not be allowed to deliver vaginally.[36] Caesarean section is therefore indicated in this setting unless delivery can be delayed until the effects of the warfarin have worn off. In general, if there is an anticipated likelihood of premature delivery, the change from oral anticoagulants to heparin should be initiated earlier.

Low molecular weight heparin

There is much interest in the use of low molecular weight heparin in pregnancy because of its ease of use and superior bioavailability. Low molecular weight heparin does not cross the placenta and also has a lower frequency of heparin-induced thrombocytopenia. In addition, there is probably a reduced risk of osteoporosis with its use. Challenges with its use include that it has a long half-life and is not easily reversed. Furthermore, a spectrum of anticoagulation tests detect measurable pharmacodynamic differences between the various currently available low molecular weight heparin preparations when they are administered so as to achieve equivalent anti-Xa doses.[37]

The data on the use of low molecular weight heparin during pregnancy in the setting of mechanical heart valves are few and confined to small groups of women.[38,39] Several case reports detailing its use have appeared in the literature, and both valve thrombosis and maternal death have been reported with its use.[39–41] Because of the risks of valve thrombosis, the manufacturers of enoxaparin issued a warning against its use in pregnant women with mechanical prosthetic heart valves (Lovenox® injection package insert, Aventis Pharmaceuticals, 2002). This warning was prompted following a study in South Africa comparing unfractionated heparin and enoxaparin given in a dose of 1 mg/kg twice daily subcutaneously. The study was discontinued after two of seven women treated with enoxaparin died from valve thrombosis.[16] Concern has been expressed about the validity of this study, however, and it has been suggested that anti-Xa levels were not achieved because of poor compliance. Some authors have subsequently suggested that low molecular weight heparin can be used effectively, but that the usual standard weight-adjusted dosing should be avoided. The American College of Chest Physicians recommendation is that women who elect to use low molecular weight heparin should have it administered twice daily, and should be dosed to achieve anti-Xa levels of 1–1.2 iu/ml 4–6 hours after subcutaneous injection. This could be used throughout pregnancy or until the 13th week, when warfarin may be substituted until the middle of the third trimester, and then heparin restarted.[23]

Because the reported series are very small, however, the value of antifactor Xa in terms of efficacy and safety remains to be established, and no large series have been published. The use of low molecular weight heparin in pregnancy with mechanical heart valves therefore remains controversial. Certainly, standard doses of low molecular weight heparin should not be used and, if low molecular weight heparin is used, the optimum dosage should be achieved using meticulous anti-Xa monitoring.

As with unfractionated heparin, low molecular weight heparin is cleared through the kidney and subject to pharmacokinetics that vary during pregnancy.[42] Because of the physiological changes in pregnancy such as increased plasma volume, increased glomerular filtration rate and production of placental heparinase, enoxaparin appears to have a higher clearance and larger volume of distribution during early pregnancy compared with that in the same women postpartum.[43] Between early and late pregnancy the maximum concentration achieved decreases, consistent with the volume expansion of pregnancy.[43] Barbour et al.[44] reported considerable variability in the anti-Xa activity with low molecular weight heparin use throughout the three trimesters, and it was noteworthy that using the manufacturer's recommended dosage for twice daily dalteparin of 100 iu/kg, only 54% of pregnancies achieved therapeutic peak anti-Xa levels.

Oran et al.[45] reviewed pregnancy data published between 1989 and 2004 regarding low molecular weight heparin. There were 74 women with 81 pregnancies, most of whom had a mitral valve prosthesis. In 60 pregnancies, low molecular weight heparin was used throughout while in 21 pregnancies low molecular weight heparin was used in the second half of the first trimester and again at term. In 51 pregnancies the anti-Xa levels were monitored to determine that dosage was adequate, while in 30 pregnancies a fixed dose was used. Thromboemboli occurred in ten of the 81 pregnancies (12%). All of these women had mitral valve prostheses, again emphasising that these valves are more vulnerable to thromboembolic complications. All the women with thromboemboli were on low molecular weight heparin throughout pregnancy and nine of the ten were on the fixed dose regimen. These results underscore the need for meticulous monitoring of anti Xa levels and the recommendation from these authors is that the anti-Xa levels 4–6 hours post-injection should be maintained at a minimum of 1 iu/ml.

The use of low molecular weight heparin thus remains profoundly problematic. There have been no very large series reported, and few data to establish the appropriate levels of anti-Xa that should be achieved. If this approach is used, it is suggested that anti-Xa activity should be measured at least every 2 weeks (both peak and trough levels), and the dosage adjusted accordingly. The heparin should be withdrawn at least

24 hours before delivery and changed to intravenous unfractionated heparin that can be terminated abruptly. This permits more controlled cessation of anticoagulation, since there is concern about bleeding and haematoma development if epidural anaesthesia is to be used.

Aspirin

Low-dose aspirin given in the second and third trimesters of pregnancy may be a useful adjunctive therapy to prevent valve thrombosis.[46] One meta-analysis of non-pregnant women reported that the addition of antiplatelet therapy to oral anticoagulants further reduces the risk of arterial embolism by about two-thirds in women with mechanical prosthetic heart valves.[47] Imperiale *et al.*[48] demonstrated that, if given in low-dose (60–150 mg/day), for pregnancy-induced hypertension or intra-uterine growth restriction, it is safe for both the mother and the fetus. Some degree of uncertainty remains, however, regarding its safety in the first trimester.

Conclusions

In summary, there is no perfect management strategy for women with prosthetic heart valves. If the mother has a tissue prosthesis, a reoperation is inevitable eventually, with its attendant risks. Mechanical prostheses are more problematic than tissue prostheses during pregnancy, particularly mitral prostheses, and especially the older generation of valves in this position. There is no perfect anticoagulant strategy and each approach has its own set of problems. Warfarin is associated with increased embryopathy and fetal loss, although less so when the dose is less than 5 mg daily. Since warfarin is a more effective anticoagulant than heparin in pregnancy, this may be the best alternative in women who are at higher risk of valve thrombosis. Alternatively, unfractionated heparin can be used in the first trimester, although APTT monitoring must be meticulous and should be maintained at least twice the control value. It is possible that the addition of periodic anti-Xa levels monitoring may be helpful in this regard although there are no prospective controlled trials to help inform this decision. Warfarin may be substituted at around 13 weeks of gestation but should be discontinued well in advance of anticipated labour. Heparin should be used from about 35 weeks, in anticipation of delivery.

There are few data regarding the use of low molecular weight heparin and while it seems an attractive option because it does not cross the placenta, maternal deaths have been reported with its use. If low molecular weight heparin is used, meticulous anti-Xa monitoring is necessary, maintaining 4 hour post-injection anti-Xa levels at around 1–1.2 iu/ml. Once organogenesis in the fetus is complete and there is no risk of embryopathy, after the first trimester it is probably preferable to discontinue heparin and substitute warfarin during the second and early third trimesters, changing back to unfractionated heparin well before delivery.

Adjunctive aspirin therapy in the second and third trimesters should be considered with any of the above regimens. Long-term anticoagulants should be resumed as soon as possible postpartum.

References

1.   Elkayam UR. Anticoagulation in pregnant women with prosthetic heart valves: a double jeopardy. *J Am Coll Cardiol* 1996;27:1704–6.

2. Warnes CA, Scott ML, Silver GM, Smith CW, Ferrans VJ, Roberts WC. Comparison of late degenerative changes in porcine bioprostheses in the mitral and aortic valve position in the same patient. *Am J Cardiol* 1983;51:965–8.

3. North RA, Sadler L, Stewart AW, McCowan LM, Kerr AR, White HD. Long-term survival and valve-related complications in young women with cardiac valve replacements. *Circulation* 1999;99:2669–76.

4. Yun KL, Miller DC, Moore KA, Mitchell RS, Oyer PE, Stinson EB, *et al.* Durability of the Hancock MO bioprosthesis compared with standard aortic valve bioprostheses. *Ann Thorac Surg* 1995;60(2 Suppl):S221–8.

5. Jamieson WR, Janusz MT, Miyagishima RT, Munro AI, Gerein AN, Allen P, *et al.* The Carpentier–Edwards standard porcine bioprosthesis: long-term evaluation of the high pressure glutaraldehyde fixed prosthesis. *J Card Surg* 1988;3(3 Suppl):321–36.

6. Badduke BR, Jamieson WR, Miyagishima RT, Munro AI, Gerein AN, MacNab J, *et al.* Pregnancy and childbearing in a population with biologic valvular prostheses. *J Thorac Cardiovasc Surg* 1991;102:179–86.

7. Jamieson WR, Miller DC, Akins CW, Munro AI, Glower DD, Moore KA, *et al.* Pregnancy and bioprostheses: influence on structural valve deterioration. *Ann Thorac Surg* 1995;60(2 Suppl):S282–6; discussion S287.

8. Elkayam U, Bitar F. Valvular heart disease and pregnancy. Part II. Prosthetic valves. *J Am Coll Cardiol* 2005;46:403–10.

9. Hung L, Rahimtoola SH. Prosthetic heart valves and pregnancy. *Circulation* 2003;107:1240–6.

10. Sbarouni E, Oakley CM. Outcome of pregnancy in women with valve prostheses. *Br Heart J* 1994;71:196–201.

11. Bortolotti U, Milano A, Mazzucco A, Valfre C, Russo R, Valente M, *et al.* Pregnancy in patients with a porcine valve bioprosthesis. *Am J Cardiol* 1982;50:1051–4.

12. Born D, Martinez EE, Almeida PA, Santos DV, Carvalho AC, Moron AF, *et al.* Pregnancy in patients with prosthetic heart valves: the effects of anticoagulation on mother, fetus, and neonate. *Am Heart J* 1992;124:413–17.

13. Sadler L, McCowan L, White H, Stewart A, Bracken M, North R. Pregnancy outcomes and cardiac complications in women with mechanical, bioprosthetic and homograft valves. *BJOG* 2000;107:245–53.

14. Avila WS, Rossi EG, Grinberg M, Ramires JA. Influence of pregnancy after bioprosthetic valve replacement in young women: a prospective five-year study. *J Heart Valve Dis* 2002;11:864–9.

15. Salazar E, Espinola N, Roman L, Casanova JM. Effect of pregnancy on the duration of bovine pericardial bioprostheses. *Am Heart J* 1999;137(4 Pt 1):714–20.

16. Elkayam U, Singh H, Irani A, Akhter MW. Anticoagulation in pregnant women with prosthetic heart valves. *J Cardiovasc Pharmacol Ther* 2004;9:107–15.

17. Meschengieser SS, Fondevila CG, Santarelli MT, Lazzari MA. Anticoagulation in pregnant women with mechanical heart valve prostheses. *Heart* 1999;82:23–6.

18. Salazar E, Izaguirre R, Verdejo J, Mutchinick O. Failure of adjusted doses of subcutaneous heparin to prevent thromboembolic phenomena in pregnant patients with mechanical cardiac valve prostheses. *J Am Coll Cardiol* 1996;27:1698–703.

19. Dahlman TC. Osteoporotic fractures and the recurrence of thromboembolism during pregnancy and the puerperium in 184 women undergoing thromboprophylaxis with heparin. *Am J Obstet Gynecol* 1993;168:1265–70.

20. Warkentin TE. Heparin-induced thrombocytopenia in patients treated with low-molecular-weight heparin or unfractionated heparin. *Can J Cardiol* 1995;11 Suppl C:29C–34C.

21. Decousus HA, Croze M, Levi FA, Jaubert JG, Perpoint BM, De Bonadona JF, et al. Circadian changes in anticoagulant effect of heparin infused at a constant rate. *Br Med J (Clin Res Ed)* 1985;290:341–4.

22. Chunilal SD, Young E, Johnston MA, Robertson C, Naguit I, Stevens P, et al. The APTT response of pregnant plasma to unfractionated heparin. *Thromb Haemost* 2002;87:92–7.

23. Bates SM, Greer IA, Hirsh J, Ginsberg JS. Use of antithrombotic agents during pregnancy: the Seventh ACCP Conference on Antithrombotic and Thrombolytic Therapy. *Chest* 2004;126(3 Suppl):627S–44S.

24. Brill-Edwards PA, Demers C, Donovan D, et al. Establishing a therapeutic range for heparin therapy. *Chest* 1993;104:1679–84.

25. Ginsberg JS, Hirsh J. Use of antithrombotic agents during pregnancy. *Chest* 1995;108(4 Suppl):305S–11S.

26. Chan WS, Anand S, Ginsberg JS. Anticoagulation of pregnant women with mechanical heart valves: a systematic review of the literature. *Arch Intern Med* 2000;160:191–6.

27. Anderson DR, Ginsberg JS, Burrows R, Brill-Edwards P. Subcutaneous heparin therapy during pregnancy: a need for concern at the time of delivery. *Thromb Haemost* 1991;65:248–50.

28. Hall JG, Pauli RM, Wilson KM. Maternal and fetal sequelae of anticoagulation during pregnancy. *Am J Med* 1980;68:122–40.

29. Ginsberg JS, Hirsh J, Turner DC, Levine MN, Burrows R. Risks to the fetus of anticoagulant therapy during pregnancy. *Thromb Haemost* 1989;61:197–203.

30. Cotrufo M, de Luca TS, Calabro R, Mastrogiovanni G, Lama D. Coumarin anticoagulation during pregnancy in patients with mechanical valve prostheses. *Eur J Cardiothorac Surg* 1991;5:300–4; discussion 305.

31. Vitale N, De Feo M, De Santo LS, Pollice A, Tedesco N, Cotrufo M. Dose-dependent fetal complications of warfarin in pregnant women with mechanical heart valves. *J Am Coll Cardiol* 1999;33:1637–41.

32. Iturbe-Alessio I, Fonseca MC, Mutchinik O, Santos MA, Zajarias A, Salazar E. Risks of anticoagulant therapy in pregnant women with artificial heart valves. *N Engl J Med* 1986;315:1390–3.

33. Sareli P, England MJ, Berk MR, Marcus RH, Epstein M, Driscoll J, et al. Maternal and fetal sequelae of anticoagulation during pregnancy in patients with mechanical heart valve prostheses. *Am J Cardiol* 1989;63:1462–5..

34. Wesseling J, Van Driel D, Heymans HS, Rosendaal FR, Geven-Boere LM, Smrkovsky M, et al. Coumarins during pregnancy: long-term effects on growth and development of school-age children. *Thromb Haemost* 2001;85:609–13.

35. Bonnar J. Haemostasis and coagulation disorders in pregnancy. In: Bloom AL, Thomas DP, editors. *Haemostasis and Thrombosis*. Edinburgh: Churchill Livingstone; 1987. p. 570–84.

36. Thorp JA, Poskin MF, McKenzie DR, Heimes B. Perinatal factors predicting severe intracranial hemorrhage. *Am J Perinatol* 1997;14:631–6.

37. White RH, Ginsberg JS. Low-molecular-weight heparins: are they all the same? *Br J Haematol* 2003;121:12–20.

38. Lee LH, Liauw PC, Ng AS. Low molecular weight heparin for thromboprophylaxis during pregnancy in 2 patients with mechanical mitral valve replacement. *Thromb Haemost* 1996;76:628–30.

39. Rowan JA, McCowan LM, Raudkivi PJ, North RA. Enoxaparin treatment in women with mechanical heart valves during pregnancy. *Am J Obstet Gynecol* 2001;185:633–7.

40. Lev-Ran O, Kramer A, Gurevitch J, Shapira I, Mohr R. Low-molecular-weight

heparin for prosthetic heart valves: treatment failure. *Ann Thorac Surg* 2000;69:264–5; discussion 265–6.

41. Mahesh B, Evans S, Bryan AJ. Failure of low molecular-weight heparin in the prevention of prosthetic mitral valve thrombosis during pregnancy: case report and a review of options for anticoagulation. *J Heart Valve Dis* 2002;11:745–50.

42. Sephton V, Farquharson RG, Topping J, Quenby SM, Cowan C, Back DJ, et al. A longitudinal study of maternal dose response to low molecular weight heparin in pregnancy. *Obstet Gynecol* 2003;101:1307–11.

43. Casele HL, Laifer SA, Woelkers DA, Venkataramanan R. Changes in the pharmacokinetics of the low-molecular-weight heparin enoxaparin sodium during pregnancy. *Am J Obstet Gynecol* 1999;181(5 Pt 1):1113–7.

44. Barbour LA, Oja JL, Schultz LK. A prospective trial that demonstrates that dalteparin requirements increase in pregnancy to maintain therapeutic levels of anticoagulation. *Am J Obstet Gynecol* 2004;191:1024–9.

45. Oran B, Lee-Parritz A, Ansell J. Low molecular weight heparin for the prophylaxis of thromboembolism in women with prosthetic mechanical heart valves during pregnancy. *Thromb Haemost* 2004;92:747–51.

46. Ginsberg JS, Chan WS, Bates SM, Kaatz S. Anticoagulation of pregnant women with mechanical heart valves. *Arch Intern Med* 2003;163:694–8.

47. Cappelleri JC, Fiore LD, Brophy MT, Deykin D, Lau J. Efficacy and safety of combined anticoagulant and antiplatelet therapy versus anticoagulant monotherapy after mechanical heart-valve replacement: a metaanalysis. *Am Heart J* 1995;130(3 Pt 1):547–52.

48. Imperiale TF, Petrulis AS. A meta-analysis of low-dose aspirin for the prevention of pregnancy-induced hypertensive disease. *JAMA* 1991;266:260–4.

Chapter 12
Aortopathies, including Marfan syndrome and coarctation

Lorna Swan

Overview of the clinical problem

The most recent confidential enquiry into maternal mortality in the UK documented eight deaths from aortic dissection in the preceding 10 years.[1] This accounts for approximately 20% of maternal cardiac fatalities – a similar proportion to that for coronary artery or pulmonary vascular disease. The exact level of morbidity associated with aortic pathology during pregnancy is unknown but is likely to be substantial. This is particularly important because many of the adverse outcomes associated with aortopathies are potentially preventable (which is not true of all forms of cardiac disease in pregnancy). We should therefore identify those women prone to dissection and tailor therapeutic options to minimise their risk

Normal aortic function during pregnancy

The haemodynamic consequences of pregnancy, such as an increase in circulating volume and a reduction in systemic vascular resistance, are well documented.[2,3] Functional and structural adaptive change is also seen in the aorta. During normal pregnancy the left ventricular outflow tract and aorta dilate a little (approximately 5%) and the aorta becomes more compliant.[4,5] These changes are most likely due to the interplay of haemodynamic and hormonal factors; however, precise mechanisms are not fully understood. Many of the changes are adaptive, to optimise cardiovascular function (for example a reduction in vascular resistance in combination with an increase in aortic compliance will assist left ventricular ejection). However, in a vulnerable aorta these same adaptive features can result in pathology.

The aorta contains oestrogen receptors and some components of protein function, such as matrix metalloproteinase (MMP) activity, are under direct hormonal influence.[6,7] Structural changes in great artery function that are documented include reticulin fibre fragmentation, loss of acid mucopolysaccharides and impaired elastic fibre corrugation. Arterial cystic medial necrosis has also been reported in healthy pregnant women.[8] Aortic dissection is most common in the third trimester and peripartum which may suggest that superimposed haemodynamic factors are predominant at this latter stage.[9]

Aortopathies and related conditions

There are a wide range of congenital and acquired pathologies that predispose to aortopathy and dissection:

- Marfan syndrome
- coarctation of the aorta (native and repaired)
- bicuspid aortic valve disease
- Turner syndrome
- other connective tissue disorders, e.g. Ehlers–Danlos syndrome type IV
- tetralogy of Fallot (rare)
- Takayasu arteritis
- trauma
- drugs (e.g crack cocaine)
- severe hypertension
- atherosclerosis
- infection (rare).

Many of the principles involved in the management of these disorders are similar irrespective of aetiology. This paper will concentrate on two of the most common disorders encountered in pregnancy – Marfan syndrome and coarctation of the aorta.

Marfan syndrome

Marfan syndrome is an inheritable connective tissue disorder with an autosomal dominant inheritance.[10] In the UK there are approximately 10 000 individuals with Marfan syndrome. Assuming a normal fertility pattern one would expect approximately 150 pregnancies in women with Marfan syndrome annually.[11] The actual number of pregnancies will probably be less, as some of these women will choose not to have a family for various reasons, including concerns over the recurrence risk and fears regarding maternal wellbeing.[12]

Only a proportion of women with Marfan syndrome will be fully aware of their diagnosis and under appropriate specialist follow-up. Knowledge of the implications of pregnancy and the opportunity for prepregnancy counselling are not universal. This is of concern as, without prepregnancy counselling, important health checks in an asymptomatic mother will be omitted, and the opportunity for informed decision making may be lost

Non-aortopathy complications of Marfan syndrome

Aortic aneurysm formation and dissection are, by far, the most concerning features of Marfan syndrome. However Marfan syndrome is a wider connective tissue disorder with other sequelae that may have an impact on all stages of pregnancy and delivery.

Mitral valve regurgitation due to a floppy or prolapsing mitral valve is another common cardiac manifestation.[13] Regurgitant lesions are usually well tolerated during pregnancy. An exception to this is when there is a degree of pre-existing ventricular dysfunction which may be adversely affected by further volume loading.

A number of obstetric complications have been described in women with Marfan syndrome:

- aortic dissection, aneurysm formation
- aortic regurgitation with or without ventricular dysfunction
- mitral valve prolapse with or without regurgitation with or without ventricular dysfunction
- early pregnancy loss – possible association with habitual abortion
- premature rupture of membranes
- pelvis instability, back pain
- cervical weakness, uterine inversion
- postpartum haemorrhage
- poor fetal outcome (and recurrence risk).

Whether these associations are genuine and causal is unclear.

Pregnancy as a risk factor for aortic disease

A relationship between pregnancy and aortic dissection was first reported in 1944.[14] However, the validity and strength of this relationship is not clear. In this respect the literature is probably misleading. A plethora of case reports, which are notoriously prone to negative publication bias (cases with an abnormal outcome are thought to be worth writing up whereas a normal outcome is thought unremarkable and is not reported), would suggest a strong relationship. Indeed, the earliest papers suggested than in women with Marfan syndrome under the age of 40 years 50% of dissections are associated with pregnancy.[15,16]

In contrast, recent cohort studies have suggested that this association is less marked than had previously been thought.[17] Meijboom et al.[18] followed a population of women with Marfan syndrome and documented surprisingly stable aortic root diameters throughout pregnancy and the puerperium (Table 12.1). They stated that in women without a history of aortic involvement, dissection during pregnancy is uncommon.

Table 12.1.   Growth of the aortic root; data from Meijboom et al.[18]

	Pregnancy group (n = 22)	Control childless group (n = 22)	P
Overall	0.28 mm/year	0.19 mm/year	0.08
Root < 40 mm at baseline	0.20 mm/year	0.20 mm/year	0.96
Root > 40 mm at baseline	0.36 mm/year	0.14 mm/year	0.001

These data are based on a mean follow-up of 6.4 years (3 years prepregnancy and 3 years post)

Table 12.2. Marfan recommendations in the public domain

Guideline	Aortic root diameter	Beta blockers	Delivery
European Society of Cardiology (ESC), 2003[19]	< 40 mm – 1% risk of dissection > 40 mm – 10% risk of dissection	Continue	> 45 mm – consider caesarean
American College of Cardiology (ACC)/American Heart Association (AHA), 1998[20]	> 50 mm – elective surgery preconception > 40 mm at booking – consider termination	Continue	Short second stage or perhaps caesarean section (under general anaesthetic)
National Marfan Foundation (USA) website[21]	> 50 mm – 'extreme' risk > 40 mm – individual risk assessment	Most patients	Dilated root – consider caesarean
Marfan Association (UK) website[22]	'Very personal decision' (no further details given)	–	–

Risk stratification

The European Society of Cardiology[19] and the American Heart Association/American College of Cardiology[20] have produced guidelines on the optimal management of women with Marfan syndrome considering pregnancy (Table 12.2). In addition, the Marfan self-help groups also distribute written and electronic information to their members.[21,22] There are small differences between these guidelines but agreement on the general principles governing management, which can be summarised as follows:

1. All women with known Marfan syndrome should be aware of the implications of pregnancy and should, if they wish, have access to expert prepregnancy advice.

2. Women with an aortic root less than 40 mm should be reassured that the risks are less than that of someone with a larger root. A figure of approximately 1% should be given for a significant adverse cardiac event. This risk may be greater if there is a positive family history of dissection.

3. Women with an aortic root above 40 mm should be aware of the increased risk of an adverse outcome. This risk increases with size, rapid rate of change and a positive family history. It should be appreciated that the risk is likely to be a continuum, increasing with increasing root diameter. The risk does not suddenly increase from low to high at a diameter of 40 mm, although this is a convenient reference value for counselling.

4. Beta blockers should be offered to all women with Marfan syndrome and consideration given to continuing these throughout pregnancy.

Although the majority of dissections occur owing to proximal root dilatation, fatal dissection can occur outwith this setting. Dissection can even occur in 'low-risk' aortas that are not dilated.[23] Although this is rare, the woman needs to be aware that a reassuring echo does not equate to 'no risk'. A positive family history of dissection or a rapid increase in the aortic diameter should also be added into the equation when discussing risk.[24,25]

Distal aortic dissection is often unpredictable. Immer *et al.*[26] have suggested that for proximal dissections, root diameter and rate of change are reliable predictors but that there are no equivalent predictors for more distal dissection. The distal aorta also has the disadvantage of being more difficult to image than the root.

Successful pregnancies have been documented in women with previous aortic root replacement but most specialists still regard these women as being at a significant risk of further events. When a composite metal valve and graft have been used, the risks associated with anticoagulation complicate care further.[27]

It should be reiterated that the absence of risk factors does not equate with no risk. In comparison with the average healthy woman in the West, where the maternal mortality is about 1 in 20 000, any Marfan pregnancy is 'high risk'.

Medical therapy

Chronic beta blockade, originally achieved with high-dose propranolol, slows the rate of aortic root enlargement and reduces the risk of aortic dissection in patients with Marfan syndrome.[28] This is thought to be due to direct blood pressure effects, changes in aortic compliance and to alterations in aortic pressure–area relationships.[29] Although patient response to beta blockers may be rather heterogeneous they remain the mainstay of medical treatment in this population.[30] Current guidelines suggest that all women with Marfan syndrome should be beta blocked irrespective of their aortic root dimensions.[19] During pregnancy the risk versus benefit needs to be discussed fully but for most women it is advisable that beta blockers be continued. Calcium channel blockers are occasionally used when patients are intolerant of beta blockers but the data for this therapy are less robust.[31]

Prenatal diagnosis

Prenatal diagnosis using gene probes, using fetally derived cells either from chorionic villus sampling at 13 weeks or from amniocentesis at 16 weeks, can be offered if the family genetic mutation is known. It is easier to identify the mutation if there are several family members affected.[32] Women should be referred to the clinical geneticist prior to pregnancy as establishing which of the multiple genes determining fibrillin development is involved may be a prolonged process.

Monitoring during pregnancy

Echocardiography is the foundation of aortic imaging for the well patient. This can simply and non-invasively track the diameters of the aortic root and assess the aortic valve. The aortic root is best measured at three levels, the 'annulus', the sinuses of Valsalva and the aorto-tubular junction, from the long-axis parasternal window. Imaging every 6–10 weeks has been suggested by several groups.[33]

Magnetic resonance imaging (MRI) can be performed during pregnancy. Some units insist on only scanning after the first trimester.[34] Computed tomography (CT) gives a significant dose of radiation exposure (in excess of 100 chest X-rays) but the benefit of the information obtained may outweigh this risk.[35]

Transoesophageal echocardiography (TOE) is an alternative method of imaging the thoracic aorta and root but is less helpful for imaging the arch. During pregnancy the increased risk of gastro-oesophageal reflux means that TOE should be done with a protected airway (i.e. under a general anaesthetic with endotracheal intubation). In practice, TOE is rarely needed in this scenario.

Symptoms of dissection

Catastrophic cardiovascular collapse may be the first sign of dissection, in which case the diagnosis is often clear. Other symptoms heralding a new event include chest and back pain, dizziness, collapse and haemoptysis. Caution should be exercised with women who present with suspected pulmonary thromboembolism and negative investigations.[1] Women with Marfan syndrome should be warned regarding symptoms of dissection and encouraged to actively request cardiac review if they present unwell to their local hospital. The Marfan associations encourage affected people to wear or carry medical alert information. A low threshold for early imaging (either MRI or CT) is essential.

Treatment of aortic dissection or 'near dissection' during pregnancy

If echocardiography demonstrates increasing aortic root diameters during pregnancy then difficult management decisions need to be faced. New aortic regurgitation may also be another indication of a developing 'unstable' situation.

If the fetus is viable, it has been suggested that the woman should be delivered promptly and then undergo urgent, or semi-urgent, root surgery.[26,36] This is usually either a composite 'root and valved' graft or a valve-sparing aortic root replacement retaining the woman's own aortic valve.[37,38] If the clinical situation allows, there should be a window between delivery and subsequent cardiac surgery (some units suggest 48 hours) to minimise the risks of postpartum bleeding. If the pregnancy is at a pre-viable stage, root surgery may need to be undertaken with the fetus *in situ*. There are cardiopulmonary bypass techniques that can minimise fetal risk but bypass is nevertheless associated with fetal loss.[39] Normotensive high-flow, high-pressure techniques can minimise the hypotensive ischaemic insult to the feto-placental bed (see Chapter 8 on invasive procedures in pregnancy for more detail).[40]

It may be possible to treat distal dissections non-surgically, assuming there is no extravasation of blood and no loss of arterial supply to a critical organ. Endovascular repairs are possible but there are no data regarding this technique during pregnancy. As with all dissections, meticulous attention to blood pressure is paramount.

Delivery issues

Obstetrician and cardiologists hold strong views regarding the optimal way to deliver mothers with cardiac disease. However, outwith the setting of breech delivery there are no randomised data to suggest either vaginal delivery or caesarean section is systematically superior.

In this population the important principles determining delivery are:

1. timing – when there is evidence of an unstable aorta, delivery may need to be before term and at short notice

2. adequate control of blood pressure with invasive monitoring

3. minimisation of the catecholamine response and reduction of aortic sheer stress; with a vaginal delivery this usually means an assisted second stage with regional analgesia.

Women with Marfan syndrome often have dural ectasia and spinal deformities. This potentially increases the likelihood of a failed or patchy epidural,[41] although this is rarely a clinical problem.

The risk of postpartum haemorrhage should be anticipated. Bolus doses of vaso-pressor agents, such as ergometrine, should be avoided. In the presence of significant valve involvement, prophylaxis against endocarditis should not be forgotten for caesarean or instrumented deliveries.

In women with a dilated aortic root the risk of dissection persists after delivery. During the puerperium meticulous blood pressure control and further cardiac assess-ment should be performed. Women with Marfan syndrome are not appropriate for early discharge.

Coarctation of the aorta

Coarctation of the aorta, a narrowing in the aorta usually at the site of the ductus arteriosus, accounts for 5–8% of congenital heart disease.[42] Although the majority of coarctations are detected in the neonatal period, they may be diagnosed at any age and can present for the first time during pregnancy. Coarctation is commonly associated with other congenital and acquired cardiovascular abnormalities which can impact on pregnancy. The following lesions are associated with coarctation of the aorta:

■ bicuspid aortic valve (with or without regurgitation/stenosis)

■ proximal aortopathy (usually with bicuspid valve)

■ patent duct – often only a neonatal problem

■ ventricular septal defect

■ hypoplasic aortic arch

■ abnormal head and neck vessels (5%)

■ intra-cerebral berry aneurysms (5%)

■ multi-level left heart obstruction (e.g. sub-aortic stenosis, aortic valve disease, parachute mitral valve known as Shone syndrome).

The following sequelae are associated with coarctation:

■ hypertension

■ aortic obstruction (native or re-coarctation)

■ lower body hypotension (affecting the placenta)

■ aortic rupture (especially if patch repair or bicuspid valve)

■ left ventricular hypertrophy with or without failure

■ late atherosclerotic disease (coronaries, cerebral)

■ endocarditis.

This chapter will focus on simple (isolated) coarctation.

In cardiac obstetric practice, the majority of mothers with coarctation will have had previous surgical intervention. In the series of Beauchesne et al.,[43] 32% had native disease.[43] However, even following successful surgical repair, important sequelae remain. The most significant of these are hypertension, re-coarctation and aneurysm formation.

Native coarctation

Women with undiagnosed coarctation may present during pregnancy. This may be the first occasion since childhood that the woman has had a clinical examination or an assessment of their blood pressure. Significant hypertension, especially systolic hypertension, in the first trimester should alert medical staff to the possibility of an occult coarctation.[1] A systolic murmur, especially over the scapulae, may also be present. Good practice should include a measurement of blood pressure in both arms and an assessment of leg pulses (and/or leg blood pressures).

Diagnosis can often be confirmed with echocardiography, although when requesting this examination specific mention of the possibility of a coarctation should be stated to ensure that appropriate images of the aortic arch are obtained. Other imaging modalities (CT or MRI) are often needed to plan treatment, if required.[44]

The presence of a significant coarctation is potentially difficult to manage during pregnancy and indeed both the fetal and maternal life may be at risk. The major concern is severe maternal hypertension that is refractory to drug therapy, and, paradoxically, hypotension of the feto-placental unit.

When severe coarctation is detected, the options include attempting to progress with medical therapy (antihypertensives), surgical repair of the coarctation with the fetus *in situ*, attempting trans-catheter coarctation stenting or terminating the pregnancy. There are no case reports to date of stenting during pregnancy and there are potential concerns regarding the quality of the aortic tissue in this setting.

Repaired coarctation

Hypertension

Late hypertension is common after coarctation repair.[45] This is an age-related phenomenon that can occur even in the absence of re-coarctation.[46] During pregnancy, hypertension may be due to pre-existing, and often unrecognised, hypertension or due to superimposed pregnancy induced hypertension with or without pre-eclampsia. Coarctation of the aorta has been quoted as a risk factor for pregnancy-induced hypertension but whether this is truly a pregnancy-induced elevation of blood pressure is unclear.[47] In the largest cohort of pregnant coarctation patients so far reported, 30% had hypertension. The majority of these had evidence of aortic obstruction (either native, residual or recurrent coarctation).[43]

All care providers (physicians, midwives, anaesthetists, etc.) should be aware that in women with repaired coarctation the left arm blood pressure may be a poor reflection of the systemic pressure owing to previous use of the subclavian artery as part of the initial repair. It is thus good practice to measure the blood pressure in both arms.

Hypertension in this setting can be at least partly controlled using beta blocker therapy, although there is little literature to support this practice. Drugs such as angiotensin-converting enzyme (ACE) inhibitors or angiotensin-receptor blockers tend to be avoided for the dual reasons of possible feto-toxicity and worsening of any coarctation gradient if present (a scenario similar to aortic stenosis).[48] The place of coarctation stenting during pregnancy to control hypertension is not clear.

Re-coarctation

The principles of managing re-coarctation are similar to those with a native lesion. Fortunately re-coarctation gradients (which reflect the severity of the narrowing) are likely to be less severe. It may be useful intermittently to assess lower limb blood pressures to assess the difference between upper and lower body perfusion. The feto-placental unit will obviously be exposed to blood pressures closer to those in the leg rather than in the arm.[49] There is little evidence to suggest that coarctation or re-coarctation increases in severity during pregnancy.[50] The standard therapy for re-coarctation outside pregnancy is stenting.

Aneurysm formation

By far the most concerning complication of coarctation is actually, at least in part, a complication of treatment rather than the lesion *per se*. Women who are of childbearing age will have had surgical repairs in an era when patch grafting was a common technique. This involved placing a diamond-shaped patch of artificial material, such as Dacron™ (polyethylene terephthalate), over the coarctation site. Unfortunately, hindsight has revealed that this technique leads to the formation of repair site pseudo-aneurysms.

Knyshov *et al.*[51] reported a large series of patients with patch repair aneurysms. In this cohort progression and rupture were common. It is therefore important to establish the type of repair a woman may have had prior to, or early on in, pregnancy. This will aid risk stratification. If this information is not available, the worst-case scenario should be assumed (a patch graft) and imaging with MRI performed as early as possible.

The principles of managing these aneurysms are similar to the Marfan aneurysm group. They include serial assessment, meticulous blood pressure control and early intervention. The option of a covered stent graft inserted via a femoral cut-down may be an alternative to re-do surgery. However, even in non-pregnant patients, treatment of such aneurysms, either surgically or by a trans-catheter approach, may be associated with significant morbidity and mortality.

Recurrence risk

The recurrence risk of a fetus having a congenital cardiac lesion if the mother has a coarctation may be up to 10%.[52] Fetal echocardiography should therefore be offered. Diagnosing fetal coarctation can be difficult. More severe left heart disease will be detected with greater ease.

Bicuspid aortic valve disease

The presence of a bicuspid aortic valve is associated with a proximal aortic aortopathy. This can occur in the absence of coarctation or a haemodynamically significant valve lesion.[53] This form of aortic root dilatation is generally more diffuse than that seen in Marfan syndrome (Figure 12.1). The risks of aneurysm formation, aortic regurgitation and aortic dissection are all present. Some centres use Marfan-type guidelines when

(a)

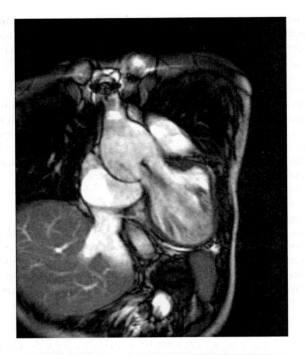

(b)

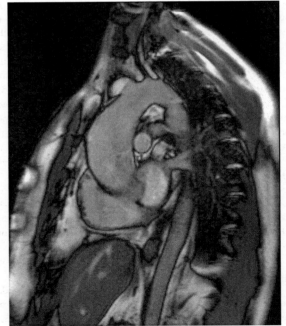

Figure 12.1. (a) Localised aortic root dilatation at the sinuses of Valsalva in Marfan syndrome; (b) diffuse aortic root dilatation in bicuspid aortic valve disease

deciding on treatment options (e.g. beta blockers or surgical referral). However, data are not available to support these practices and it has been suggested that for equivalent root diameters the 'bicuspid aorta' might be less vulnerable.

Turner syndrome

Assisted fertility techniques are now able to facilitate pregnancy in women with Turner syndrome. This has highlighted the potential for dissection in this population. In the non-pregnant Turner population about 16–33% have a degree of aortic root enlargement.[54] The equivalent risk in pregnancy is not known but there are several case reports in the literature of dissection.[43,55] Women should be encouraged to seek cardiology review prior to embarking on such treatment.

Ehlers–Danlos syndrome

Ehlers–Danlos syndrome type IV produces a widespread vasculopathy in addition to its more generalised connective tissue effects. Large artery rupture and significant peripartum bleeding are well recognised.[56] Uterine rupture and pneumothoraces have also been reported and maternal mortality may be up to 20%.[57] Fortunately type IV is relatively rare and other more common forms have a more benign course.

References

1. Lewis G, editor. *Why Mothers Die 2000–2002: The Sixth Report of Confidential Enquiries into Maternal Deaths in the United Kingdom.* London: RCOG Press; 2004.
2. Mabie WC, DiSessa TG, Crocker LG, Sibai BM, Arheart KL. A longitudinal study of cardiac output in normal human pregnancy. *Am J Obstet Gynecol* 1994;170:849–56.
3. Katz R, Karliner JS, Resnik R. Effects of a natural volume overload state (pregnancy) on left ventricular performance in normal human subjects. *Circulation* 1978;58:434–41.
4. Robson SC, Hunter S, Boys RJ, Dunlop W. Serial study of factors influencing changes in cardiac output during pregnancy. *Am J Physiol* 1989;256:H1060–5.
5. Poppas A, Shroff SG, Korcarz CE, Hibbard JU, Berger DS, Lindheimer MD, *et al.* Serial assessment of the cardiovascular system in normal pregnancy. Role of arterial compliance and pulsatile arterial load. *Circulation* 1997;95:2407–15.
6. Campisi D, Cutolo M, Carruba G, Lo Casto M, Comito L, Granata OM, *et al.* Evidence for soluble and nuclear site I binding of estrogens in human aorta. *Atherosclerosis* 1993;103:267–77.
7. Wingrove CS, Garr E, Godsland IF, Stevenson JC. 17beta-oestradiol enhances release of matrix metalloproteinase-2 from human vascular smooth muscle cells. *Biochim Biophys Acta* 1998;1406:169–74.
8. Manallo-Estrella P, Barker AE. Histopathologic findings in human aortic media associated with pregnancy. *Arch Path* 1967;83:336–41.
9. Pedowitz P, Perell A. Aneurysms complicated by pregnancy. I. Aneurysms of the aorta and its major branches. *Am J Obstet Gynecol* 1957;73:720–35.
10. Pyeritz RE. The Marfan syndrome. *Annu Rev Med* 2000;51:481–510.
11. Lind J, Wallenburg HC. The Marfan syndrome and pregnancy: a retrospective study in a Dutch population. *Eur J Obstet Gynecol Reprod Biol* 2001;98:28–35.
12. Meijboom LJ, Drenthen W, Pieper PG, Groenink M, van der Post JA, Timmermans J, *et al.*; On behalf of the ZAHARA investigators. Obstetric complications in Marfan syndrome. *Int J Cardiol* 2006;110:53–9.

13. Pini R, Roman MJ, Kramer-Fox R, Devereux RB. Mitral valve dimensions and motion in Marfan patients with and without mitral valve prolapse. Comparison to primary mitral valve prolapse and normal subjects. *Circulation* 1989;80:915–24.

14. Schnitker MA, Bayer CA. Dissection aneurysm of the aorta in young individuals, particularly in association with pregnancy. *Ann Intern Med* 1944;29:486–511.

15. Williams GM, Gott VL, Brawley RK, Schauble JF, Labs JD. Aortic disease associated with pregnancy. *J Vasc Surg* 1988;8:470–5.

16. Hirst AE, Johns VJ, Kime SW. Dissecting aneurysm of the aorta: a review of 505 cases. *Medicine (Baltimore)* 1958;37:217–79.

17. Oskoui R, Lindsay J. Aortic dissection in women < 40 years of age and the unimportance of pregnancy. *Am J Cardiol* 1994;73:821–3.

18. Meijboom LJ, Vos FE, Timmermans J, Boers GH, Zwinderman AH, Mulder BJ. Pregnancy and aortic root growth in the Marfan syndrome: a prospective study. *Eur Heart J* 2005;26914–20.

19. Oakley C, Child A, Jung B, Presbitero P, Tornos P, Klein W, *et al.* The task force on the management of cardiovascular diseases during pregnancy of the European Society of Cardiology. *Eur H J* 2003;24:761–81.

20. Bonow RO, Carabello B, de Leon AC, Edmunds LH, Junior, Fedderly BJ, Freed MD, *et al.* ACC/AHA guidelines for the management of patients with valvular heart disease. A report of the American College of Cardiology/American Heart Association. Task Force on Practice Guidelines (Committee on Management of Patients with Valvular Heart Disease). *J Am Coll Cardiol* 1998;32:1486–588.

21. Rossiter JP. *Obstetric Concerns.* National Marfan Foundation [www.marfan.org].

22. Marfan Association UK. *Fact Sheet* [www.marfan.org.uk].

23. Groenink M, Lohuis TA, Tijssen JG, Naeff MS, Hennekam RC, van der Wall EE, *et al.* Survival and complication free survival in Marfan's syndrome: implications of current guidelines. *Heart* 1999;82:499–504.

24. Silverman DI, Gray J, Roman MJ, Bridges A, Burton K, Boxer M, *et al.* Family history of severe cardiovascular disease in Marfan syndrome is associated with increased aortic diameter and decreased survival. *J Am Coll Cardiol* 1995;26:1062–7.

25. Legget ME, Unger TA, O'Sullivan CK, Zwink TR, Bennett RL, Byers PH, *et al.* Aortic root complications in Marfan's syndrome: identification of a lower risk group. *Heart* 1996;75:389–95.

26. Immer FF, Bansi AG, Immer-Bansi AS, McDougall J, Zehr KJ, Schaff HV, *et al.* Aortic dissection in pregnancy: analysis of risk factors and outcome. *Ann Thorac Surg* 2003;76:309–14.

27. Williams A, Child A, Rowntree J, Johnson P, Donnai P. Marfan's syndrome: successful pregnancy after aortic root and arch replacement. *BJOG* 2002;109:1187–8.

28. Shores J, Berger KR, Murphy EA, Pyeritz RE. Progression of aortic dilatation and the benefit of long-term beta-adrenergic blockade in Marfan's syndrome. *N Engl J Med* 1994;330:1335–41.

29. Groenink M, de Roos A, Mulder BJ, Spaan JA, van der Wall EE. Changes in aortic distensibility and pulse wave velocity assessed with magnetic resonance imaging following beta-blocker therapy in the Marfan syndrome. *Am J Cardiol* 1998;82:203–8.

30. Rios AS, Silber EN, Bavishi N, Varga P, Burton BK, Clark WA, *et al.* Effect of long-term beta-blockade on aortic root compliance in patients with Marfan syndrome. *Am Heart J* 1999;137:1057–61.

31. Rossi-Foulkes R, Roman MJ, Rosen SE, Kramer-Fox R, Ehlers KH, O'Loughlin JE, *et al.* Phenotypic features and impact of beta blocker or calcium antagonist therapy on aortic lumen size in the Marfan syndrome. *Am J Cardiol* 1999;83:1364–8.

32. Harton GL, Tsipouras P, Sisson ME, Starr KM. Mahoney BS, Fugger EF, et al. Preimplantation genetic testing for Marfan syndrome. *Mol Hum Reprod* 1996;2:713–15.

33. Rossiter JP, Repke JT, Morales AJ, Murphy EA, Pyeritz RE. A prospective longitudinal evaluation of pregnancy in the Marfan syndrome. *Am J Obstet Gynecol* 1995;173:1599–606.

34. Colletti PM, Platt LD, Obstetric MRI acceptable under specific criteria. *Diagn Radiol* 1989;11:84.

35. Aroua A, Bize R, Buchillier-Decka I, Vader JP, Valley JF, Schnyder P. X-ray imaging of the chest in Switzerland in 1998: a nationwide survey. *Eur Radiol* 2003;13:1250–9.

36. Zeebregts CJ. Schepens MA, Hameeteman TM, MorshuisWJ, de la Riviere AB. Acute aortic dissection complicating pregnancy. *Ann Thorac Surg* 1997;64:1345–8.

37. Bentall H, De Bono A. A technique for complete replacement of the ascending aorta. *Thorax* 1968;23:338–9.

38. David TE, Feindel CM. An aortic valve-sparing operation for patients with aortic incompetence and aneurysm of the ascending aorta. *J Thorac Cardiovasc Surg* 1992;103:617–21.

39. Parry AJ, Westaby S. Cardiopulmonary bypass during pregnancy. *Ann Thorac Surg* 1996;61:1865–9.

40. Mahli A, Izdes S, Coskun D. Cardiac operations during pregnancy: review of factors influencing fetal outcome. *Ann Thorac Surg* 2000;69:1622–6.

41. Lacassie HJ, Millar S, Leithe LG, Muir HA, Montana R, Poblete A. Dural ectasia: a likely cause of inadequate spinal anaesthesia in two parturients with Marfan's syndrome. *Br J Anaesth* 2005;94:500–4.

42. Kaemmerer H. Aortic coarctation and interrupted aortic arch. In: Gatzoulis MA, Webb GD, Daubeney PEF, editors. *Diagnosis and Management of Adult Congenital Heart Disease.* London: Churchill Livingstone; 2003. p. 253–65.

43. Beauchesne LM, Connolly HM, Ammash NM, Warnes CA. Coarctation of the aorta: outcome of pregnancy. *J Am Coll Cardiol* 2001;38:1728–33.

44. Stern HC, Locher D, Wallnofer K, Weber F, Scheid KF, Emmrich P, et al. Noninvasive assessment of coarctation of the aorta: comparative measurements by two-dimensional echocardiography, magnetic resonance, and angiography. *Pediatr Cardiol* 1991;12:1–5.

45. Stewart AB, Ahmed R, Travill CM, Newman CG. Coarctation of the aorta life and health 20–44 years after surgical repair. *Br Heart J* 1993;69:65–70.

46. Presbitero P, Demarie D, Villani M, Perinetto EA, Riva G, Orzan F, et al. Long term results (15–30 years) of surgical repair of aortic coarctation. *Br Heart J* 1987;57:462–7.

47. Siu SC, Sermer M, Colman JM, Alvarez AN, Mercier LA, Morton BC, et al. Prospective multicenter study of pregnancy outcomes in women with heart disease. *Circulation* 2001;104:515–21.

48. Barr M. Teratogen update: angiotensin-converting enzyme inhibitors. *Teratology* 1994;50:399–409.

49. Kupferminc MJ, Lessing JB, Jaffa A, Vidne BA, Peyser MR. Fetomaternal blood flow measurements and management of combined coarctation and aneurysm of the thoracic aorta in pregnancy. *Acta Obstet Gynecol Scand* 1993;72:398–402.

50. Kelly D, Amadi A. Serial pressure gradients across a thoracic coarctation of the aorta during pregnancy. *Eur J Echocardiogr* 2005;6:288–90.

51. Knyshov GV, Sitar LL, Glagola MD, Atamanyuk MY. Aortic aneurysms at the site of the repair of coarctation of the aorta: a review of 48 patients. *Ann Thorac Surg* 1996;61:935–9.

52. Rose V. Gold RJM, Lindsay G, Allen M. A possible increase in the incidence of congenital heart defects among the offspring of affected parents. *J Am Coll Cardiol* 1985;6:376–82.

53. Cecconi M, Manfrin M, Moraca A, Zanoli R, Colonna PL, Bettuzzi MG, *et al.* Aortic dimensions in patients with bicuspid aortic valve without significant valve dysfunction. *Am J Cardiol* 2005;95:292–4.
54. Ostberg JE, Brookes JA, McCarthy C, Halcox J, Conway GS. A comparison of echocardiography and magnetic resonance imaging in cardiovascular screening of adults with Turner syndrome. *J Clin Endocrinol Metab* 2004;89:5966–71.
55. Nagel TC, Tesch LG. ART and high risk patients. *Fertil Steril* 1997;68:748–9.
56. Germain DP, Herrera-Guzman Y, Vascular Ehlers–Danlos syndrome. *Ann Genet* 2004;47:1–9.
57. Lurie S, Manor M, Hagay ZJ. The threat of type IV Ehlers–Danlos syndrome on maternal well-being during pregnancy: early delivery may make the difference. *J Obstet Gynaecol* 1998;18:245–8.

Table 13.1. Mitral valve area and severity of mitral stenosis (MS)

MS severity	Mitral valve area (cm²)
Mild	≥1.5
Moderate	1.1–1.5
Severe	≤1.0

Treatment

The mainstay of medical management is to reduce heart rate to allow time for left ventricular filling. This is achieved in women with mild and moderate MS by bedrest, oxygen therapy, beta blockade and a diuretic. If atrial fibrillation occurs, therapeutic-dose low molecular weight heparin anticoagulation should be given, and sinus rhythm restored promptly (see Chapter 18).

If the woman's condition continues to deteriorate treatment depends on the gestational stage of the pregnancy. If the fetus is viable it should be delivered first and then definitive treatment for the MS carried out. If the fetus cannot be delivered with a reasonable prognosis, attempts can be made to relieve the stenosis in the presence of a continuing pregnancy. The cut-off gestation for such decisions has to be individualised, based on the circumstances in each case, but is likely to be somewhere between 26 and 30 weeks.

Balloon mitral valvotomy is the treatment of choice if, as is the case in most young women, the morphology of the valve is suitable. In experienced hands, the procedure has about a 95% success rate[3-5] and carries little risk to the mother or fetus. Radiation doses to the fetus can be reduced somewhat with maternal abdominal screening, and fluoroscopy times should be limited to 5–8 minutes[4-6] (see Chapter 8). The risk of developing acute mitral regurgitation such that emergency mitral valve replacement is necessary is low in centres with high-volume experience; however, on-site facilities for emergency cardiac surgery must be available.

It should be noted that all the publications reporting large numbers of cases come from centres in developing countries (such as India and South America) or those with a high immigrant population. UK data from the British Cardiovascular Intervention Society (BCIS) show that, of the 33 centres that together performed a total of 165 balloon mitral valvotomies in 2004, only six performed more than eight in that year and 13 centres performed only one or two (Figure 13.2). Mitral valvotomy in pregnancy should only be undertaken by an experienced operator and women should be referred to a centre where the procedure is performed frequently.

Where balloon mitral valvotomy is not available, closed mitral valvotomy is a safe alternative, since it avoids the need for cardiopulmonary bypass.[7] This situation will rarely arise in the UK, firstly because catheter techniques are now widely available and secondly because few surgeons now have experience of closed mitral valvotomy.

Any valve replacement during or soon after pregnancy carries a high risk to mother and fetus; cardiac surgery in pregnancy and the puerperium are discussed below.

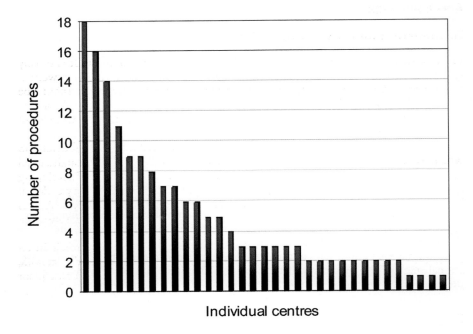

Figure 13.2. Number of mitral balloon valvotomies performed per UK centre in 2004 (total = 165); modified with permission from Peter Ludman and the British Cardiovascular Intervention Society (BCIS)

Mode of delivery

Vaginal delivery, with epidural analgesia, is preferred for the majority of women. Invasive monitoring should be used in symptomatic women and those with severe MS. Antibiotic prophylaxis should be given.

Risk factors for poor outcome in mitral stenosis

The major risk factors for maternal morbidity are severe MS and a history of any prepregnancy cardiac event.[2] The risk of maternal complications rises from 26% in mild MS, to 38% and 67% for moderate and severe MS, respectively. Maternal mortality may be up to 2%.[2,8] Other cardiac and non-cardiac conditions should also be considered when assessing risk. It should be noted that coexisting severe mitral and aortic regurgitation does not increase the risks of pregnancy in mild MS.[2]

The risk of an adverse fetal outcome, including prematurity, intrauterine growth restriction and death, is directly related to the severity of MS.

Aortic stenosis

Introduction and pathophysiology

In the UK, significant AS in women of childbearing age is uncommon. It is usually secondary to bicuspid aortic valve disease, which is four times less common in women than in men. Coexisting congenital cardiac lesions such as coarctation should be considered when assessing the risk and management of pregnancy. Severe rheumatic AS is not common in women of childbearing age; if it is present, there will almost certainly also be severe rheumatic mitral valve disease.

Pregnancy is usually well tolerated in women with isolated mild and moderate AS with good ventricular function. However, the increasing cardiac output through a fixed obstructive lesion means that pregnant women with severe AS are at risk of developing symptoms for the first time, including dyspnoea, angina, syncope, pulmonary oedema, left ventricular failure and sudden death. The risk of maternal death in severe AS has been quoted as 17%, with a fetal mortality of 30%,[9] although more recent data are more encouraging.[10]

The increased circulating volume and stroke volume of pregnancy result in an increase in left ventricular pressure and in the pressure gradient across the stenotic aortic valve. This may result in failure to increase coronary blood flow with consequent compromise to myocardial perfusion, leading to ventricular failure.

Prepregnancy assessment

An asymptomatic woman with isolated AS is likely to tolerate pregnancy well if:

- the resting ECG shows no left ventricular strain pattern
- left ventricular function is normal
- the prepregnancy mean Doppler derived aortic valve pressure gradient is less than 50 mmHg, and the peak gradient less than 80 mmHg
- exercise capacity is normal, with formal exercise testing showing a normal blood pressure rise and no ST segment changes.

Table 13.2 shows the classification of the severity of AS according to ECG assessment.

Table 13.2. Echocardiographic assessment of severity of aortic stenosis (AS)[a]

AS severity	Peak Doppler gradient (non-pregnant) (mm Hg)	Mean Doppler gradient (non-pregnant) (mm Hg)	Valve area (cm²)
Mild	≤ 30	≤ 15	> 1.5
Moderate	31–79	16–49	0.8–1.5
Severe	≥ 80	≥ 50	≤ 0.7

[a] All these estimates are influenced by ventricular function; the severity of aortic stenosis may be underestimated in the presence of impaired ventricular function

Antenatal monitoring

Termination of pregnancy should be discussed as an option for women with severe AS, depending on the gestational age at diagnosis/presentation, and on the wishes and views of the mother and her family.

Signs and symptoms of decompensation during pregnancy include:

■ more dyspnoea or tachycardia than would be expected for a normal pregnancy
■ new-onset angina
■ pulmonary oedema and syncope
■ new ECG changes (ST segment depression).

During pregnancy the aortic valve Doppler gradient should increase as the cardiac output increases. A fall in echo Doppler derived aortic valve gradient suggests that left ventricular function is impaired, and this should be assessed by echocardiography.

Medical management

As with MS, medical treatment is aimed at reducing the heart rate to allow time for left ventricular ejection and coronary filling. Bedrest with oxygen therapy and beta blockade may allow the pregnancy to progress until the fetus can be safely delivered.

Intervention

If the woman's condition deteriorates and the gestational age does not allow for delivery of a baby with a reasonable prognosis, intervention without interrupting the pregnancy can be considered. The options are balloon aortic valvotomy, surgical aortic valvotomy or aortic valve replacement. Compared with the extensive litera-ture on balloon valvotomy for MS, there are only a few case reports of balloon aortic valvotomy during pregnancy, probably reflecting both the rarity of severe AS in pregnancy and the widely accepted poor results of balloon aortic valvotomy in adults.[11]

Aortic balloon valvotomy is usually a palliative procedure in adults, and in pregnant women should be seen as a bridge to aortic valve replacement, allowing sufficient relief of the stenosis to permit the pregnancy to progress. Careful echocardiographic assessment is needed to assess the suitability of the valve for balloon valvotomy since it may result in severe aortic regurgitation or aortic rupture requiring high-risk emergency surgery, tamponade and embolism.

Cardiopulmonary bypass surgery during pregnancy

If surgery for AS is necessary during pregnancy, valve replacement is likely to be necessary, since (as with balloon valvotomy) surgical valvotomy is unlikely to result in adequate relief of stenosis while at the same time leaving a competent valve.

Cardiopulmonary bypass in pregnancy carries a high risk of maternal and fetal demise. The risk of maternal death is up to 15% and that of fetal death between 19% and 33%.[12-14] A number of factors contribute to the high maternal and fetal risk. Operations may need to be performed as an emergency with a haemodynamically unstable woman and at a time when the most experienced team may be unavailable. The hormonal effects of pregnancy render maternal tissues more elastic and friable than in the non-pregnant state, contributing to maternal risk. While the woman is on cardiopulmonary bypass there is a risk of heparin-induced placental bleeding. Low-pressure, non-pulsatile perfusion during bypass reduces placental perfusion. Pulsatile pressure is thought to reduce uterine contractions by inducing nitric oxide release. Cardiopulmonary bypass with pulsatile perfusion has been reported[15] as a possible technique to improve fetal outcome (in four cases, there was one fetal death, with no maternal deaths). For more details on cardiac interventions in pregnancy see Chapter 8.

Labour and delivery in aortic stenosis

Vaginal birth is usually the safest mode of delivery, unless there is an obstetric indication for a caesarean section. Slow and incremental low-dose epidural analgesia is appropriate, taking care to avoid vasodilatation.[16] Women with severe AS should be monitored invasively (with an arterial line and external pressure transducer and central venous access) and careful fluid balance maintained. Antibiotic prophylaxis should be given.

References

1. Lewis G, editor. *Why Mothers Die 2000–2002: The Sixth Report of Confidential Enquiries into Maternal Deaths in the United Kingdom.* London: RCOG Press; 2004.
2. Silversides CK, Colman JM, Sermer M, Siu SC. Cardiac risk in pregnant women with rheumatic mitral stenosis. *Am J Cardiol* 2003;91:1382–5.
3. Nercolini DC, da Rocha Loures Bueno R, Eduardo Guerios E, Tarastchuk JC, Pacheco AL, Pia de Andrade PM, *et al.* Percutaneous mitral balloon valvuloplasty in pregnant women with mitral stenosis. *Catheter Cardiovasc Interv* 2002;57:318–22.
4. Routray SN, Mishra TK, Swain S, Patnaik UK, Behera M. Balloon mitral valvuloplasty during pregnancy. *Int J Gynaecol Obstet* 2004;85:18–23.
5. Gupta A, Lokhandwala YY, Satoskar PR, Salvi VS. Balloon mitral valovotomy in pregnancy: maternal and fetal outcomes. *J Am Coll Cardiol* 1998;187:409–15.
6. Sivadasanpillai H, Srinivasan A, Sivasubramoniam S, Mahadevan KK, Kumar A, Titus T, *et al.* Long term outcome of patients undergoing balloon mitral valvotomy in pregnancy. *Am J Cardiol* 2005;95:1504–6.
7. Aggarwal N, Suri V, Goyal A, Malhotra S, Manoj R, Dhaliwal RS. Closed mitral valvotomy in pregnancy and labour. *Int J Gynecol Obstet*;2205:118–21.
8. Hameed A, Karaalp IS, Tummala PP, Wani OR, Canetti M, Akhter MW, *et al.* The effects of valvular heart disease on maternal and fetal outcome of pregnancy. *J Am Coll Cardiol* 2001;37:893–9.
9. Aria F, Pineda J. Aortic stenosis and pregnancy. *J Reprod Med* 1978;20:229–32.
10. Silversides C, Colman J, Sermer M, Farine D, Siu SC. Early and intermediate-term outcomes of pregnancy with congenital aortic stenosis. *Am J Cardiol* 2003;91:1386–9.
11. Radford D, Walters DL. Balloon aortic valvotomy in pregnancy. *Aust N Z J Obstet Gynaecol* 2004;44:577–9.
12. Gopal K, Hudson IM, Ludmir J, Braffman MN, Ewing S, Bavaria JE, *et al.* Homograft aortic root replacement during pregnancy. *Ann Thorac Surg* 2002;74:243–5.
13. Parry AJ, Westaby S. Cardiopulmonary bypass during pregnancy. *Ann Thorac Surg* 1996;61:1865–9.
14. Chambers CE, Clark SL. Cardiac surgery during pregnancy. *Clin Obstet Gynecol* 1994;37:316–23.

15. Jahangiri M, Clarke J, Prefumo F, Pumphrey C, Ward D. Cardiac surgery during pregnancy: pulsatile or non-pulsatile perfusion? *J Thorac Cardiovasc Surg* 2003;126:894–5.

16. Suntharalingam G, Dob D, Yentis SM. Obstetric epidural analgesia in aortic stenosis: a low-dose technique for labour and instrumental delivery. *Int J Obstet Anesth* 2001;10:129–34.

Chapter 14
Right heart lesions

Anselm Uebing and Michael A Gatzoulis

Introduction

Congenital heart disease (CHD) is the most common inborn defect, with an incidence of 0.8% among infants around the world. The continual improvement in medical and surgical therapy over the past five decades has led to more than 85% of children with congenital heart lesions now surviving into adulthood.[1,2] There are currently about 250 000 adults with congenital heart lesions living in the UK.[3] Half of these are women, mostly of reproductive age. About 40–45% of people born with congenital heart defects have lesions predominantly affecting the right heart.[4] Right heart lesions increase the risks of pregnancy to both the mother and the fetus, and the women affected require specific care to minimise maternal and fetal morbidity and mortality.

This chapter highlights some key issues that women with right-sided congenital heart lesions face. It first summarises some general considerations related to their management and then focuses on specific lesions that predominantly affect the right heart and how these may affect women going through pregnancy.

General considerations

Preconception evaluation and counselling

The management of women with congenital right heart lesions should ideally begin before conception.[5] A careful assessment of functional capacity is needed to estimate the likelihood that the women will tolerate the haemodynamic burden of pregnancy and the potential complications. Preconception evaluation should include a careful history and physical examination, an echocardiogram, electrocardiography (ECG) and a cardiopulmonary exercise test. Cardiac magnetic resonance imaging should be a routine part of this evaluation in women with systemic right ventricles (transposition of the great arteries (TGA) after an atrial switch operation, or congenitally 'corrected' transposition of the great arteries (ccTGA)) and functional univentricular hearts with or without a Fontan-type operation because transthoracic echocardiography often only provides a limited amount of detailed information on ventricular function. The potential risks of pregnancy on the basis of this evaluation should be discussed with the woman and her family, ideally in a joint clinic involving at least a cardiologist specialising in CHD and an obstetrician specialising in high-risk pregnancy.

The risk for pregnant women with CHD of suffering adverse cardiovascular events such as symptomatic arrhythmia, stroke, pulmonary oedema, overt heart failure or death increases with the anatomical complexity of the congenital heart lesion, the degree of cyanosis, myocardial dysfunction, poor functional class and the severity of systemic outflow tract obstruction. Based on retrospective and prospective data from a total of 851 pregnancies among women with heart disease, the following four independent predictors of maternal adverse cardiac events were identified:[6,7]

- poor functional class prior to pregnancy (NYHA class higher than II (see Appendix A)) or cyanosis
- impaired systemic ventricular function (ejection fraction below 40%)
- left heart obstruction (mitral valve area less than 2 cm^2, aortic valve area less than 1.5 cm^2, left ventricular outflow tract peak Doppler gradient more than 30 mmHg prior to pregnancy)
- preconception history of adverse cardiac events such as symptomatic arrhythmia, stroke, transient ischaemic attack and pulmonary oedema.

The need for thorough assessment of individual women with CHD before pregnancy cannot be overemphasised. This assessment then forms the basis for risk stratification, advice and decision making.

Antenatal care

Antenatal care should involve both obstetricians and cardiologists. The frequency of evaluations during pregnancy should be decided on the basis of the severity of the cardiac disease and the woman's functional status. It should be noted that the normal anatomical and functional changes of pregnancies can complicate the clinical evaluation of women with CHD, especially if the right heart is affected. Physical signs such as raised jugular venous pulsation, mild ankle oedema or right ventricular heave do not necessarily indicate right heart failure.

Labour and delivery and the postpartum period

The timing and mode of delivery should be discussed and decided jointly by obstetricians, cardiologists and anaesthetists. Decisions should be made well in advance and be communicated appropriately to the woman and the tertiary and local team members. In our practice we copy all notes, investigations and the recommended delivery plan to the woman.

In principle, vaginal delivery carries a lower risk of complications for both the mother and the fetus. Compared with caesarean section, vaginal delivery causes smaller volume shifts, less haemorrhage, fewer clotting complications and fewer infections.[8] With appropriate anaesthesia and shortening of the second stage of labour, vaginal delivery can be performed safely in most women with right heart congenital lesions. Maternal monitoring during labour and delivery should be individualised and usually includes continuous ECG monitoring and pulse oximetry, and, occasionally, invasive blood pressure recording (intra-arterial line connected to a pressure transducer).

All women with congenital right heart lesions should be warned against lying flat during pregnancy, and especially in labour, to avoid aortocaval compression. Left decubitus position is the position of choice during labour, as it is during pregnancy.

The early postpartum period (third stage of labour and delivery of the placenta) is also a potentially high-risk period. It is associated with large shifts in venous return to the right heart. Uterine contraction and decreased caval compression can increase venous return rapidly. Conversely, blood loss from uterine haemorrhage can reduce venous return. Rapid haemodynamic changes during this period can lead to haemodynamic compromise and management should aim to limit blood volume and blood pressure shifts as much as possible.

Antibiotic prophylaxis

Although not generally recommended by the American Heart Association (AHA)/ American College of Cardiology (ACC) guidelines for uncomplicated vaginal delivery,[9] antibiotic prophylaxis for labour and delivery should be considered for women with congenital right heart lesions because there is a significant risk of bacteraemia at delivery.[10] Antibiotic prophylaxis should certainly be prescribed for all operative deliveries because of the potentially devastating effects of endocarditis.

Congenital right heart lesions

Right heart lesions usually lead to abnormal loading conditions of the right ventricle and can generally be divided into those where the ventricle is predominantly subjected to volume overload or pressure overload.

Volume overload to the right ventricle results from lesions where the pulmonary or tricuspid valve is regurgitant or where additional volume is delivered to the right heart and the pulmonary circulation resulting from left to right shunting (more at the atrial than at the ventricular level). Volume overload is typically increased in lesions such as:

■ atrial septal defect (ASD)
■ pulmonary regurgitation (isolated (rare) or resulting from repair of tetralogy of Fallot (ToF) or relief of pulmonary valve stenosis)
■ Ebstein anomaly of the tricuspid valve.

Pressure overload to the right ventricle results from lesions such as:

■ pulmonary stenosis (isolated or following repair of ToF)
■ ccTGA
■ TGA after Mustard or Senning repair.

The latter two lesions have the right ventricle supporting the systemic circulation. They thus represent an extreme form of right ventricular pressure overload.

In addition, 'univentricular' hearts palliated with a Fontan-type operation can be considered right heart lesions as there is no substantial ventricle to support the pulmonary circulation, although the right heart may not be anatomically involved from the outset. This group of women will thus also be discussed in this chapter.

Furthermore, chronic cyanosis (without pulmonary arterial hypertension) is often a feature of right heart lesions such as pulmonary atresia with ventricular septal defect (VSD) and multiple aortopulmonary collateral arteries (MAPCAs). This lesion will also be discussed in this chapter to highlight some general concepts of care for women with cyanotic heart disease without pulmonary arterial hypertension.

Atrial septal defect

Atrial septal defects account for about 7–10% of cases of CHD and are two to three times more common in women than men.[11] Various forms of ASD exist with respect to their anatomical position in the inter-atrial septum (Figure 14.1). The defect may be located in the region of the oval fossa, forming the ostium secundum ASD, or in the lower part of the inter-atrial septum, forming the ostium primum ASD. The sinus venosus ASD is located in the cranial part of the inter-atrial septum with the superior vena cava overriding the defect. The ostium secundum ASD is by far the most common type. An ostium primum ASD is often associated with regurgitation of the left-sided atrioventricular valve.

Regardless of the anatomical position, any ASD permits blood flow from the left to the right atrium, which leads to enlargement of the right atrium and ventricle and increased pulmonary blood flow (Figure 14.2).

Indications for ASD closure depend mostly on the size of the defect and the degree of left to right shunting. A small defect without any evidence of right atrial or right ventricular enlargement does not warrant closure (unless there is previous history of transient ischaemic attack or stroke). An ASD leading to right heart enlargement (ratio of pulmonary to systemic blood flow usually greater than 1.5) should ideally be closed before pregnancy. Pulmonary hypertension is not common in patients with ASDs but obviously has to be excluded before closure. Anticipated benefits from ASD closure are improved functional class and overall quality of life as well as risk reduction for atrial arrhythmia and right heart failure.[12–15]

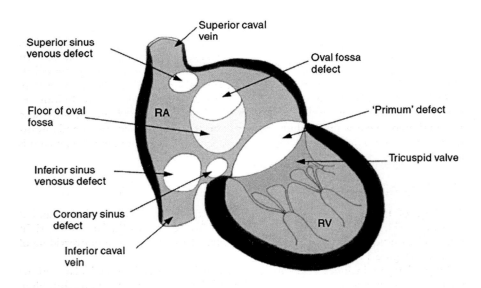

Figure 14.1.   Anatomy of the most common types of atrial septal defect, viewed from the right atrium; RA = right atrium, RV = right ventricle; reproduced with permission from Gatzoulis *et al.*[37]

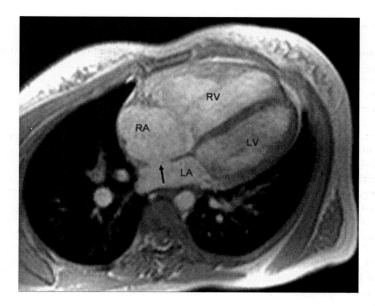

Figure 14.2.   Cardiac magnetic resonance image of an atrial septal defect (ASD) (arrow); ASDs result in left to right shunting; blood from the pulmonary veins enters the left atrium (LA), after which some of it crosses the ASD into the right atrium (RA), subsequently leading to enlargement of the RA and right ventricle (RV); LV = left ventricle; reproduced with permission from Gatzoulis *et al.*[37]

In the absence of pulmonary hypertension and right ventricular dysfunction, pregnancy is well tolerated in a woman with an ASD. A decrease in systemic vascular resistance reduces the magnitude of left to right shunting. Consequently, the effects of increases in cardiac output and blood volume on the right ventricle are attenuated.

Atrial arrhythmias (from right atrial distension) and paradoxical embolism are potential hazards during pregnancy, although the latter is uncommon. Low-dose aspirin should be considered to reduce the risk of thromboembolic events, and thromboprophylaxis with low molecular weight heparin should be commenced if bed rest is required.

Tetralogy of Fallot

Tetralogy of Fallot is the most common cyanotic congenital heart lesion and it constitutes about 3.5% of the cases of CHD.[16] ToF consists of a large VSD, right ventricular outflow tract obstruction, right ventricular hypertrophy and overriding of the aorta (Figure 14.3).

Surgical repair includes VSD closure and relief of the right ventricular outflow tract obstruction, and may involve patching of the pulmonary valve annulus, often leading to pulmonary regurgitation. Pulmonary regurgitation in turn may lead to right ventricular enlargement and dysfunction and is associated with ventricular tachycardia and sudden cardiac death.[17] Atrial arrhythmias are not uncommon after repair of ToF, especially if right atrial enlargement is present.

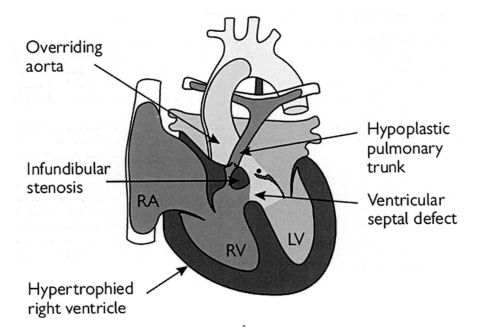

Figure 14.3. Tetralogy of Fallot is characterised by a large ventricular septal defect (VSD), an aorta that overrides the left and right ventricles, obstruction of the right ventricular outflow tract, and right ventricular hypertrophy; with substantial obstruction of the right ventricular outflow tract, blood is shunted through the VSD from right to left; reproduced from Uebing *et al.*, with permission from Oxford University Press.[38]

Nevertheless, pregnancy is a relatively low-risk endeavour for most women with repaired ToF. The risks of pregnancy depend largely on the status of the repair. Mild to moderate right ventricular outflow tract obstruction is well tolerated and so is pulmonary regurgitation, provided that right ventricular function is maintained. Severe pulmonary regurgitation after ToF repair has, however, been reported as a maternal risk factor during pregnancy and this mirrors our own anecdotal experience on changes in right ventricular size related to pregnancy long after ToF repair.[18] Furthermore, the risk for adverse maternal events associated with pregnancy increases if right or left ventricular dysfunction or pulmonary hypertension due to small pulmonary arteries is present in women with ToF.[19,20] The latter is uncommon, however. During pregnancy, periodic assessment should focus on signs of right and left heart dysfunction and clinical arrhythmia.

Tetralogy of Fallot can be part of the DiGeorge syndrome (present in 15% of ToF patients). Genetic testing should be offered before pregnancy as the recurrence risk of DiGeorge syndrome is 50%. In its absence, the risk for recurrence of CHD in the fetus is about 2–3%.[21]

Antibiotic prophylaxis should be considered for all women and be administered for operative delivery.

Ebstein anomaly of the tricuspid valve

Ebstein anomaly is a malformation of the tricuspid valve and consists of apical displacement of the tricuspid valve with resultant tricuspid regurgitation and enlargement of the right heart chambers. Because of inefficient right heart function, patients have reduced cardiac output, which can be further compromised by atrial re-entry tachycardia. Chest radiography to assess heart size prior to conception (Figure 14.4) is an approximate but reproducible marker of severity of disease.

Ebstein anomaly is frequently associated with an ASD that allows right to left shunting leading to cyanosis and with Wolff–Parkinson–White syndrome (in about 15% of patients). Survival into adulthood is common but patients can present with right heart failure, supraventricular arrhythmias or cyanosis.

In women without cyanosis or signs of heart failure, pregnancy is usually well tolerated. However, in cyanotic women in particular, pregnancy is associated with an increased risk of prematurity and fetal loss.[22,23] Monitoring during pregnancy should focus on the potential development of cyanosis, heart failure and arrhythmias. If an ASD is present, low-dose aspirin should be considered to reduce the risk of thromboembolic events, and thromboprophylaxis with low molecular weight heparin should be commenced if bed rest is required.

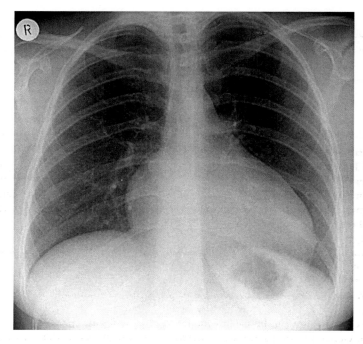

Figure 14.4.   Typical chest X-ray of moderate Ebstein anomaly of the tricuspid valve; note a large heart with normal and not increased pulmonary vascular markings and a small pedicle of the heart (small pulmonary artery and aorta) indicative of the low cardiac output status

Pulmonary stenosis

Pulmonary stenosis is an isolated congenital obstruction of the right ventricular outflow tract, usually at the level of the pulmonary valve, and occasionally at the sub- or supravalvular level. It constitutes about 10% of the cases of CHD. Pulmonary stenosis is also part of ToF and can be a residuum after ToF repair. Catheter interventional or surgical relief of pulmonary stenosis is recommended for patients with a peak to peak pressure gradient across the stenosis of more than 50 mmHg or a peak right ventricular pressure of more than 75 mmHg. Ideally, it should be performed before pregnancy.[24] Adult patients with pulmonary stenosis are mostly asymptomatic but when the stenosis is severe and longstanding they can develop right heart failure or atrial arrhythmia. If an inter-atrial communication is present, cyanosis can occur resulting from right to left shunting at atrial level. Isolated right ventricular outflow tract obstruction – even when severe – is usually well tolerated during pregnancy when right heart function is preserved.[25] Nevertheless, women with severe pulmonary stenosis may experience right heart failure or atrial arrhythmias. In cases of early right heart failure, balloon valvuloplasty should be considered (see Chapter 8).[26] Antibiotic prophylaxis should be recommended for labour and delivery in affected women.

Pulmonary stenosis can be part of Noonan syndrome (clinical features: short stature, a short webbed neck, pectus excavatum, hypertelorism and low-set ears). Noonan syndrome is of autosomal dominant inheritance and therefore carries a recurrence risk of 50%. Genetic testing should be offered before pregnancy if Noonan syndrome is clinically suspected. Furthermore, patients with Noonan syndrome have a more myxomatous type of pulmonary stenosis often involving the supravalvular area and usually do not respond well to balloon valvuloplasty.

Congenitally corrected transposition of the great arteries

In ccTGA the ventricles and the great arteries are 'inverted'. Systemic venous return enters the left ventricle which then ejects into the pulmonary artery. Pulmonary venous return enters the right ventricle which fills the aorta. The circulation is therefore 'physiologically corrected' but the right ventricle supports the systemic circulation (Figure 14.5).

Congenitally corrected transposition of the great arteries is often associated with the following heart defects, which impact on prognosis:

- ■ systemic (tricuspid) atrioventricular valve abnormalities (Ebstein-like) with valve insufficiency
- ■ VSD
- ■ subpulmonary stenosis
- ■ complete heart block (acquired)
- ■ Wolff–Parkinson–White syndrome.

Successful pregnancy can be achieved in many women with ccTGA and a systemic right ventricle. The overall risk for this group depends largely on associated lesions, systemic ventricular function, function of the systemic atrioventricular valve (tricuspid valve) and the woman's functional class.[27] While the long-term impact of successful and completed pregnancy on right ventricular function in women with ccTGA is somewhat unclear, a mortality rate of up to 4% has been reported in a small

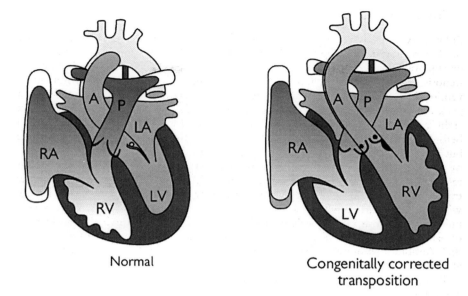

Normal   Congenitally corrected
                          transposition

Figure 14.5.   The ventricles are inverted in congenitally corrected transposition of the great arteries
(ccTGA); systemic venous return enters the left ventricle (LV), which ejects into the
pulmonary circulation (P); pulmonary venous return enters the right ventricle, which
supports the systemic circulation; A = aorta, RA = right atrium, LA = left atrium;
reproduced from Uebing *et al.*, with permission from Oxford University Press.[38]

series of women with systemic right ventricles, and this needs to be discussed in
preconception counselling.[6]

Cardiac magnetic resonance imaging should be performed as part of the prepregnancy evaluation as it provides invaluable data on the function of the systemic right
ventricle and the function of the tricuspid valve. A treadmill exercise test should also
be performed before pregnancy to document the woman's functional status and her
ability to increase heart rate during exercise. Monitoring during pregnancy should
include serial assessment of ventricular and tricuspid valve function and of heart
rhythm. Ventricular and valve function may deteriorate when blood volume and
cardiac output increase during pregnancy.

Transposition of the great arteries

Transposition of the great arteries accounts for 5–7% of all congenital heart malformations. In TGA the right ventricle gives rise to the aorta and the left ventricle gives
rise to the pulmonary artery (Figure 14.6). The majority of adults with this condition
will have had an 'atrial switch operation' (Mustard or Senning operation) in childhood. After atrial switch operations, patients have a right ventricle supporting the

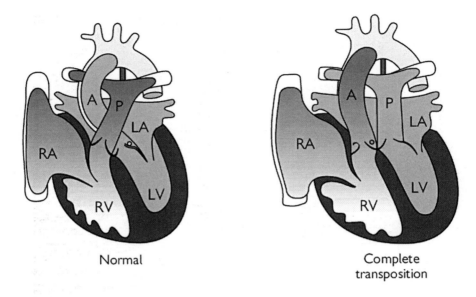

Normal

Complete
transposition

Figure 14.6. Transposition of the great arteries (TGA) and atrial switch operation; in TGA (complete transposition), systemic venous blood returns to the right atrium (RA), from which it goes to the right ventricle (RV) and then to the aorta (A); pulmonary venous blood returns to the left atrium (LA), from which it goes to the left ventricle (LV) and then to the pulmonary artery (P); reproduced from Uebing *et al.*, with permission from Oxford University Press.[38]

systemic circulation, as with ccTGA. Late complications following the atrial switch operation include sinus node dysfunction with bradycardia, atrial arrhythmias and dysfunction of the systemic right ventricle. Women with good or only mildly impaired right ventricular function and no history of arrhythmia have a relatively low risk during pregnancy.[28,29] Prepregnancy evaluation should include thorough assessment of ventricular function. Patency of the atrial baffles redirecting blood flow to the pulmonary and systemic ventricle has also to be demonstrated before pregnancy to ensure that an increased cardiac output can be accommodated (Figure 14.7). Both ventricular function and patency of the baffles should ideally be assessed with cardiovascular magnetic resonance imaging.

As tachycardia is part of the physiological adaptation of the circulatory system to pregnancy, chronotropic competence should be assessed before pregnancy, with exercise testing.

During pregnancy, clinical assessment should focus on early signs of heart failure and arrhythmias. If atrial tachycardia occurs, sinus rhythm should be restored without delay. Direct current (DC) cardioversion is usually effective and safe when needed during pregnancy.

There is an increased risk of thromboembolic events during pregnancy in women who have undergone the atrial switch procedure, mainly as a consequence of atrial tachycardia and/or systemic ventricular dysfunction. Low-dose aspirin should be given to all affected women.

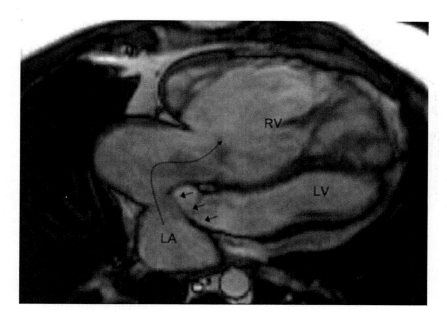

Figure 14.7. Cardiac magnetic resonance imaging of a patient with transposition of the great arteries (TGA) and atrial switch operation; a baffle (small arrows) is created in the atria to redirect blood from the left atrium (LA) into the systemic right ventricle (RV); systemic venous blood returns to the subpulmonary left ventricle (LV); the systemic RV is markedly enlarged, squashing the LV; reproduced with kind permission from Dr Philip Kilner, CMR Unit, Royal Brompton & Harefield NHS Trust, London, UK

Early evidence suggests that pregnancy may have an adverse long-term effect on ventricular function and on the functional class of women with TGA and previous atrial procedures, and this needs to be investigated further.[30]

Univentricular hearts after Fontan–type operations

Many adults with functional 'univentricular hearts' have undergone Fontan–type operations. Following the Fontan operation the systemic venous return is diverted directly to the pulmonary circulation without the incorporation of a subpulmonary ventricle. Blood flow to the lungs is driven only by systemic venous pressure. The 'single' ventricle supports the systemic circulation (Figure 14.8).

Several Fontan–type operations exist, connecting either the right atrium or the caval veins with the pulmonary arteries, the latter called total cavopulmonary connection (TCPC) (Figure 14.9). All 'Fontan patients' are at risk of various complications related to surgery and/or the abnormal circulatory physiology persisting after surgery ('low cardiac output status'):

■ atrial arrhythmias related to scarring from surgery or to atrial distension from high venous pressure are common and can cause profound haemodynamic deterioration

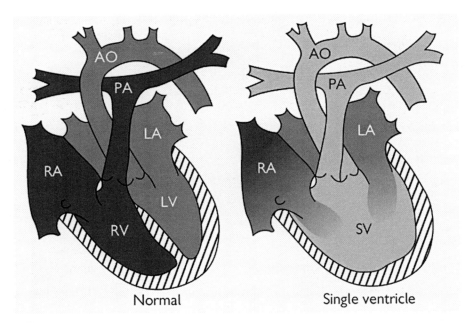

Figure 14.8. As opposed to the normal heart, a 'single' ventricle (SV) collects blood from the right atrium (RA) and the left atrium (LA); PA = pulmonary artery, AO = aorta, RV = right ventricle, LV = left ventricle; reproduced from Uebing *et al.*, with permission from Oxford University Press.[38]

- thrombosis diathesis is present as a consequence of sluggish blood flow in the systemic venous pathways and/or in the right atrium
- impairment of ventricular function is part of the 'natural' history in these patients, especially if the systemic ventricle is of right ventricular morphology
- cyanosis can result from persistent systemic venous to left-sided bypass tracts leading to right to left shunting.

Although data are limited, it can be assumed that the overall risks of pregnancy for women with single-ventricle physiology palliated with a Fontan-type procedure are moderate or moderate to severe. Legitimate concerns mainly relate to the effect of pregnancy on ventricular function, a prothrombotic circulatory system and a tendency to poorly tolerated atrial arrhythmias.

The risks of pregnancy mainly relate to the woman's functional status, her history of arrhythmias, her ventricular function and the degree of cyanosis.[31] The maternal risk is acceptable if the woman is in NYHA class I or II, ventricular function is good, there is no cyanosis at rest or during exercise and there is no history of arrhythmia.

Prepregnancy evaluation should include cardiac magnetic resonance imaging and cardiopulmonary exercise testing to assess ventricular function and functional status, as well as the woman's ability to increase cardiac output and oxygen saturation during exercise. Affected women should have the high risk of miscarriage and preterm delivery explained to them carefully before pregnancy. As the 10 year survival rate

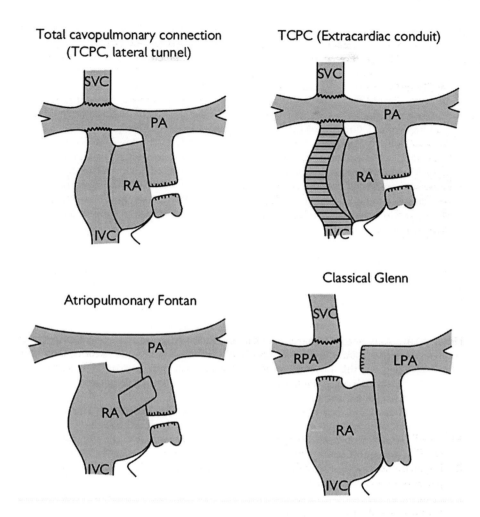

Figure 14.9. Various Fontan-type operations exist as palliative operations for patients with univentricular hearts; in all of them, systemic venous return is diverted to the lung without interposition of a subpulmonary ventricle; the operations differ regarding the type of connection between the systemic veins and the pulmonary arteries; IVC = inferior vena cava; LPA = left pulmonary artery; PA = pulmonary artery; RA = right atrium; RPA = right pulmonary artery; SVC = superior vena cava; TCPC = total cavopulmonary connection; modified with permission from Gatzoulis et al.[37]

following a Fontan operation is only 60–80%, it is important to discuss maternal long-term prognosis during preconception counselling as the woman's limited life expectancy is clearly likely to have a major impact on the long-term care of her child.

Close cardiovascular monitoring is mandatory throughout pregnancy, delivery and the postpartum period. Monitoring should focus on early signs of heart failure, arrhythmia, thromboembolic complications and cyanosis. Low-dose aspirin should be given until the 35th week of pregnancy, and then replaced by low molecular weight heparin for the remainder of pregnancy. Depending on the woman's clinical status, inpatient bed rest and oxygen supplementation should be considered during the third trimester. If bed rest is necessary, anticoagulation with low molecular weight heparin should be administered instead of aspirin for thromboprophylaxis.

Women should lie in the lateral position to avoid supine hypotension from compression of the vena cava and the aorta, particularly during labour. Dehydration should be avoided. Growth of the fetus should be monitored frequently.

Vaginal delivery should be the aim as it usually carries the lowest risk of complications such as haemorrhage, thromboembolism or infection. To avoid pain and anxiety leading to an additional increase in cardiac output during delivery, epidural anaesthesia should be introduced early as it has minimal effects on haemodynamic performance. After delivery, the risk of thromboembolic complications persists and anticoagulation with low molecular weight heparin should be continued until the woman is fully mobilised.

Pulmonary atresia with VSD and MAPCAs

Pulmonary atresia with VSD is characterised by the absence of a direct connection between the heart and the pulmonary artery tree, a large VSD and two good-sized ventricles. Pulmonary blood supply is provided via MAPCAs, a patent ductus arteriosus or both (Figure 14.10). A proportion of patients with this condition can be repaired surgically with closure of the VSD and reconstruction of the right ventricular outflow tract with a conduit (e.g. homograft). This renders them acyanotic. They then more or less have the physiology of a repaired ToF. The remainder, however, in particular those with a complex anatomy and non-confluent pulmonary arteries, are not suitable for repair and remain cyanotic.

Provided that pulmonary hypertension (which may be segmental) is excluded in these women, pregnancy does not carry a prohibitively high risk for the mother. The incidence of fetal complications, including fetal loss, low birth weight and prematurity, however, is high and related to severity of cyanosis. Cyanosis *per se* often worsens during pregnancy as right to left shunting increases, compromising pulmonary blood flow and thus oxygenation.

Maternal complications in cyanotic women relate to thrombosis, bleeding diathesis and the risk of arrhythmia and heart failure.[32] Ventricular function and the degree of cyanosis are the major determinants for maternal and fetal outcome in this group.[33] Both must be monitored carefully throughout pregnancy, delivery and the postpartum period. To reduce maternal oxygen consumption and thus cyanosis, bed rest with low molecular weight heparin and continuous nasal oxygen administration should be considered. Fetal growth needs to be monitored closely. Vaginal delivery should be the aim as it usually carries the lowest risk of complications such as haemorrhage, clotting complications and infections. Antibiotic prophylaxis should be administered for labour and delivery in affected women.

Summary

As in CHD in general, the risks associated with pregnancy and delivery in women with right heart lesions increase with poor functional class prior to pregnancy, impairment of ventricular function and a history of arrhythmia, stroke or transient ischaemic attack and cyanosis.[6,7] Preconception evaluation and lesion-specific risk stratification are

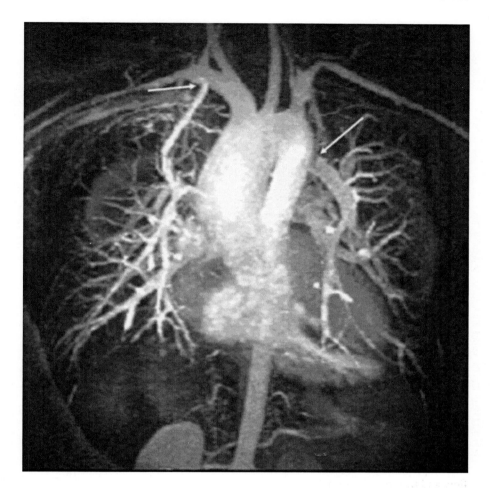

Figure 14.10. Cardiac magnetic resonance angiography with gadolinium contrast enhancement for visualisation of the pulmonary blood supply in a patient with pulmonary atresia with ventricular septal defect (VSD); there is no antegrade blood flow from the heart into the pulmonary artery system as the pulmonary valve is atretic; the aorta is the only vessel arising from the heart; pulmonary blood flow – out of necessity – comes from various major aortopulmonary collateral arteries (MAPCAs, arrows); reproduced with kind permission from Dr Philip Kilner, CMR Unit, Royal Brompton & Harefield NHS Trust, London, UK

essential and should result in an individualised management plan to prevent avoidable complications and crisis management.

Cardiovascular morbidity related to pregnancy in these women consists mainly of arrhythmia (mainly atrial), right heart failure, thromboembolic events and occasionally death (Table 14.1). Spontaneous vaginal delivery should be the aim for the majority of women unless obstetric or specific cardiac reasons determine otherwise.

Table 14.1. Maternal and fetal outcome of pregnancy in women with right heart lesions; values are numbers of pregnancies

Lesion	Pregnancies	Maternal outcome			Fetal deaths	Fetal outcome	
		Maternal deaths	Maternal adverse events (other than deaths)	Total		Fetal adverse events (other than deaths)[a]	Total
Atrial septal defect[34]	126 (mainly repaired)	0	1 (TE 1)	1/126 (0.8%)	0	21 (SUT 16; SGA 5)	21/126 (16%)
Pulmonary stenosis[6,7,35]	35	0	0	0/58 (0%)	0	0	0/58 (0%)
	6	0	0		0	0	
	17	0	0		0	0	
Tetralogy of Fallot[6,7,19,20]	112 (8 unrepaired)	0	0 (A 2; CHF 2; TE 1; RHD 1)	17/248 (7%)	1	31 (SUT 30; PM 1)	70/248 (28%)
	63		7 (A 5; CHF 2)		0	25 (SUT 12; PM 5; SGA 8)	
	20		2 (A 2)		0	2 (PM 2)	
	53		2 (CHF 2)	0	0	11[b]	
Ebstein anomaly[6,7,22,23]	11	0	0	8/68 (12%)	2	42 (PM 23; SUT 19)	64/169 (38%)
	41	0	2 (A 1; Cy 1)		1	14 (PM 5; SUT 5; SGA 4)	
	12	0	4 (A 3; CHF 1)		0	4[b]	
	4	0	2 (A 1; CHF 1)		0	1 (SGA 1)	
Transposition of the great arteries after atrial switch[6,7,28-30]	28	0	3 (A 2; CHF 1)	25/140 (17%)	0	0	53/140 (38%)
	69	0	13 (A 11; TE 2)		0	46 (SUT 17; PM 16; TE 2; SGA 11)	
	15	0	0		1	2 (SUT 2)	
	25	1	8 (A 4; CHF 3; TE 1)		0	3[b]	
	3	0	0		0	1 (PM 1)	
Congenitally corrected transposition of the great arteries[6,7,27,36]	45	0	5 (CHF 3; TE 1; Cy 1)	11/113 (10%)	0	17 (SUT 12; PM 5)	30/113 (26%)
	60	0	2 (CHF 2)		1	11 (SUT 10; PM 1)	
	6	0	4 (CHF 2; A 2)		0	0	
	2	0	0		0	1(PM1)	
Pulmonary atresia[32]	26	1	2 (TE 1; CHF 1)	3/26 (8%)	2	18 (SUT 13; PM 5)	20/26 (77%)
Fontan[31]	33	0	2 (A 2; CHF 1)	2/33 (6%)	0	14 (SUT 13; PM 1)	14/33 (42%)
Total	**812**	**2/812 (0.2%)**	**65 (A 35; CHF 21; TE 7; Cy 2; RHD 1)**	**67/812 (8%)**	**8/812 (1%)**	**264 (SUT 149; PM 66; SGA 29; TE 2; 18[a])**	**272/812 (33%)**

[a] Fetal (> 20 weeks of gestation) and neonatal death; [b] Adverse event not further specified
A = arrhythmia; CHF = congestive heart failure; Cy = worsening of cyanosis; PM = premature delivery (<37 weeks); RHD = right heart dilatation; SGA = small for gestational age (<2500 g birthweight); SUT = spontaneous unplanned termination of pregnancy; TE = thromboembolic event

Regurgitant or volume overload lesions are on the whole better tolerated than stenotic lesions or single-ventricle physiology, although more data are required to confirm this view. Most women with right heart lesions can have their own children at relatively low risk provided they are supported by a multidisciplinary team with suitable facilities.

References

1. Nieminen HP, Jokinen EV, Sairanen HI. Late results of pediatric cardiac surgery in Finland: a population-based study with 96% follow-up. *Circulation* 2001;104:570–5.
2. Thorne S, Deanfield J. Long-term outlook in treated congenital heart disease. *Arch Dis Child* 1996;75:6–8.
3. Wren C, O'Sullivan JJ. Survival with congenital heart disease and need for follow up in adult life. *Heart* 2001;85:438–43.
4. Hoffman JIE. Incidence, mortality and natural history. In: Anderson RH, Baker EJ, Macartney FJ, Rigby ML, Shinebourne EA, Tynan M, editors. *Paediatric Cardiology*. London, New York, Toronto: Churchill Livingstone; 2002. p. 111–39.
5. Uebing A, Steer PJ, Yentis SM, Gatzoulis MA. Pregnancy and congenital heart disease. *BMJ* 2006;332:401–6.
6. Siu SC, Sermer M, Colman JM, Alvarez AN, Mercier LA, Morton BC, et al. Prospective multicenter study of pregnancy outcomes in women with heart disease. *Circulation* 2001;104:515–21.
7. Siu SC, Sermer M, Harrison DA, Grigoriadis E, Liu G, Sorensen S, et al. Risk and predictors for pregnancy-related complications in women with heart disease. *Circulation* 1997;96:2789–94.
8. Steer PJ. Pregnancy and contraception. In: Gatzoulis MA, Swan L, Therrien J, Pantely GA, editors. *Adult Congenital Heart Disease: a Practical Guide*. Oxford: BMJ Publishing Group, Blackwell Publishing Ltd; 2005. p. 16–35.
9. Baddour LM, Wilson WR, Bayer AS, Fowler VG Jr, Bolger AF, Levison ME, et al.; Committee on Rheumatic Fever, Endocarditis, and Kawasaki Disease; Council on Cardiovascular Disease in the Young; Councils on Clinical Cardiology, Stroke, and Cardiovascular Surgery and Anesthesia; American Heart Association; Infectious Diseases Society of America. Infective endocarditis: diagnosis, antimicrobial therapy, and management of complications: a statement for healthcare professionals from the Committee on Rheumatic Fever, Endocarditis, and Kawasaki Disease, Council on Cardiovascular Disease in the Young, and the Councils on Clinical Cardiology, Stroke, and Cardiovascular Surgery and Anesthesia, American Heart Association: endorsed by the Infectious Diseases Society of America. *Circulation* 2005;111:e394–434.
10. Boggess KA, Watts DH, Hillier SL. Krohn MA, Benedetti TJ, Eschenbach DA. Bacteremia shortly after placental separation during cesarean delivery. *Obstet Gynecol* 1996;87(5 Pt 1):779–84.
11. Feldt RH, Avasthey P, Yoshimasu F, Kurland LT, Titus JL. Incidence of congenital heart disease in children born to residents of Olmsted County, Minnesota, 1950–1969. *Mayo Clin Proc* 1971;46:794–9.
12. Brochu MC, Baril JF, Dore A, Juneau M, De Guise P, Mercier LA. Improvement in exercise capacity in asymptomatic and mildly symptomatic adults after atrial septal defect percutaneous closure. *Circulation* 2002;106:1821–6.
13. Attie F, Rosas M, Granados N, Zabal C, Buendia A, Calderon J. Surgical treatment for secundum atrial septal defects in patients >40 years old. A randomized clinical trial. *J Am Coll Cardiol* 2001;38:2035–42.

14. Gatzoulis MA, Freeman MA, Siu SC, Webb GD, Harris L. Atrial arrhythmia after surgical closure of atrial septal defects in adults. *N Engl J Med* 1999;340:839–46.

15. Murphy JG, Gersh BJ, McGoon MD, Mair DD, Porter CJ, Ilstrup DM, *et al.* Long-term outcome after surgical repair of isolated atrial septal defect. Follow-up at 27 to 32 years. *N Engl J Med* 1990;323:1645–50.

16. Mitchell SC, Korones SB, Berendes HW. Congenital heart disease in 56,109 births. Incidence and natural history. *Circulation* 1971;43:323–32.

17. Gatzoulis MA, Balaji S, Webber SA, Siu SC, Hokanson JS, Poile C, *et al.* Risk factors for arrhythmia and sudden cardiac death late after repair of tetralogy of Fallot: a multicentre study. *Lancet* 2000;356:975–81.

18. Khairy P, Ouyang DW, Fernandes SM, Lee-Parritz A, Economy KE, Landzberg MJ. Pregnancy outcomes in women with congenital heart disease. *Circulation* 2006;113:517–24.

19. Veldtman GR, Connolly HM, Grogan M, Ammash NM, Warnes CA. Outcomes of pregnancy in women with tetralogy of Fallot. *J Am Coll Cardiol* 2004;44:174–80.

20. Meijer JM, Pieper PG, Drenthen W, Voors AA, Roos-Hesselink JW, van Dijk AP, *et al.* Pregnancy, fertility, and recurrence risk in corrected tetralogy of Fallot. *Heart* 2005;91:801–5.

21. Nora JJ. From generational studies to a multilevel genetic–environmental interaction. *J Am Coll Cardiol* 1994;23:1468–71.

22. Connolly HM, Warnes CA. Ebstein's anomaly: outcome of pregnancy. *J Am Coll Cardiol* 1994;23:1194–8.

23. Donnelly JE, Brown JM, Radford DJ. Pregnancy outcome and Ebstein's anomaly. *Br Heart J* 1991;66:368–71.

24. Brickner ME, Hillis LD, Lange RA. Congenital heart disease in adults. First of two parts. *N Engl J Med* 2000;342:256–63.

25. Elkayam U, Bitar F. Valvular heart disease and pregnancy Part I. Native valves. *J Am Coll Cardiol* 2005;46:223–30.

26. Loya YS, Desai DM, Sharma S. Mitral and pulmonary balloon valvotomy in pregnant patients. *Indian Heart J* 1993;45:57–9.

27. Connolly HM, Grogan M, Warnes CA. Pregnancy among women with congenitally corrected transposition of great arteries. *J Am Coll Cardiol* 1999;33:1692–5.

28. Clarkson PM, Wilson NJ, Neutze JM, North RA, Calder AL, Barratt-Boyes BG. Outcome of pregnancy after the Mustard operation for transposition of the great arteries with intact ventricular septum. *J Am Coll Cardiol* 1994;24:190–3.

29. Drenthen W, Pieper PG, Ploeg M, Voors AA, Roos-Hesselink JW, Mulder BJ, *et al.* Risk of complications during pregnancy after Senning or Mustard (atrial) repair of complete transposition of the great arteries. *Eur Heart J* 2005;26:2588–95.

30. Guedes A, Mercier LA, Leduc L, Berube L, Marcotte F, Dore A. Impact of pregnancy on the systemic right ventricle after a Mustard operation for transposition of the great arteries. *J Am Coll Cardiol* 2004;44:433–7.

31. Canobbio MM, Mair DD, van der Velde M, Koos BJ. Pregnancy outcomes after the Fontan repair. *J Am Coll Cardiol* 1996;28:763–7.

32. Neumayer U, Somerville J. Outcome of pregnancies in patients with complex pulmonary atresia. *Heart* 1997;78:16–21.

33. Presbitero P, Somerville J, Stone S, Aruta E, Spiegelhalter D, Rabajoli F. Pregnancy in cyanotic congenital heart disease. Outcome of mother and fetus. *Circulation* 1994;89:2673–6.

34. Zuber M, Gautschi N, Oechslin E, Widmer V, Kiowski W, Jenni R. Outcome of pregnancy in women with congenital shunt lesions. *Heart* 1999;81:271–5.

35. Hameed A, Yuodim K, Mahboob A, Goodwin T, Wing D, Elkayam U. Effect of the severity of pulmonary stenosis on pregnancy outcome: a case control study. *Am J Obstet Gynecol* 2004;191:93.

36. Therrien J, Barnes I, Somerville J. Outcome of pregnancy in patients with congenitally corrected transposition of the great arteries. *Am J Cardiol* 1999;84:820–4.

37. Gatzoulis MA, Swan L, Therrien J, Pantely GA, editors. *Adult Congenital Heart Disease: a Practical Guide*. Oxford: BMJ Publishing Group, Blackwell Publishing Ltd; 2005.

38. Uebing A, John A, Gatzoulis MA. Adult congenital heart disease. In: Myerson SG, Choudhury RP, Mitchell A, editors. *Emergencies in Cardiology*. Oxford, New York: Oxford University Press; 2006. p. 217–46.

Chapter 15

Pregnancy and pulmonary hypertension: new approaches to the management of a life-threatening condition

David G Kiely, Charles A Elliot, Victoria J Webster and Peter Stewart

Introduction

Pulmonary hypertension (PH) was previously thought to be a rare condition with a relentlessly progressive course and few treatment options. However, it is increasingly recognised in association with other conditions and recent advances have resulted in the development of effective therapies. As a consequence, people with PH have an increased life expectancy and more women of childbearing age with known PH are considering pregnancy.

In women with PH, pregnancy is associated with a high risk of maternal death. Reports exist in the literature advocating a variety of approaches to the management of PH during pregnancy but despite this the mortality of the condition remains high. A recent single-centre series reported a maternal mortality of 36% despite expert conventional management. Alternative strategies involving the use of new pulmonary vasodilator therapies have raised the possibility of an improved outcome in a selected group of women although excess maternal mortality remains.

It is currently recommended that women with PH should be strongly advised against pregnancy and given clear contraceptive advice, and, if needed, early termination of pregnancy. When women who are fully informed and understand the risks of doing so choose to continue their pregnancies, early treatment with targeted pulmonary vascular therapy represents a realistic treatment option and may improve the chances of maternal survival. With timely admission to hospital and close cooperation among a multidisciplinary team, a successful outcome for mother and fetus is possible, although maternal mortality remains high.

This chapter provides an overview of the epidemiology, natural history and treatment of PH and of the challenge of managing a woman with PH during pregnancy, labour and the postpartum period.

Definition of PH

Pulmonary hypertension is defined at cardiac catheterisation as a mean pulmonary artery pressure (MPAP) of 25 mmHg or more at rest or 30 mmHg on exercise, although the diagnosis is usually suggested following echocardiography.[1]

Classification of PH

The World Health Organization (WHO) reclassified PH in 2003 into the following five major groups:[1]

- pulmonary arterial hypertension (PAH)
- PH with left heart disease
- PH with lung disease and/or hypoxaemia
- PH due to thrombotic and/or embolic disease
- miscellaneous group

(In the second and third groups above, treatment is best aimed at the underlying disease and these women usually do not require specialist assessment. However, it is increasingly recognised that women with certain forms of lung disease may respond to targeted pulmonary vascular therapy.)

This classification illustrates the importance of identifying the cause of PH in defining the natural history and in determining treatment. Women with chronic thromboembolic pulmonary hypertension (CTEPH) can potentially be cured by surgery (pulmonary endarterectomy).[2]

Pulmonary arterial hypertension (PAH) can be classified as follows:

- idiopathic PAH:
  - ☐ sporadic
  - ☐ familial
- PAH (sporadic or familial), which is associated with:
  - ☐ collagen vascular disease
  - ☐ congenital systemic to pulmonary shunts
  - ☐ portal hypertension
  - ☐ HIV infection
  - ☐ drugs/toxins
- persistent PH of the newborn
- PAH with significant venous or capillary involvement.

Women with PAH can be improved with selective pulmonary arterial vasodilators.[3] This includes those women with idiopathic pulmonary arterial hypertension (IPAH, formerly known as primary pulmonary hypertension), PH associated with systemic to pulmonary shunts, and PH associated with connective diseases such as systemic sclerosis.

Pathophysiology of PH

The hallmark of PH is an increase in the pulmonary vascular resistance resulting in an increased workload placed on the right side of the heart. The precise pathological changes leading to this are to some degree dependent on disease aetiology. In IPAH, typical changes are seen in the small arterioles, with medial smooth muscle hypertrophy, thickening or fibrosis of the intima of the vessels with *in situ* thrombosis, and in some cases plexiform lesions, which are all histological features shared with other forms of PAH.[4] In CTEPH, the increase in pulmonary vascular resistance is brought about partly by obstruction of the pulmonary vascular bed due to an 'organised' thrombus that has become incorporated into the vessel wall, although interestingly these patients also have the histological changes of PAH.[5] This is the rationale for treating some of these women with pulmonary arterial vasodilators as a bridge to pulmonary endarterectomy or as a definitive treatment in inoperable disease. In women with left-sided heart disease (such as impaired left ventricular function or mitral valve disease), the primary problem is that of pulmonary venous hypertension. The disease process and clinical features are that of the underlying cardiac problem and treatment should be directed at this underlying problem rather than solely at the pulmonary arterial circulation. A rare cause of PH is pulmonary vaso-occlusive disease (PVOD) (previously known as pulmonary veno-occlusive disease but renamed to reflect the involvement of both pulmonary arterial and venous circulations), which has a particularly poor prognosis.[6] This may be worsened by pulmonary arterial vasodilators because they can precipitate pulmonary oedema.[7]

This chapter concerns the management of PH involving the pre-capillary circulation (i.e. PAH and CTEPH) and does not discuss the management of those women with post-capillary PH (PH associated with left-sided heart disease), where the natural history, management issues and, in particular, the treatment are different.

Clinical features of PH

The cardinal symptoms of PH are fatigue and breathlessness due to inability of the right heart to generate a sufficient cardiac output. This may initially be mild and occur only on strenuous exertion but it is progressive and may later be accompanied by chest pains (similar to angina and reflecting right ventricular ischaemia) and pre-syncope or syncope on exercise. Syncope usually reflects a low cardiac output and indicates severe disease. In addition to elevated pulmonary vascular resistance and decreases in the right-sided cardiac output, this is due to impaired filling of the left ventricle due to compression by an enlarging right ventricle. As right heart failure develops, women may develop ascites and ankle oedema. It should be noted that ankle swelling can occur very late in the natural history of the disease, and, in young women, may never occur. In women with right to left shunts, either via a patent foramen ovale or intracardiac defect, 'classical features' of right heart failure may not appear despite severe elevations of pulmonary artery pressure. Signs on examination may be very few initially and in particular may be difficult to identify in pregnant women, where a hyperdynamic circulation, loud second heart sound and flow murmurs are common. The clinical signs in advanced PH are the following:

- tachycardia
- elevated jugular venous pressure (JVP)
- right ventricular heave
- pulmonary flow murmur
- tricuspid regurgitation
- loud pulmonary component of the second heart sound
- hepatomegaly with or without pulsation

- ascites
- peripheral oedema.

Making the diagnosis of PH

The non-specific nature of the symptoms and the subtle nature of the signs of pulmonary vascular disease often delay diagnosis.[8] The chest X-ray (CXR) and/or electrocardiogram (ECG) are said to be abnormal in 80% of patients with established disease.[9] The most common non-invasive investigation suggesting PH is a transthoracic echocardiogram (TTE). With TTE an estimate of the systolic pulmonary artery pressure (SPAP) can be derived from the jet of tricuspid regurgitation (when present). This is calculated using the modified Bernoulli equation ($p = 4v^2$ where p = pressure gradient between the right atrium and ventricle and v = peak tricuspid jet velocity) and adding an estimate of right atrial pressure. In addition, other features may suggest PH (dilated right-sided chambers, right ventricular hypertrophy) and other causes of PH can be diagnosed (valvular heart disease, left ventricular dysfunction, intracardiac shunts). Subsequent investigation aims to confirm or refute the presence of PH and, where present, identify the aetiology and severity. This requires extensive investigation (Table 15.1) and usually right heart catheterisation. In pregnant women one may instinctively wish to delay investigation, and have concerns regarding radiation exposure and the finite risk of invasive investigation, particularly where the mother wishes to continue with the pregnancy regardless of the risk to her health. However, it should be remembered that PH in pregnancy carries a grave prognosis and having more information available will help in making difficult management decisions. The need for investigation can be tailored dependent on the individual woman's presentation. Where features are classical this may avoid the need for the standard battery of investigations.

Table 15.1. Investigations for assessing pulmonary hypertension

Modality/system	Investigation
Imaging	Chest X-ray
	Ventilation perfusion scanning
	High-resolution computed tomography (HRCT) of the lungs
	Contrast-enhanced helical CT of pulmonary arteries
	Magnetic resonance angiography
	Pulmonary angiogram (in selected cases)
Pulmonary	Lung function
	Nocturnal oxygen saturation monitoring
	Exercise test (6 minute walk/shuttle)
Cardiology	ECG
	Echocardiography
	Cardiac catheterisation
Blood	Arterial blood gases
	Routine haematology and biochemistry
	Thrombophilia screen
	Autoimmune screen
	HIV testing

Epidemiology and treatment of PH

Pulmonary hypertension is a challenging disease to diagnose, classify accurately and treat. Pulmonary arterial hypertension and CTEPH are rare, with an estimated prevalence of only 50 cases per million of the population (1 in 20 000). Idiopathic pulmonary arterial hypertension is a severe and progressive disease but is even rarer, with an incidence of only 1–2 cases per million of the population per year. However, it is three times more common in women than in men.[9] With 'conventional' treatment, patients have a median survival of only 2.8 years from diagnosis.[10] In systemic sclerosis, PH has a profound effect on the prognosis, with an 80% two-year survival in the absence of PH, in contrast to only 40% with the development of PH.[11] In the setting of congenital heart disease, the presence of PH also has an adverse effect on prognosis, although the presence of an intracardiac defect confers a real survival benefit compared with other forms of PAH. This is due to the intracardiac defect allowing blood to shunt from the right to left side in the face of high pulmonary artery pressures, thereby offloading the right ventricle.

Until the advent of transplantation in the 1980s, no specific treatment was available for patients with PH. The novel therapies that have been developed since than have been shown to improve symptoms and survival of patients with PH. Those with severe disease have a five-year survival of only 27% with supportive treatment alone but this is increased to 54% with certain targeted therapies.[12] These therapies include orally active agents such as endothelin blockers such as bosentan,[13] sitaxsentan[14] and ambrisentan,[15] and phosphodiesterase inhibitors such as sildenafil.[16] More complex therapies include nebulised (iloprost),[17] subcutaneous (treprostinil)[18] and intravenous (epoprostenol (prostacyclin), iloprost, treprostinil) prostaglandin therapy.[12,19,20] Owing to the relatively recent advent of these therapies there is little experience of their use during pregnancy. Some of them have, however, been demonstrated to have teratogenic effects in animal studies.

These treatments are often complex and their use and monitoring requires significant expertise. As such, investigation and treatment of certain forms of PH (particularly PAH and CTEPH) are currently focused at nationally designated specialist centres. In the UK, centres currently exist in Sheffield, London, Cambridge, Newcastle and Glasgow. There is also a specialist centre in Dublin, Ireland.

The challenges of managing pregnant women with PH

The pre-existence or gestational occurrence of PH is considered to pose an extreme risk of maternal death owing to the additional cardiovascular stresses that pregnancy places on an overburdened right ventricle. Although the physiological effects of pregnancy on the cardiovascular system are well documented,[21] the low prevalence of PH coupled with the historically low survival of such women means that clinical experience is very limited, particularly in IPAH. The sporadic nature of this illness and (until recently) the fragmented nature of the delivery of specialised pulmonary vascular care around the world have meant that reports have been largely anecdotal. Even in large pulmonary vascular centres, the experience has been relatively limited. Owing to the improved prognosis of patients with Eisenmenger syndrome, much of the literature is based on this patient population, although the physiology is very different from IPAH. Even in this group, the data are limited and point to a poor prognosis. Although systematic reviews exist on the management of pregnancy in women with PH there are inherent flaws in interpreting such a varied data set.

As experience in the management of PH develops so will evidence-based guidelines. However, in the short term, management is likely to remain pragmatic and steps should be taken to centralise the management of these women.

Cardiovascular adaptations during pregnancy, labour and the postpartum period

Pregnancy results in major hormonal and haemodynamic changes to meet the metabolic demands of both the fetus and the mother. Hormonal changes and the release of various vasoactive substances normally result in a reduction in systemic and pulmonary vascular resistance. The blood volume usually exceeds the non-pregnant level by 10% in the eighth week of gestation, reaching a peak that is 40–50% above prepregnancy levels between the 32nd and 36th week,[22] and then remaining essentially unchanged until term. Oxygen consumption rises by approximately 30% during pregnancy. Cardiac output increases steadily during the first two trimesters owing to increases in both heart rate and stroke volume, reaching a peak at approximately 28 weeks. In the third trimester it may plateau, increase or decrease slightly, until further major changes occur at the onset of labour.[23–25] Uterine contractions release up to 500 ml of blood into the circulation with an increase in cardiac output of a further 10–40%, to 60–80% above prepregnancy levels,[26] although this can be attenuated (but not completely abolished) by regional analgesia. These changes in cardiac output are modified by body posture, particularly in the third trimester. Delivery results in aortocaval decompression and redistribution of blood volume with a transient increase in cardiac output, although variable amounts of blood loss due to vaginal lacerations, poor uterine contractility or caesarean section lead to unpredictable changes in circulating blood volume, cardiac output and blood pressure. Whereas blood volume rapidly returns to normal following delivery, it takes up to 2 weeks for the major haemodynamic changes induced by pregnancy to return to prepregnancy levels after vaginal delivery (and longer after caesarean section).[27] It can take over 6 months for the more subtle haemodynamic changes to return to the non-pregnant state.

In women with severe PAH and a low cardiac output state (less than 3 litres per minute in some cases), the demands of increasing blood volume and cardiac output may not be met by an already compromised right ventricle. In addition, it is not known what direct effects pregnancy may have on the pulmonary vasculature and whether hormonal changes or the release of vasoactive mediators may have adverse effects on pulmonary vascular tone.

It is clear that women with severe PAH may fail to cope with these haemodynamic demands. In a recent series from France[28] that included three women who deteriorated between 12 and 23 weeks of gestation, two women died and one woman survived following termination of pregnancy. Certainly in our experience, any major decline in cardiac performance in the second trimester of pregnancy is a life-threatening event for the mother, although we have been able transiently to improve one mother's condition prior to delivery with intravenous prostaglandin (Table 15.2).[29] Deterioration early in pregnancy undoubtedly reflects either an inability to cope with the haemodynamic requirements of pregnancy and/or intense pulmonary vasoconstriction occurring as a direct consequence of pregnancy. In support of a role for the latter, at least in part, is the observation of haemodynamic improvement following prostaglandin therapy in some of these women while continuing with the pregnancy.

The peri- and postpartum period is also a fraught time for these women. Significant mortality occurs immediately following delivery,[21] which presumably reflects the large changes in blood volume (with concomitant shifts in fluid) and the inability of a compromised cardiovascular system to respond to this. Indeed, volume overload in the immediate postpartum period can result in a negative Starling response,[30] which may be avoided by augmenting the physiological diuresis following delivery.

Management of PH in pregnancy: a historical perspective

In efforts to minimise risks to the mother, a number of different approaches have been taken with respect to the timing of hospital admission and delivery, the mode of delivery (vaginal versus caesarean) and the choice of anaesthesia (regional versus general). The approach taken is likely to have reflected the individual needs of the woman as well as the preference of the supervising clinician. The lack of systematic prospective evaluation, however, does not allow any definite conclusions to be made regarding the benefits of each strategy. Nevertheless, it is clear that even with expert care the mortality remains high and has not changed substantially during the last three decades.[21,28,31,32]

In a retrospective review spanning four decades to 1978, Gleicher et al.[31] found that 30% of all pregnancies in women with Eisenmenger syndrome resulted in maternal death. Lower mortality rates have been seen in single- or two-centre studies, with for example an 11% mortality in the London–Torino study,[33,34] similarly low mortality rates in an Indian study,[35] and survival of all five women with Eisenmenger syndrome in a study[36] of eight women with PH in Canada. These series raised the possibility that the mortality in this form of PH had improved, particularly where the experience was concentrated in large centres. One the other hand, the UK national survey by Yentis et al.[37] that was published in 1998 reported that overall mortality remained about 40%, with little evidence of any improvement during the previous 30 years.

Table 15.2. Haemodynamic status of a 23-year-old pregnant woman with a diagnosis of idiopathic pulmonary arterial hypertension (IPAH) made 3 years previously in NYHA class II who decompensated over a period of a few days before presenting with a cardiopulmonary arrest from which she was subsequently resuscitated (day 1); the results demonstrate severe disease that improved with intravenous prostaglandin therapy with further haemodynamic improvement seen following delivery (operative delivery day 5)

	Day 1	Day 5 (delivery)	Day 5 (delivery) + 4 h
FiO$_2$	0.6%	0.45%	0.45%
MAP (mmHg)	114	102	101
MPAP (mmHg)	68	42	34
RA (mmHg)	18	3	1
TPR ((dyn s)/cm^5)	1265	533	451
CO (l/min)	4.3	6.3	6

FiO$_2$ = fraction inspired oxygen; MAP = mean arterial pressure; MPAP = mean pulmonary artery pressure; RA = right atrial pressure; TPR = total pulmonary resistance; CO = cardiac output

Weiss et al.[21] systematically reviewed all journals and book chapters using MEDLINE from 1978 to 1996. They identified reports of 73 women with Eisenmenger syndrome, 30 women with 'primary pulmonary hypertension' (now renamed IPAH) and 25 women with 'secondary vascular pulmonary hypertension' (now reclassified). This represents a large but heterogeneous population from many countries and centres. Unfortunately, in contrast to a prospective study, no validation of the diagnosis was possible and there was no suggestion of any uniformity in clinical practice. These investigators identified a mortality of 36% in Eisenmenger syndrome (similar to that in the Yentis et al. study[37]), 30% in 'primary pulmonary hypertension' and 56% in women with 'secondary pulmonary hypertension'. In those with Eisenmenger syndrome, 47% delivered at term, 33% at between 32 and 36 weeks of gestation and 20% before 31 weeks. Three women died during pregnancy but the mortality was even higher postpartum with 23 women dying within 30 days of delivery (and 14 of these dying between 2 and 7 days following delivery). The cause of death was described as 'pulmonary hypertensive crisis' and 'therapy-resistant heart failure' in 13 cases, with sudden death in seven. Autopsy identified thromboembolism in three cases although it should be noted that chronic thrombosis may often be seen in proximal pulmonary arteries in clinically stable patients with longstanding Eisenmenger syndrome. This does not necessarily imply that these women died of acute thrombosis. In women with 'primary pulmonary hypertension', 41% delivered at term, 37% at between 32 and 36 weeks and 22% before 31 weeks. All eight deaths in the postpartum group were within 35 days of delivery (mostly between 2 and 7 days postpartum) and were due to 'therapy-resistant heart failure'. The mortality of women with 'secondary vascular pulmonary hypertension' was also high at 56%, although this group was very heterogeneous. It included women with connective tissue disease and unusual disease processes such as Takayasu arteritis, peripheral pulmonary artery stenosis, hepatitis and dwarfism with congenital hypothyroidism. This was a very different population of women to those with pre-capillary forms of PH that are usually seen in a pulmonary vascular clinic. Mortality was high in the immediate postpartum period, with six of 14 deaths occurring within the first 24 hours. Death was due to progressive 'heart failure' in seven women and was sudden in the other seven.

Interestingly, adverse events were noted in two women in the Eisenmenger group who received oxytocic drugs, and 'pulmonary hypertensive crises' were also noted in one woman from each of the other two groups.[21] This class of drugs does have a potentially adverse effect on the pulmonary vasculature. Although they can be used safely in selected individuals, their use should be carefully controlled, and small boluses given initially to assess the effect on systemic and pulmonary vasculatures.

Weiss et al.[21] acknowledged the study's limitations but it did allow them to identify a number of risk factors for death in this patient population. These include late diagnosis, elevated diastolic pulmonary artery pressure and late hospital admission. It is difficult to validate the importance of these factors as the data set is incomplete, with a variety of confounding factors and physician preference at different centres influencing treatment. In particular, although operative delivery is identified as a risk factor for maternal death, this may simply reflect the fact that that the more symptomatic women were delivered early because of the severity of their underlying condition. In addition, although the postpartum period is well recognised as a period when women are at high risk of acute decompensation, this study was unusual in that death during pregnancy was rare. This may in part reflect publication bias.

In a recent publication from a major pulmonary vascular centre in France,[28] a retrospective review of women managed at the centre between 1992 and 2002 was reported. Again, a heterogeneous population of women was identified, but not surprisingly it was more in keeping with the disease spectrum seen by physicians with a primary interest in pulmonary vascular disease. Of 14 women and 15 pregnancies managed during this period, six cases were associated with congenital heart disease, four with IPAH, two with CTEPH, one with mixed connective tissue disease-associated PAH, one with HIV-associated PAH and one with fenfluramine-associated PAH. In this population, two women died during pregnancy at 12 and 23 weeks of gestation and another who had deteriorated had an elective termination of pregnancy at 21 weeks and subsequently improved. All three of these women had PAH with no evidence of an intracardiac shunt (which may be expected to confer a survival advantage in the setting of rising pulmonary artery pressures). There were three additional deaths at 1 week, 3 weeks and 3 months following delivery, respectively. The death 1 week following delivery was of a woman with a systemic to pulmonary shunt. Significantly, the five women who remained stable during pregnancy were in NYHA class II (New York Heart Association classification, see Appendix A) with relatively well-preserved exercise capacities whereas the women who deteriorated during pregnancy and died were either in NYHA class III before pregnancy or presented for the first time during pregnancy in NYHA class IV (breathless at rest). Only one woman in this study was on targeted pulmonary vascular therapy with an oral prostaglandin analogue although three women who deteriorated in the postpartum period were treated with intravenous epoprostenol (prostacyclin). In this series a number of approaches were used to manage delivery: caesarean section and regional anaesthesia in five cases, caesarean section and general anaesthesia in four cases and vaginal delivery with regional anaesthesia in four cases. There was no significant difference in outcome associated with these different approaches. The authors concluded that, despite expert treatment in a specialist centre, PH complicating pregnancy had a high mortality rate at 36% and although a scheduled caesarean delivery using combined spinal–epidural analgesia remained an attractive option there was no clear evidence of benefit from this approach.

In summary, reviews of published series and systematic reviews going back over 50 years of managing pregnant women with PH using conventional therapy show that the maternal mortality remains high. Most authors suggest that the mortality has remained unchanged over recent decades but several large series from single centres that are expert in the management of congenital heart disease report a lower mortality than that seen in a recent systematic review of the experience of various centres. This seems to support the widely held belief that expert management and assessment can improve the prognosis of these women. However, such a conclusion must remain tentative. Moreover, in the setting of severe PAH in the absence of an intracardiac shunt, the maternal mortality of pregnancy-associated PH appears to have changed little, despite a variety of approaches to mode of delivery and anaesthesia, even where the clinicians concerned are expert in the management of PH.[21,28]

Management of PH in pregnancy: a new approach

A review of the current literature on the outcome of pregnancy in women with PH identifies that, despite different approaches at the time of delivery, mortality remains high, particularly in women with severe PAH. Interestingly, women may deteriorate early (usually in the second trimester when the mortality without the intervention of early delivery is extremely high) or in the immediate postpartum period. Although the mode of death is variable in women deteriorating during pregnancy, the vast majority dying in the immediate postpartum period are identified as dying from a 'pulmonary hypertensive crisis' or 'heart failure'. This raises the possibility of directing treatment specifically at the pulmonary vasculature to reduce the degree of pulmonary vasoconstriction.

It should be remembered that 'heart failure' does not necessarily equate to rising pulmonary artery pressures, although this is the usual cause. It is important to be aware of changes in blood volume and fluid shifts, particularly postpartum. In the setting of significant PAH for example, immediately following delivery when myocardial contractility is reduced, volume overload may result in an adverse effect on the Starling curve.[30] Of course, this can be treated by diuretics, but the advent of a number of new pulmonary vasodilator therapies raises the possibility of pre-emptive intervention in women with PAH who are pregnant, in order to prevent decompensation occurring. Another important issue relates to the timing of commencement of therapy. This must balance the potential benefits to the mother with the potential risks of the treatment to the fetus and the mother. Although the health of the mother is paramount, decisions regarding the risk to benefit ratio of a new therapy are often difficult, particularly when the evidence base is lacking. Furthermore, certain therapies such as bosentan have been associated with teratogenicity in animal studies, which has limited their use in early pregnancy.[38]

A number of cases have recently been reported in the literature of successful pregnancies using inhaled pulmonary vasodilators,[39] intravenous vasodilators[30,40] or a combination of the two routes of administration during both the third trimester and the postpartum period. As well as successful reports, there are cases where maternal death was not avoided despite specialist intensive treatment.[30,41] These are a stark reminder that, although newer therapies may provide an option, they do not represent the complete answer to the difficulty of PH in pregnancy.

We have recently published our experience of the early introduction of pulmonary arterial vasodilator therapy with the prostaglandin analogue, nebulised iloprost.[29] In the absence of any published data we were keen to identify a drug and mode of delivery that we felt would minimise the risk to mother and fetus. Intravenous therapy, although potent, introduces the risk of potentially life-threatening line infections. In a clinically stable woman where the aim of drug therapy was to reduce pulmonary artery pressure and also ameliorate any potential rises in pulmonary artery pressure due to non-specific stimuli, particularly around the time of delivery, we were keen to minimise potential adverse effects of therapy and life-threatening iatrogenic problems.

Our three cases treated with nebulised iloprost demonstrated a highly variable presentation and natural history of PH and its progress in pregnancy. Two women presented in the first trimester and the other early in the second, without any increase in breathlessness. The decision to commence iloprost in two women (one with familial PAH and the other with PAH associated with an atrial septal defect) not receiving pulmonary arterial vasodilator therapy was based on their worsening breathlessness through previous pregnancies. In the woman receiving bosentan therapy (IPAH) it was felt necessary to continue treatment because of the unstable nature of her disease prior to pulmonary vascular therapy.

The introduction of inhaled iloprost (as early as the eighth week of gestation) was tolerated without any adverse events and all three infants were free from congenital birth defects. In one case the route of iloprost administration was switched to intravenous delivery at 25 weeks because of symptom progression and this resulted in an immediate clinical improvement. However, early delivery at 25 weeks + 5 days was still necessary. In all cases delivery was by caesarean section with regional anaesthetic, at gestations ranging between 25 weeks + 5 days and 36 weeks. Delivery was performed without haemodynamic compromise or adverse effect on the PH. One case, involving a placenta praevia, did result in significant intraoperative and postoperative blood loss but this was dealt with swiftly by blood replacement and surgical control of the bleeding.

In our group of women, the use of iloprost seems to have been associated with a better outcome than would be expected and is was also associated with symptomatic improvement in two women. One woman deteriorated despite nebuliser therapy but she was rescued with the addition of intravenous treatment, which in this case we believe was life saving. The potential for iloprost use raises further questions such as the optimal timing of treatment initiation, the route of administration and the optimum dose to be used. In these matters we are guided by the individuals' progress in previous pregnancies along with their current clinical symptoms. The route of drug administration can be debated, with some considering the intravenous route (via an indwelling central venous catheter) to be more effective than the inhaled route. Nebulised iloprost has been demonstrated to be an effective treatment for PH[17] and it avoids the potential complications of intravenous lines, such as infections that can result in life-threatening sepsis. We initiated nebulised iloprost and continued this where there was a favourable response, converting to intravenous drug if there was clinical deterioration. Based on our limited experience, we suggest that in the absence of specific contraindications a pregnant woman deteriorating on nebulised treatment should be immediately converted to intravenous therapy pending delivery.

The women in our group saw the physician responsible for the care of their pulmonary vascular disease and their obstetrician regularly and frequently throughout their pregnancies. They were also in close contact with specialist nurses for support and advice and were encouraged to report any change in their symptoms. Key to the process was the early involvement of anaesthetic, haematological and critical care teams with advanced preparation and clear planning for the peripartum period.

Subsequently, Bendayan et al.[42] from Israel published a case series based on their experience of three women (IPAH, Eisenmenger syndrome and PAH related to systemic lupus erythematosus) treated with intravenous prostacyclin therapy. Two women conceived while on intravenous therapy and the other commenced therapy at 16 weeks of gestation. These women were delivered by caesarean section with general anaesthesia at between 28 and 32 weeks with no neonatal or maternal mortality. In addition, eight other women were identified from the literature who were treated with epoprostenol therapy (three long term[30,40,43] and five receiving it for a short period preoperatively or perioperatively[30,41,44,45]) and one other woman treated with iloprost in the preoperative period.[46] Of these 12 pregnancies, there were two maternal deaths.

The advent of targeted pulmonary vascular therapy provides clinicians with the option of a variety of therapies and modes of administration. Although the results of these recent publications make positive reading one must always be aware of publication bias, with less successful outcomes often not being reported. Nonetheless, this new approach raises important issues such as the choice of therapy, at what stage it should be introduced and at what level of disease severity.

Management of PH in pregnancy: a pragmatic approach

Preconception counselling

Owing to the high mortality associated with PH in pregnancy, we advise strongly against pregnancy in women with this condition. We provide clear contraceptive advice and, if needed, offer early termination of pregnancy. However, owing to improvements in drug therapy, women are living longer with better exercise capacity and improved quality of life. As a consequence, a number of women may still express a wish to become pregnant. Easterling et al.[30] have recommended a year of successful therapy and near-normal right ventricular function following an initial positive response to vasodilator therapy before pregnancy is considered. It should be noted that such women represent the minority and even in women who are clinically stable the course of their disease can be difficult to predict. Women with more severe PH in NYHA class III are at particularly high risk but those in NYHA class II still face a significant risk of death. Indeed, in our series a young woman in NYHA class II who was clinically stable on therapy with a good exercise capacity and good right ventricular function before pregnancy had a cardiorespiratory arrest at 25 weeks of gestation despite having been stable until a few days prior to her arrest (Figure 15.1). Although she was successfully resuscitated, responded to intravenous therapy and ultimately delivered a live infant, her case demonstrated the difficulty of predicting the natural history of PH during pregnancy.

Initiation of targeted pulmonary vascular therapy and anticoagulation

In women in NYHA class III with significant PAH or CTEPH who wish to proceed with pregnancy, our current approach is to offer therapy with nebulised iloprost and, if there is subsequent deterioration, switch to intravenous prostaglandin therapy. We explain the lack of evidence and the unknown potential effects on the fetus. Owing to the teratogenic effects of bosentan in animal studies, we would not advocate the use of this drug in early pregnancy.[38] The effects of other therapies such as sildenafil are not yet known. It is likely that over the coming years experience with different therapies will grow and evolve.

Assessment and follow-up during pregnancy

Assessment and follow-up depends on the individual woman, her progress and the proximity of her home to the supervising centre. As a minimum, we advocate an assessment every 4 weeks until 28 weeks of gestation, then fortnightly until 32 weeks and then weekly until delivery. Depending on the individual woman, early admission to hospital for bed rest and observation may be appropriate. The timing of this depends on several variables. Assessing disease progress is difficult but requires a clear history, examination and ECG at every visit. We also routinely assess exercise capacity using the incremental shuttle walking test,[47] which correlates with cardiac output and also with mortality in non-pregnant women with PH.[48] Echocardiography also provides additional information although deterioration is often detectable clinically simply by taking a careful history at each clinic visit. We do not routinely perform cardiac catheterisation (except for diagnostic purposes, and even in a woman presenting for the first time with PH this is not always mandatory). It is important

(a)

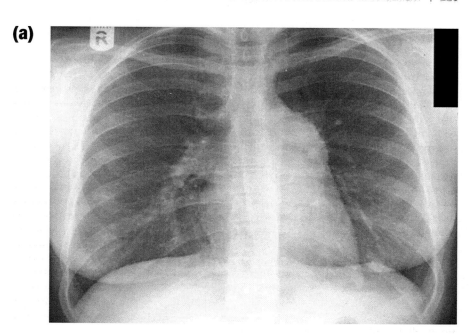

(b)

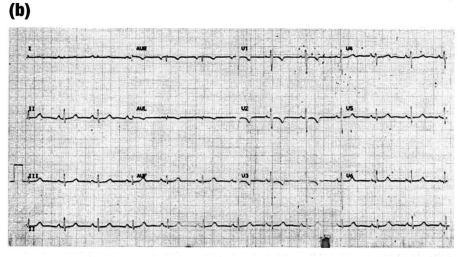

Figure 15.1. (a) Chest X-ray and (b) electrocardiograph in a 23-year-old pregnant woman with idiopathic pulmonary arterial hypertension (IPAH)

early on in pregnancy for the woman and her family to meet members of the multidisciplinary team (in particular the anaesthetic staff, obstetrician, neonatologist and intensivist). It is also important at this time that the necessary plans are made to cover the management of the rest of the pregnancy, including procedures such as sterilisation at delivery if this is appropriate.

Timing of delivery

The timing of delivery is dependent on the progress of the woman and the condition of the baby. The health of the mother is appropriately paramount to her medical advisers. It is clear that early deterioration in the first two trimesters of pregnancy is associated with a very poor outcome and, if this occurs, the mother should be advised that in order to safeguard her health, her pregnancy should be terminated. Some women, however, decide to continue with pregnancy despite the significant risks that this poses. If pregnancy proceeds and the woman is clinically stable a judgement should be made regarding the optimal time for delivery from the perspective of both the mother and the baby. The survival and progress of the baby is usually close to normal if they are delivered at or after 34 weeks of gestation. Cognitive and behavioural development, however, may be delayed.[49] A woman with moderately severe disease, limited exercise capacity and slowly progressive symptoms should be advised that early delivery is probably in their best interests, balancing the health of the mother with that of her much-wanted child. Women with good exercise capacity may choose to proceed to term, although this exposes the mother to additional risk. It is not known whether early delivery reduces the risk of problems for the mother occurring early in the postpartum period.

Monitoring of the mother at delivery and in the early postpartum period

Continuous ECG, pulse oximetry and invasive arterial blood pressure monitoring are essential during delivery. Like other groups, we use radial or femoral arterial access, an internal jugular central venous line, additional peripheral venous access and, in selected cases, Swan–Ganz catheterisation. We have used the latter in two cases and it is particularly helpful in assessing causes of hypotension, enabling us to distinguish between blood loss and a rise in pulmonary artery pressure. Measurement of pulmonary capillary wedge pressure (PCWP) is not essential in these women and our practice has been to leave the tip of the catheter in the main pulmonary artery, thus avoiding complications associated with catheter displacement. This form of invasive monitoring is associated with an increased risk of complications and we do not advocate its routine use in women with underlying systemic to pulmonary shunts. We have recently found that lithium dilution cardiac output monitoring (LiDCO™; LiDCO, London, UK) can be helpful in managing women with PH undergoing anaesthetic procedures. It requires central venous and arterial access and allows continuous measurement of cardiac output, systemic blood pressure and systemic vascular resistance.[50] Figure 15.2 illustrates the utility of this technique in identifying the cause of hypotension in a woman with PH, an atrial septal defect and a placenta praevia, immediately following delivery.

Women should ideally be managed in a high-dependency area for up to 7 days following delivery, with regular clinical review. Care should be taken to avoid fluid overload, with prompt treatment using diuretics if it occurs. Special care should be taken if blood transfusion is necessary. If the woman is clinically stable, we remove the arterial lines and central venous access as quickly as the clinical state allows, to avoid iatrogenic complications.

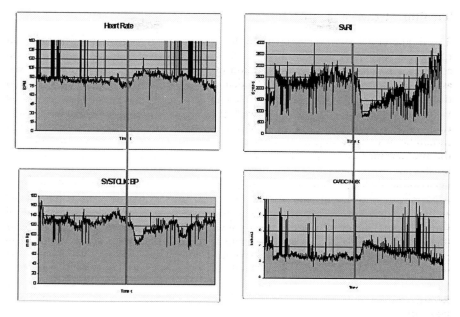

Figure 15.2.   Continuous real-time tracings of heart rate, systemic vascular resistance index (SVRI), systolic blood pressure and cardiac index in a woman with pulmonary arterial hypertension (PAH) and an atrial septal defect immediately following delivery; the vertical line identifies a period of tachycardia and hypotension due to haemorrhage; the use of lithium dilution cardiac output monitoring (LiDCO™) clearly shows a rise in cardiac index, suggesting that the hypotension is due to haemorrhage with an appropriate cardiovascular response rather than hypotension due to a 'pulmonary hypertensive crisis'

Mode of delivery and anaesthetic management

Vaginal delivery has been advocated by some groups.[36] If this is contemplated, it is essential that regional anaesthesia is used as it decreases the adverse haemodynamic consequences of labour. Our experience, however, is limited to elective caesarean section. This, in our view, is preferable as delivery is usually preterm. Preterm induction of labour is often difficult, and labour is likely to be prolonged. Bearing down in the second stage of labour is contraindicated because of the reduction in venous return and hence decreased right heart preload. An emergency caesarean after a long unsuccessful labour is the most difficult situation. An elective procedure has the advantages of taking place on a predetermined date and under optimal circumstances, with all members of the extended multidisciplinary team present. Importantly, the availability of intensive/high-dependency beds for the immediate post-delivery period can be arranged. The caesarean should be performed by an experienced surgeon. Surgery also has the advantage of allowing direct access to the uterus if excessive haemorrhage occurs. Surgical techniques such as elective uterine compression sutures can be used to minimise blood loss.[51] Controlling the intravascular volume changes at delivery is vitally important. Caesarean section inevitably increase the risks of thromboembolism, but these women are invariably anticoagulated, thus minimising the risk. Oxytocic drugs may have potentially adverse effects and should be reserved for circumstances where they are essential.[21,52] They should be given in small doses initially, to assess the haemodynamic effect.

A number of deliveries under regional anaesthesia have been reported.[39,43,46,53] We have used epidural anaesthesia with small incremental doses, and have also used combined spinal–epidural anaesthesia. The latter provides the advantages of a spinal anaesthetic with a denser sensory block but by using low doses of spinal anaesthesia avoids the hypotension associated with single-shot spinal anaesthesia. Single-shot spinals are not advocated in these women because of the risk of profound hypotension and the inability of the failing right ventricle to mount an appropriate cardiovascular response. General anaesthesia has been used by a number of centres[41,44] but increases in pulmonary artery pressure have been noted at tracheal intubations.[54,55] Additionally, positive-pressure ventilation has adverse effects on venous return and can have deleterious effects on cardiovascular performance in women with reduced cardiovascular reserve. Regional anaesthesia also has the advantage of good post-operative analgesia and in women needing to return to theatre it allows easy top-up of anaesthesia. As mentioned earlier, oxytocic drugs may have adverse effects. They can be given safely in some women but it is advisable to use small doses initially to assess the haemodynamic effect. In the case of Syntocinon® (Alliance, Chippenham, Wilts), a continuing low-dose infusion using small volumes of fluid is preferable to bolus injections.

Other issues

The requirements of autonomy dictate that the views of the woman are paramount. One should never underestimate the risks that some individuals will take to achieve motherhood even in the face of overwhelming danger. Additionally, although regular antenatal care is important, the woman may be unable or unwilling to follow the management plan that seems appropriate to the clinician. The other family members are also important and the psychological impact of an adverse outcome on them should always be borne in mind. Pregnancy can result in the death of the mother and the unborn child and this possibility is an emotional burden that needs to be shared by all those supporting the mother in her endeavour

Conclusion

Women with PH should be advised against pregnancy and provided with clear contraceptive advice and, if needed, early termination of pregnancy. When women who are fully informed and understand the risks of doing so choose to continue their pregnancy, treatment with targeted pulmonary vascular therapy represents a realistic option and may improve the chances of maternal survival. With timely admission to hospital and close cooperation among a multidisciplinary team, a successful outcome for mother and baby is possible.

References

1.   Simonneau G, Galie N, Rubin LJ, Langleben D, Seeger W, Domenighetti G, *et al*. Clinical classification of pulmonary hypertension. *J Am Coll Cardiol* 2004;43(12 Suppl S):5S–12S.

2. Jamieson SW. Pulmonary thromboendarterectomy. *Heart* 1998;79:118–20.

3. Humbert M, Sitbon O, Simonneau G. Treatment of pulmonary arterial hypertension. *N Engl J Med* 2004;351:1425–36.

4. Humbert M, Morrell NW, Archer SL, Stenmark KR, MacLean MR, Lang IM, et al. Cellular and molecular pathobiology of pulmonary arterial hypertension. *J Am Coll Cardiol* 2004;43(12 Suppl S):13S–24S.

5. Moser KM, Bloor CM. Pulmonary vascular lesions occurring in patients with chronic major vessel thromboembolic pulmonary hypertension. *Chest* 1993;103:685–92.

6. Shackelford GD, Sacks EJ, Mullins JD, McAlister WH. Pulmonary venoocclusive disease: case report and review of the literature. *AJR: Am J Roentgenol* 1977;128:643–8.

7. Palmer SM, Robinson LJ, Wang A, Gossage JR, Bashore T, Tapson VF. Massive pulmonary edema and death after prostacyclin infusion in a woman with pulmonary veno-occlusive disease. *Chest* 1998;113:237–40.

8. British Cardiac Society Guidelines and Medical Practice Committee. Recommendations on the management of pulmonary hypertension in clinical practice. *Heart* 2001;86 Suppl 1:i1–13.

9. Rich S, Dantzker DR, Ayres SM, Bergofsky EH, Brundage BH, Detre KM, et al. Primary pulmonary hypertension. A national prospective study. *Ann Intern Med* 1987;107:216–23.

10. D'Alonzo GE, Barst RJ, Ayres SM, Bergofsky EH, Brundage BH, Detre KM, et al. Survival in patients with primary pulmonary hypertension. Results from a national prospective registry. *Ann Intern Med* 1991;115:343–9.

11. Stupi AM, Steen VD, Owens GR, Barnes EL, Rodnan GP, Medsger TA Jr. Pulmonary hypertension in the CREST syndrome variant of systemic sclerosis. *Arthritis Rheum* 1986;29:515–24.

12. Rubin LJ, Mendoza J, Hood M, McGoon M, Barst R, Williams WB, et al. Treatment of primary pulmonary hypertension with continuous intravenous prostacyclin (epoprostenol). Results of a randomized trial. *Ann Intern Med* 1990;112:485–91.

13. Rubin LJ, Badesch DB, Barst RJ, Galie N, Black CM, Keogh A, et al. Bosentan therapy for pulmonary arterial hypertension. *N Engl J Med* 2002;346:896–903.

14. Barst RJ, Langleben D, Frost A, Horn EM, Oudiz R, Shapiro S, et al. Sitaxsentan therapy for pulmonary arterial hypertension. *Am J Respir Crit Care Med* 2004;169:441–7.

15. Galie N, Badesch D, Oudiz R, Simonneau G, McGoon MD, Keogh AM, et al. Ambrisentan therapy for pulmonary arterial hypertension. *J Am Coll Cardiol* 2005;46:529–35.

16. Galie N, Ghofrani HA, Torbicki A, Barst RJ, Rubin LJ, Badesch D, et al. Sildenafil citrate therapy for pulmonary arterial hypertension. *N Engl J Med* 2005;353:2148–57.

17. Olschewski H, Simonneau G, Galie N, Higenbottam T, Naeije R, Rubin LJ, et al. Inhaled iloprost for severe pulmonary hypertension. *N Engl J Med* 2002;347:322–9.

18. Simonneau G, Barst RJ, Galie N, Naeije R, Rich S, Bourge RC, et al. Continuous subcutaneous infusion of treprostinil, a prostacyclin analogue, in patients with pulmonary arterial hypertension: a double-blind, randomized, placebo-controlled trial. *Am J Respir Crit Care Med* 2002;165:800–4.

19. Barst RJ, Rubin LJ, Long WA, McGoon MD, Rich S, Badesch DB, et al. A comparison of continuous intravenous epoprostenol (prostacyclin) with conventional therapy for primary pulmonary hypertension. The Primary Pulmonary Hypertension Study Group. *N Engl J Med* 1996;334:296–302.

20. Higenbottam TW, Butt AY, Dinh-Xaun AT, Takao M, Cremona G, Akamine S. Treatment of pulmonary hypertension with the continuous infusion of a prostacyclin analogue, iloprost. *Heart* 1998;79:175–9.

21. Weiss BM, Zemp L, Seifert B, Hess OM. Outcome of pulmonary vascular disease in pregnancy: a systematic overview from 1978 through 1996. *J Am Coll Cardiol* 1998;31:1650–7.

22. Weiss BM, Hess OM. Pulmonary vascular disease and pregnancy: current controversies, management strategies, and perspectives. *Eur Heart J* 2000;21:104–15.

23. Bonica JJ. Maternal anatomic and physiologic alterations during pregnancy and parturition. In: Bonica JJ, editor. *Practice of Obstetric Analgesia and Anesthesia*, 2nd edn. Baltimore: Williams & Wilkins; 1995. p. 45–82.

24. Poppas A, Shroff SG, Korcarz CE, Hibbard JU, Berger DS, Lindheimer MD, *et al.* Serial assessment of the cardiovascular system in normal pregnancy. Role of arterial compliance and pulsatile arterial load. *Circulation* 1997;95:2407–15.

25. van Oppen AC, Stigter RH, Bruinse HW. Cardiac output in normal pregnancy: a critical review. *Obstet Gynecol* 1996;87:310–18.

26. Hunter S, Robson SC. Adaptation of the maternal heart in pregnancy. *Br Heart J* 1992;68:540–3.

27. Cheek TG, Gutsche BB. Maternal physiologic alteration during pregnancy. In: Hugues SC, editor. *Shnider and Levinson's Anesthesia for Obstetrics*. Philadelphia: Lippincott Williams & Wilkins; 2001. p. 3–18.

28. Bonnin M, Mercier FJ, Sitbon O, Roger-Christoph S, Jais X, Humbert M, *et al.* Severe pulmonary hypertension during pregnancy: mode of delivery and anesthetic management of 15 consecutive cases. *Anesthesiology* 2005;102:1133–7.

29. Elliot CA, Stewart P, Webster VJ, Mills GH, Hutchinson SP, Howarth ES, *et al.* The use of iloprost in early pregnancy in patients with pulmonary arterial hypertension. *Eur Respir J* 2005;26:168–73.

30. Easterling TR, Ralph DD, Schmucker BC. Pulmonary hypertension in pregnancy: treatment with pulmonary vasodilators. *Obstet Gynecol* 1999;93:494–8.

31. Gleicher N, Midwall J, Hochberger D, Jaffin H. Eisenmenger's syndrome and pregnancy. *Obstet Gynecol Surv* 1979;34:721–41.

32. Avila WS, Grinberg M, Snitcowsky R, Faccioli R, da Luz PL, Bellotti G, *et al.* Maternal and fetal outcome in pregnant women with Eisenmenger's syndrome. *Eur Heart J* 1995;16:460–4.

33. Presbitero P, Somerville J, Stone S, Aruta E, Spiegelhalter D, Rabajoli F. Pregnancy in cyanotic congenital heart disease. Outcome of mother and fetus. *Circulation* 1994;89:2673–6.

34. Presbitero P, Rabajoli F, Somerville J. Pregnancy in patients with congenital heart disease. *Schweiz Med Wochenschr* 1995;125:311–15.

35. Saha A, Balakrishnan KG, Jaiswal PK, Venkitachalam CG, Tharakan J, Titus T, *et al.* Prognosis for patients with Eisenmenger syndrome of various aetiology. *Int J Cardiol* 1994;45:199–207.

36. Smedstad KG, Cramb R, Morison DH. Pulmonary hypertension and pregnancy: a series of eight cases. *Can J Anaesth* 1994;41:502–12.

37. Yentis, SM, Steer PJ, and Plaat F. Eisenmenger's syndrome in pregnancy: maternal and fetal mortality in the 1990s. *Br J Obstet Gynaecol* 1998;105:921–2.

38. Actelion Pharmeceuticals. (Data on file). *3rd Trax PMS Data Report to CPMP for the Period from 24 May to 19 February 2003*; 2003.

39. Weiss BM, Maggiorini M, Jenni R, Lauper U, Popov V, Bombeli T, *et al.* Pregnant patient with primary pulmonary hypertension: inhaled pulmonary vasodilators and epidural anesthesia for cesarean delivery. *Anesthesiology* 2000;92:1191–4.

40. Stewart R, Tuazon D, Olson G, Duarte AG. Pregnancy and primary pulmonary hypertension: successful outcome with epoprostenol therapy. *Chest* 2001;119:973–5.

41. Monnery L, Nanson J, Charlton G. Primary pulmonary hypertension in pregnancy; a role for novel vasodilators. *Br J Anaesth* 2001;87:295–8.

42. Bendayan D, Hod M, Oron G, Sagie A, Eidelman L, Shitrit D, *et al.* Pregnancy outcome in patients with pulmonary arterial hypertension receiving prostacyclin therapy. *Obstet Gynecol* 2005;106(5 Pt 2):1206–10.

43. Badalian SS, Silverman RK, Aubry RH, Longo J. Twin pregnancy in a woman on long-term epoprostenol therapy for primary pulmonary hypertension. A case report. *J Reprod Med* 2000;45:149–52.

44. O'Hare R, McLoughlin C, Milligan K, McNamee D, Sidhu H. Anaesthesia for caesarean section in the presence of severe primary pulmonary hypertension. *Br J Anaesth* 1998;81:790–2.

45. Geohas C, McLaughlin VV. Successful management of pregnancy in a patient with Eisenmenger syndrome with epoprostenol. *Chest* 2003;124:1170–3.

46. Wong PS, Constantinides S, Kanellopoulos V, Kennedy CR, Watson D, Shiu MF. Primary pulmonary hypertension in pregnancy. *J R Soc Med* 2001;94:523–5.

47. Billings C, Waterhouse J, Armstrong IJ, Elliot CA, Phillips J, Smith I, *et al.* The incremental shuttle walking test safely assesses exercise capacity in pulmonary hypertension *Eur Respir J* 2004;24(S48):137.

48. Elliot CA, Armstrong IJ, Billings C, Waterhouse J, Hamilton N, Kiely DG. Incremental shuttle walking test distance predicts poor prognosis in pulmonary hypertension. *Eur Respir J* 2004;24(S48):138.

49. Huddy CL, Johnson A, Hope PL. Educational and behavioural problems in babies of 32–35 weeks gestation. *Arch Dis Child Fetal Neonatal Ed* 2001;85:F23–8.

50. Jonas MM, Tanser SJ. Lithium dilution measurement of cardiac output and arterial pulse waveform analysis: an indicator dilution calibrated beat-by-beat system for continuous estimation of cardiac output. *Curr Opin Crit Care* 2002;8:257–61.

51. Hema KR, Johanson R. Techniques for performing caesarean section. *Best Pract Res Clin Obstet Gynaecol* 2001;15:17–47.

52. Pinder AJ, Dresner M, Calow C, Shorten GD, O'Riordan J, Johnson R. Haemodynamic changes caused by oxytocin during caesarean section under spinal anaesthesia. *Int J Obstet Anesth* 2002;11:156–9.

53. Ghai B, Mohan V, Khetarpal M, Malhotra N. Epidural anesthesia for cesarean section in a patient with Eisenmenger's syndrome. *Int J Obstet Anesth* 2002;11:44–7.

54. Weeks SK, Smith JB. Obstetric anaesthesia in women with primary pulmonary hypertension. *Can J Anaesth* 1991;38:814–16.

55. Blaise G, Langleben D, Hubert B. Pulmonary arterial hypertension: pathophysiology and anesthetic approach. *Anesthesiology* 2003;99:1415–32.

Chapter 16
Cardiomyopathy

Catherine Nelson-Piercy

Introduction

This chapter will discuss the relevant issues regarding cardiomyopathies in pregnancy, of which the most important are peripartum cardiomyopathy (PPCM) and hypertrophic cardiomyopathy (HCM). Restrictive cardiomyopathies will not be discussed.

The advent of objective criteria for the definition of PPCM has enabled researchers to better define the incidence and prognosis of this rare, often fatal, pregnancy-specific condition. Although certain demographic risk factors are well described, the aetiology remains unknown. Possible underlying pathophysiological mechanisms include viral myocarditis and immunologically mediated damage. Improvements in diagnosis, the management of heart failure, use of automatic implantable defibrillators, advances in the use of mechanical circulatory support and cardiac transplantation have all led to improved survival. Non-invasive assessments of cardiac contractile reserve using stress echocardiography may allow more refined counselling for those who recover and are considering future pregnancy.

Women with other forms of dilated cardiomyopathies (DCM) may present for prepregnancy counselling, or in pregnancy. Systemic ventricular dysfunction associated with symptoms (New York Heart Association (NYHA) class III–IV (see Appendix A)) or left ventricular ejection fraction (LVEF) under 30% is a contraindication to pregnancy. Management is the same as for PPCM.

As HCM is now diagnosed more commonly as a result of increased clinical awareness and familial screening, it is now also being recognised more commonly in pregnancy. Most women with HCM tolerate pregnancy well. However, rare complications can occur, particularly in those already symptomatic before pregnancy.

Peripartum cardiomyopathy

Definition

Peripartum cardiomyopathy is defined as the development of cardiac failure between the last month of pregnancy and 5 months postpartum, in the absence of an identifiable cause or recognisable heart disease prior to the last month of pregnancy, and with left ventricular systolic dysfunction demonstrated by the following echocardiographic criteria:[1]

■ LVEF less than 45% or

■ fractional shortening less than 30%.

Some workers[2] have suggested an additional criterion of left ventricular end–diastolic diameter (LVEDD) greater than 2.7 cm/m[2] (for a 70–80 kg woman, this is 4.3–4.8 cm).

Incidence

Peripartum cardiomyopathy is rare but the true incidence is unknown as mild cases probably go unrecognised. The reported incidence of PPCM varies between 1:100 and 1:15 000 live births,[3] although the higher values relate to studies without echo-cardiographic confirmation of left ventricular dysfunction where other causes of pulmonary oedema such as fluid overload have not been excluded. A more realistic estimate is probably 1:5000 to 1:10 000.[4]

Risk factors

Recognised associations of PPCM include multiple pregnancy, hypertension (be it pre-existing or related to pregnancy or pre-eclampsia), multiparity, increased maternal age and black race. It also has been linked to betasympathomimetic tocolytic therapy and cocaine abuse.[2]

Clinical features

The severity of PPCM varies from catastrophic to subclinical (when it may be discovered only fortuitously through echocardiography). The presenting features are usually those of left ventricular failure but less acute cases may be heralded by the symptoms and signs of right heart failure. The diagnosis should be suspected in any woman in the third trimester of pregnancy, peripartum, or postpartum who presents with breathlessness, tachycardia, orthopnoea, paroxysmal nocturnal dyspnoea or signs of heart failure. Of particular concern are women who complain of cough and breathlessness and who may also have audible wheeze, where there is a risk of misdiagnosing asthma.

Presentation can be with collapse, due either to severe pulmonary oedema, ventricular arrhythmias or pulmonary embolism, or to systemic emboli from mural thrombus. Heart failure precipitated by fluid overload is a common form of presentation and is often caused by the use of oxytocin (Syntocinon® (Alliance, Chippenham, Wilts)) or by fluids given to maintain cardiac output during spinal anaesthesia for delivery. The combination of a twin pregnancy, tocolytic therapy with betasympathomimetics, pre-eclampsia, steroids to induce fetal lung maturation and then Syntocinon postpartum is not uncommonly encountered in women who subsequently present with PPCM.

The chest X-ray shows an enlarged heart with pulmonary congestion or oedema and often bilateral pleural effusions.

Diagnosis

Diagnosis of PPCM involves exclusion of other causes of heart failure such as sepsis, severe anaemia or thyrotoxicosis. Transthoracic echocardiography is important to exclude other cardiac causes such as mitral stenosis, congenital heart disease or chronic hypertension with systolic dysfunction and allows fulfilment of the above echo-cardiographic diagnostic criteria.[1,2]

Echocardiography will show cardiac dilatation that usually involves all four chambers but is dominated by left ventricular hypokinesia. This may be global or most marked in a particular territory of the ventricle. Peripartum cardiomyopathy does not differ clinically from DCM except in its temporal relationship to pregnancy and the fact that women with PPCM are usually younger.

The differential diagnosis includes pre-existing DCM, pulmonary thromboembolism, amniotic fluid embolism, myocardial infarction and beta$_2$ agonist-associated pulmonary oedema.

The ejection fraction at diagnosis is fairly consistent across studies, as shown in Table 16.1.

Although presentation within the last month of pregnancy is a diagnostic criterion for PPCM, the clinical presentation and outcome of women with pregnancy-associated cardiomyopathy diagnosed early in pregnancy are similar to those of women with traditional PPCM. These two conditions may represent a continuum of a spectrum of the same disease.[5]

Aetiology

Various studies have suggested a role for infection or inflammation in the aetiology of PPCM. Invasive endomyocardial biopsy has been used for more specific diagnosis and prognosis. There is often non-specific evidence of myofibre hypertrophy, degeneration and fibrosis.[2] In one study,[6] 14 of 18 women (78%) with PPCM showed evidence of myocarditis. Of these, ten were treated with immunosuppressive therapy. Nine of these had both subjective and objective improvement. Follow-up endomyocardial biopsies showed resolution or substantial improvement in the myocardial inflammation. However, four women with myocarditis not treated with immunosuppressives also improved. In another American study[7] of 42 cases of women with PPCM who all had endomyocardial biopsy, 26 (62%) had myocarditis.

Molecular pathological investigation of endomyocardial biopsy specimens from 26 women with PPCM in Germany[8] revealed viral genomes (parvovirus B19, human herpesvirus 6, Epstein–Barr virus and human cytomegalovirus) in eight women (31%) that were associated immunohistologically with interstitial inflammation. The authors concluded that their findings supported a high prevalence of virus-associated inflammatory changes in PPCM.

In a recent study[9] of 100 African women with PPCM, levels of C-reactive protein at presentation correlated positively with baseline left ventricular (LV) end-diastolic and end-systolic diameters and inversely with LVEF. Women who died presented with significantly lower mean ejection fractions and higher plasma levels of Fas/Apo-1 (a cell surface molecule that induces apoptosis in susceptible cells).

Table 16.1. Left ventricular ejection fraction (LVEF) at presentation and follow-up in three published cohorts of women with peripartum cardiomyopathy

Study	n	LVEF at presentation	Follow-up period	LVEF at follow-up
Dorbala et al.[18]	6	25.3 ± 9.5%	5 months	53.0 ± 16.4%
Elkayam et al.[5]	100	29 ± 11%		46 ± 14%
Sliwa et al.[9]	100	26.2 ± 8.2%	6 months	42.9 ± 13.6%

Cardiac myocyte apoptosis plays a causal role in the pathogenesis of cardiomyopathy in a murine model of PPCM.[10]

In DCM there is selective upregulation of immunoglobulins against cardiac myosin of the G3 subclass (IgG3's are immunoglobulins with proinflammatory characteristics). However, in women with PPCM[11] the class G and all subclass (G1, G2, G3) immunoglobulins were raised. IgG3-positive women were in a higher NYHA class at initial presentation. The authors concluded that, unlike DCM, the impact of PPCM on humoral immunity is not subclass restricted. However, raised levels of IgG3's may be of prognostic value in clinical PPCM.

Peripartum cardiomyopathy is associated with unique sets of autoantibodies and autoantigens and some workers have suggested a model of PPCM that depends on the interaction of several factors including haemodynamic stress, genetics, immune dysregulation and fetal microchimerism, possibly leading to the breakdown of self-tolerance.[12]

Mortality and prognosis

Peripartum cardiomyopathy is one of the most common causes of maternal death in the UK and the US.[13,14] In the UK, cardiomyopathy, of which the vast majority in pregnancy is PPCM, caused 25% of the maternal deaths due to cardiac disease in the period 1991–2002.[13]

The mortality rate from PPCM has been reported at 25–50%,[2] although mortality is probably decreasing[15] and recent series from Africa[9] and California[5] give lower figures (15% and 9%, respectively). In a study comparing PPCM with other causes of cardiomyopathy, 5 year survival was 94%.[7]

Most deaths occur within the first 3 months after diagnosis.[2] Women who die usually do so rapidly after presentation. Death is from intractable heart failure, arrhythmia or pulmonary or systemic thromboembolism. Poor NYHA functional class at presentation is a predictor of death.[9]

About 30–50% recover normal (more than 50%) LV function, although there may be regional and racial variations. The percentage recovering to normal was 55% in a population in Chicago[3] and 54–64% in California[4,5] but only 23% in South Africa.[3] In a recent study,[5] normalisation of LVEF was more likely in women with LVEF greater than 30% at diagnosis.

Those women who recover usually begin to do so early (within 1 month) and recover completely within 6 months. Most studies have shown that long-term prognosis correlates with the degree of LV dysfunction at diagnosis. Women who survive PPCM have higher ejection fractions and fractional shortening and smaller LV end-diastolic diameters than those who die, and poor prognosis is related to greater LV chamber dimensions. However Witlin et al.[16] noted no association between fractional shortening and long-term survival and documented a trend toward increased LV diameters in women with progressive disease. Witlin et al.[17] also reported that women with an LV end-diastolic dimension greater than 60 mm and a fractional shortening of less than 21% were unlikely to regain normal cardiac function on follow-up echocardiograms. It has recently been shown that inotropic contractile reserve during dobutamine stress echocardiography accurately correlates with subsequent recovery of LV function and indicates a benign prognosis.[18]

Management

Women with proven or suspected PPCM should be managed by cardiologists with expertise in heart failure. In pregnant and puerperal women this should be in close collaboration with obstetricians and obstetric anaesthetists with expertise in cardiac disease in pregnancy. For undelivered women the high-dependency area or unit of the delivery suite is the most appropriate place to care for the fetus and the mother. Following delivery, the coronary or intensive care unit may be more appropriate for all but the mildest cases.

Management is the same as for other causes of heart failure and should include oxygen, diuretics and vasodilators in the first instance. Angiotensin-converting enzyme (ACE) inhibitors are used in the postpartum period and a cogent argument could be made that in the preterm infant the risks from severe prematurity outweigh the risk of renal impairment from ACE inhibitors (although preterm onset of PPCM is uncommon).

Thromboprophylaxis is imperative because of the increased risk of thrombo-embolism. A high prophylactic dose of low molecular weight heparin (LMWH) (e.g. enoxaparin 40 mg subcutaneously twice daily or dalteparin 5000 iu subcutaneously twice daily) is appropriate, unless there has been suspected or proven associated thromboembolic events or documented mural thrombus, in which case a full treatment dose of LMWH is indicated.

The cautious addition of a cardioselective beta-adrenergic blocking drug (such as bisoprolol) or a beta blocker (such as carvedilol) that has vasodilator properties may be helpful if tachycardia persists, particularly if the cardiac output is well preserved. The most gravely ill women will need intubation, ventilation and monitoring with use of inotropes and sometimes temporary support from an intra-aortic balloon pump or ventricular assist device. Heart transplantation may be the only chance of survival in severe cases and early liaison with the regional cardiac transplant centre is advisable for women with severe PPCM.

Recurrence and risks in future pregnancies

Women should remain on an ACE inhibitor for as long as LV function remains abnormal. Prognosis and recurrence depend on the normalisation of LV size within 6 months of delivery. As discussed above, women with severe myocardial dysfunction, defined as an LV end-diastolic dimension of 60 mm or more and a fractional shortening less than or equal to 21% are unlikely to regain normal cardiac function on follow-up.[17]

Recurrence rates for PPCM in a subsequent pregnancy are 50–100% in older reports.[2] Demakis et al.[19] noted a 25–50% risk of recurrence. Witlin et al.[16] reported a recurrence rate of 67% in subsequent pregnancies.

Two studies by the same group have looked at outcome in subsequent pregnancies in women with previous PPCM depending on whether they recovered normal cardiac function or not.[4] The first study[4] examined 67 pregnancies in 63 women but relied on questionnaires to physicians rather than notes review. The more recent study considered 60 subsequent pregnancies in 44 women in the USA and South Africa.[20] The women were divided into two groups depending on whether LV function and size returned to normal (LVEF 50% or greater) before a subsequent pregnancy, and the outcomes of the next pregnancy were examined. Twenty-eight (64%) of the 44 women recovered. A significant decrease in LVEF was seen in the study population as a whole. For those who had recovered, the risk of symptoms of heart failure during a subsequent pregnancy was 21%, the risk of a greater than 20% fall in LVEF either during the subsequent pregnancy or postpartum was 21%, and the risk of a persistent fall in LVEF greater than 20% was 14%. Of the women who had persistent impaired LV function before their next pregnancy, 44% developed symptoms of heart failure, 25% had a greater than 20% fall in LVEF, 31% had persistent impaired cardiac function, and 19% died. If the data are analysed excluding women who had a termination in their next pregnancy and only those who opted to continue their next pregnancy are considered, the figures are as shown in Table 16.2.

These data argue for directive counselling against subsequent pregnancies in women whose LV function has not recovered.[4] Most authorities agree that such women should be offered appropriate contraception and termination of pregnancy in the event of an unplanned pregnancy. However, for women who have recovered, the picture is less clear-cut. Certainly, some of these women may suffer recurrent PPCM[16] or a substantial reduction in LVEF that may not recover, so although the risk of death is probably low, significant morbidity may be caused by embarking on another pregnancy.[4]

Some workers have tried to refine this risk in an attempt to identify which of the women with 'recovered' LVEF are likely to deteriorate during a pregnancy. In an important study by Lampert and co-workers,[3] it was postulated that mimicking the cardiovascular stress of gestation in non-pregnant women recovered from PPCM would provide more objective data to counsel them on prognosis for future pregnancies. The study was designed quantitatively to assess LV contractile reserve in seven women with histories of PPCM. A modification of routine dobutamine stress echocardiography was employed. Left ventricular afterload was initially altered with methoxamine, an alpha$_1$-specific agonist that increases afterload by arterial vasoconstriction without direct cardiac effects. Before the initiation of the methoxamine infusion, the women were pre-medicated with atropine sulphate (0.01 mg/kg body weight) to abolish reflex cardiac slowing. The ventricular response to arterial vasoconstriction was assessed with recordings taken every 1–2 minutes until peak systolic pressure had increased 20–40 mmHg above baseline. Dobutamine (5 μg/kg per minute), a synthetic sympathomimetic amine that directly stimulates beta$_1$ receptors in the myocardium to increase myocardial contractility, with only a mild increase in heart rate and a small decrease in peripheral arterial resistance, was then infused. The dose was less than standard but enough to challenge the left ventricle, in an attempt to mimic the cardiovascular changes of normal pregnancy,

Table 16.2. Pregnancy outcome in the next pregnancy following an index pregnancy complicated by peripartum cardiomyopathy; figures exclude women who opted for termination of pregnancy; data from Elkayam *et al.*[20]

	n	Symptoms of heart failure	> 20% fall in LVEF	Persistent > 20% fall in LVEF	Prematurity	Death
Recovered	23	26%	17%	9%	13%	0
LVEF < 50%	12	50%	33%	42%	50%	25%

LVEF = left ventricular ejection fraction

especially increased cardiac output (on average 25%) and heart rate, and decreased total peripheral vascular resistance. Contractile reserve, or LV systolic reserve capacity, was quantified using the change in rate-corrected velocity of fibre shortening. The results showed that contractile reserve, or change in LV contractility over baseline values, was significantly less in the women with recovered PPCM and normal routine echocardiography than in a group of normal matched control subjects.[3]

Subclinical systolic dysfunction might explain the reported high incidence of recurrent PPCM with new pregnancies in those women, and might indicate a continuing decreased ventricular contractile reserve unmasked by the haemodynamic stress induced by pregnancy, and not a true exacerbation of the disorder. Lampert *et al.*[3] thus advised against further pregnancies even in these women with apparent unstressed full recovery of cardiac function.

This of course does not help predict those women whose reserve is truly normal but who suffer a reactivation of whatever process caused the initial cardiomyopathy. As with so many fields in obstetric medicine, the clinician is left with no clear recommendation to share with the woman. Having explained the risks of possible recurrence and possible temporary or permanent loss of cardiac function, the woman should be supported in whatever decision she makes and if she embarks on, or continues with an unplanned, pregnancy then serial echocardiograms are vital to her management.

Dilated cardiomyopathy

Idiopathic dilated cardiomyopathy refers to congestive cardiac failure secondary to dilatation and systolic (and/or diastolic) dysfunction of the ventricles (predominantly left) in the absence of congenital, valvular or coronary artery disease or any systemic disease known to cause myocardial dysfunction. The established causes of DCM are shown in Table 16.3 but in the majority of women no identifiable cause is found — hence the term 'idiopathic' DCM.[21]

The diagnostic criteria are similar to PPCM, i.e. an ejection fraction below 45% and/or a fractional shortening of less than 25%, and an LV end-diastolic dimension of more than 112% predicted value corrected for age and body surface area.[21]

On echocardiography, all four cardiac chambers are dilated and the left ventricle is usually affected more often than the right ventricle. The cardiac valves are normal, although the mitral and tricuspid valve rings are dilated and the valve leaflets do not appose each other in systole, giving rise to varying degrees of mitral and/or tricuspid regurgitation. Persistent mitral regurgitation leads to thickening of the mitral valve leaflets. As with PPCM, mural thrombus can form secondary to the low-flow cardiac output state and is most often seen in the LV apex or atria. Occasionally, the right ventricle is preferentially involved in the cardiomyopathic process. When this is noted, it may have a familial basis such as arrhythmogenic right ventricular cardiomyopathy.

Three major factors have been implicated in the pathogenesis of myocardial damage in DCM: preceding viral or infective myocarditis, autoimmunity and underlying genetic predisposition. Epidemiological, serological and molecular studies have detected evidence of enteroviral infection and, in particular, coxsackievirus B in 20–25% of patients. The mechanism of myocardial damage (rapid destruction or a long-term slowing of cardiomyocyte function) following viral infection remains unclear. Animal studies have shown that DCM is an autoimmune disease in genetically predisposed strains of mice. Approximately 30–40% of adult patients with DCM have organ-specific and disease-specific autoantibodies. The absence of these

Table 16.3. Causes of dilated cardiomyopathy; adapted from Elliott[21]

Causes	Examples
Viral infections (myocarditis)	Coxsackievirus B, HIV, echovirus, rubella, varicella, mumps, Epstein–Barr virus, measles, polio
Other infections	Bacteria (diphtheria, *Mycoplasma*), tuberculosis, septicaemia, rickettsia (psittacosis), parasites, fungi, eosinophilic (Churg–Strauss syndrome)
Neuromuscular disorders	Duchenne muscular dystrophy, Friedreich ataxia, other muscular dystrophies
Nutritional factors	Kwashiorkor, pellagra, thiamine deficiency, selenium deficiency
Collagen vascular diseases	Rheumatic fever, rheumatoid arthritis, systemic lupus erythematosus, dermatomyositis, Kawasaki disease
Haematological diseases	Thalassaemia, sickle cell disease, iron deficiency anaemia
Coronary artery diseases	Anomalous left coronary artery from pulmonary artery
Drugs	Alcohol, anthracycline, cyclophosphamide, chloroquine, iron overload
Endocrine diseases	Hypothyroidism, hyperthyroidism, hypoparathyroidism, phaeochromocytoma, hypoglycaemia
Metabolic disorders	Haemochromatosis, glycogen storage diseases, carnitine deficiency, fatty acid oxidation defects, mucopolysaccharidoses
Others	Mitochondrial, arrhythmogenic right ventricular cardiomyopathy

antibodies in the remaining patients may be related to the stage of disease progression. It has been postulated that an insult such as viral myocarditis initiates an autoimmune process with superantigen-triggered immune responses resulting in massive T-lymphocyte activation and myocardial damage.

Genetic causes account for more than 25–30% of DCM.[21] There is an increased frequency of human leucocyte antigen (HLA)-DR4 in patients with familial DCM. Autosomal dominant and recessive inheritance, X-linked transmission and polygenic and mitochondrial inheritance have all been documented.

Women with impaired LV function are tradiationally advised against pregnancy.[22] NYHA class greater than II and LVEF less than 40% are both predictors of adverse cardiac events in pregnancy.[23] Women with severe impairment may decompensate as a result of the increased intravascular volume and cardiac output during pregnancy that is poorly tolerated by these women. Pregnancy in women with primary DCM can be extremely hazardous, resulting in cardiac failure and even death. A multidisciplinary approach and consideration of termination of pregnancy may be required in the management of such women.[24]

There is conflicting evidence in the literature regarding the relative prognosis of DCM compared with PPCM. A US study[7] followed 1230 patients with cardio-myopathy of different causes, including a majority with idiopathic cardiomyopathy (50%) and 51 with PPCM. Other causes of cardiomyopathy included myocarditis, ischaemic heart disease, infiltrative myocardial disease, hypertension, HIV infection, connective-tissue disease, substance abuse and therapy with doxorubicin. After a mean follow-up of 4.4 years, 417 patients had died and 57 had undergone cardiac transplantation. Compared with the patients with idiopathic cardiomyopathy, those women with PPCM had better survival even when adjusted for age, sex and race (adjusted hazard ratio for death 0.31, 95% CI 0.09–0.98), and survival was significantly worse among those with cardiomyopathy due to infiltrative myocardial disease (adjusted hazard ratio 4.40, 95% CI 3.04–6.39), HIV infection (adjusted hazard ratio 5.86, 95% CI 3.92–8.77), therapy with doxorubicin (adjusted hazard ratio 3.46, 95% CI 1.67–7.18) and ischaemic heart disease (adjusted hazard ratio 1.52, 95% CI 1.07–2.17).[7]

Conversely, a 10 year retrospective comparative cohort study[25] of eight women with cardiomyopathy diagnosed prior to pregnancy (DCM group) and 23 with PPCM found that maternal outcomes in the PPCM group were significantly worse than in the DCM group, with three maternal deaths and four women undergoing heart transplants ($P = 0.05$). In the DCM group, one woman with a prepregnancy ejection fraction of 16% underwent transplantation after termination of pregnancy for genetic indications. None of the other women in the DCM group had a significant decline in cardiac status. The authors concluded that women with stable DCM may do well during pregnancy without significant deterioration in their cardiac status.[25]

Hypertrophic cardiomyopathy

Hypertrophic cardiomyopathy, which was previously thought to be rare, may affect up to two in 1000 people. Up to 70% of cases are familial with autosomal dominant inheritance. The diagnostic criteria for HCM are unexplained asymmetrical myocardial hypertrophy on echocardiography with a maximal wall thickness exceeding two standard deviations for age in the absence of another explanation for hypertrophy. Diagnosis is usually made in the third or fourth decade as the result of echocardiography to investigate symptoms, a heart murmur or as part of familial screening.

Many women encountered in pregnancy are asymptomatic. Clinical features do not relate to LV outflow tract obstruction and include chest pain, breathlessness, presyncope, syncope, atrial or ventricular arrhythmias, heart failure and sudden death. The overall risk of disease-related complications such as sudden death, end-stage heart failure and fatal stroke is roughly 1–2% per year.[26] Risk factors for sudden death include a positive family history (two or more sudden cardiac deaths below age 40 years), abnormal blood pressure response to exercise (failure of systolic blood pressure to rise by more than 25 mmHg from baseline values) and ventricular tachycardia. Most sudden deaths occur in patients with LV wall thickness less than 30 mm, so the presence of mild hypertrophy cannot be used to reassure women that they are at low risk.

Treatment includes medical therapy with beta blockers, antidysrhythmics, septal myectomy, dual chamber pacing and implantable cardiac defibrillators.

Several series of pregnancies in women with HCM have been reported. A retrospective questionnaire study from St George's Hospital in London[27] looked at cardiac symptoms and complications in 40 women with HCM diagnosed prior to pregnancy and 87 women in whom it was diagnosed after their first pregnancy. Although 28% of women reported cardiac symptoms in pregnancy, over 90% of these had been symptomatic before pregnancy and symptoms only deteriorated in 10%. There were no maternal deaths, although two women developed pulmonary oedema postpartum. No echocardiographic or clinical feature was found to be a useful indicator of pregnancy-related complications.[27]

An Italian study[28] examined 100 women with HCM and 199 live births. There were two pregnancy-related deaths, giving a maternal mortality rate of 10 per 1000 live births (95% CI 1.1–36.2 per 1000), which was in excess of the expected mortality in the general Italian population (relative risk 17.1, 95% CI 2.0–61.8). In a subset of 40 women where pregnancy-related morbidity was assessed, progression to NYHA functional class III or IV during pregnancy was noted in one (4%) of the 28 women who were previously asymptomatic and five (42%) of the 12 women with symptoms ($P < 0.01$). One woman had atrial fibrillation and one had syncope, both of whom had already experienced similar and recurrent events before their pregnancy. The authors concluded that outcome is likely to be good in asymptomatic women.[28]

Similar reassuring findings have been reported by a French group[29] in another retrospective questionnaire study of 150 pregnancies in 41 women with HCM, of whom 31% had symptoms prior to pregnancy. There were no maternal deaths and no deterioration in functional class. However, those with symptoms had an increased rate (18%) of preterm delivery.

In pregnancy, beta blockers should be started in women with symptoms, and continued in women already taking them. Caution is needed with regional anaesthesia/analgesia since vasodilation may be poorly tolerated. Interestingly, two of 11 women known to have HCM prior to pregnancy and receiving epidural anaesthesia in one study[27] had dizziness and one had documented hypotension (a drop in systolic blood pressure of 30 mmHg). No complications were described in women receiving general anaesthesia. Any hypovolaemia or blood loss should be aggressively corrected and the woman kept 'well filled' during labour and delivery. Asymptomatic HCM is not an indication for caesarean section and most of these women can deliver in their local units.

Conclusions

■ Women with severe PPCM in pregnancy should be managed by cardiologists, obstetricians and obstetric anaesthetists with expertise in this condition. Referral to tertiary units and regional transplantation centres should not be delayed.

■ Women who do not recover LVEF greater than 50% should be advised against future pregnancies and offered appropriate contraception or termination in the event of an unplanned pregnancy.

■ Women whose LVEF recovers to greater than 50% should be offered estimation of contractile reserve with dobutamine stress echocardiography or exercise echocardiography before a subsequent pregnancy.

■ Women with DCM may decompensate in pregnancy and should be advised against pregnancy if there is severe impairment of LV function.

■ Women with HCM usually tolerate pregnancy well and can usually remain under the care of their local units.

References

1. Pearson GD, Veille JC, Rahimtoola S, Hsia J, Oakley CM, Hosenpud JD, et al. Peripartum cardiomyopathy: National Heart, Lung, and Blood Institute and Office of Rare Diseases (National Institutes of Health) workshop recommendations and review. JAMA 2000;283:1183–8.

2. Hibbard JU, Lindheimer M, Lang RM. A modified definition for peripartum

cardiomyopathy and prognosis based on echocardiography. *Am J Obstet Gynecol* 1999;94:311–16.

3. Lampert MB, Weinert L, Hibbard J, Korcarz C, Lindheimer M, Lang RM. Contractile reserve in patients with peripartum cardiomyopathy and recovered left ventricular function. *Obstet Gynecol* 1997;176:189–95.

4. Elkayam U. Pregnant again after peripartum cardiomyopathy: to be or not to be? *Eur Heart J* 2002;23:753–6.

5. Elkayam U, Akhter MW, Singh H, Khan S, Bitar F, Hameed A, et al. Pregnancy-associated cardiomyopathy: clinical characteristics and a comparison between early and late presentation. *Circulation* 2005;111:2050–5.

6. Midei MG, DeMent SH, Feldman AM, Hutchins GM, Baughman KL. Peripartum myocarditis and cardiomyopathy. *Circulation* 1990;81:922–8.

7. Felker GM, Thompson RE, Hare JM, Hruban RH, Clemetson DE, Howard DL, et al. Underlying causes and long-term survival in patients with initially unexplained cardiomyopathy. *N Engl J Med* 2000;342:1077–84.

8. Bultmann BD, Klingel K, Nabauer M, Wallwiener D, Kandolf R. High prevalence of viral genomes and inflammation in peripartum cardiomyopathy. *Am J Obstet Gynecol* 2005;193:363–5.

9. Sliwa K, Forster O, Libhaber E, Fett JD, Sundstrom JB, Hilfiker-Kleiner D, et al. Peripartum cardiomyopathy: inflammatory markers as predictors of outcome in 100 prospectively studied patients. *Eur Heart J* 2006;27:441–6.

10. Hayakawa Y, Chandra M, Miao W, Shirani J, Brown JH, Dorn GW 2nd, et al. Inhibition of cardiac myocyte apoptosis improves cardiac function and abolishes mortality in the peripartum cardiomyopathy of Galpha(q) transgenic mice. *Circulation* 2003;108:3036–41.

11. Warraich RS, Sliwa K, Damasceno A, Carraway R, Sundrom B, Arif G, et al. Impact of pregnancy-related heart failure on humoral immunity: clinical relevance of G3-subclass immunoglobulins in peripartum cardiomyopathy. *Am Heart J* 2005;150:263–9.

12. Sundstrom JB, Fett JD, Carraway RD, Ansari AA. Is peripartum cardiomyopathy an organ-specific autoimmune disease? *Autoimmun Rev* 2002;1:73–7.

13. de Swiet M, Nelson-Piercy C. Cardiac disease. In: Lewis G, editor. *Why Mothers Die 2000–2002: The Sixth Report of Confidential Enquiries into Maternal Deaths in the United Kingdom*. London: RCOG Press; 2004. p. 137–50.

14. Deneux-Tharaux C, Berg C, Bouvier-Colle MH, Gissler M, Harper M, Nannini A, et al. Underreporting of pregnancy-related mortality in the United States and Europe. *Obstet Gynecol* 2005;106:684–92.

15. Murali S, Baldisseri MR. Peripartum cardiomyopathy. *Crit Care Med* 2005;33(10 Suppl):S340–6.

16. Witlin AG, Mabie WC, Sibai BH. Peripartum cardiomyopathy: An ominous diagnosis. *Am J Obstet Gynecol* 1997;176:182–8.

17. Witlin AG, Mabie WC, Sibai BM. Peripartum cardiomyopathy: a longitudinal echocardiographic study. *Am J Obstet Gynecol* 1997;177:1129–32.

18. Dorbala S, Brozena S, Zeb S, Galatro K, Homel P, Ren JF, et al. Risk stratification of women with peripartum cardiomyopathy at initial presentation: a dobutamine stress echocardiography study. *J Am Soc Echocardiogr* 2005;18:45–8.

19. Demakis JG, Rahimtoola SH, Sutton GC, Meadows WR, Szanto PB, Tobin JR, et al. Natural course of peripartum cardiomyopathy. *Circulation* 1971;44:1053–61.

20. Elkayam U, Tummala PP, Rao K, Akhter MW, Karaalp IS, Wani OR, et al. Maternal and fetal outcomes of subsequent pregnancies in women with peripartum cardiomyopathy. *N Engl J Med* 2001;344:1567–71.

21. Elliott P. Cardiomyopathy. Diagnosis and management of dilated cardiomyopathy. *Heart* 2000;84:106–12.

22. Thorne SA, Nelson-Piercy C, MacGregor A, Gibbs S, Crowhurst J, Panay N, *et al.* Pregnancy and contraception in heart disease and pulmonary arterial hypertension. *J Fam Plann Reprod Health Care* 2006;32:75–81.

23. Siu SC, Sermer M, Colman JM, Alvarez AN, Mercier LA, Morton BC, *et al.*; Cardiac Disease in Pregnancy (CARPREG) Investigators. Prospective multicenter study of pregnancy outcomes in women with heart disease. *Circulation* 2001;104:515–21.

24. Yacoub A, Martel MJ. Pregnancy with primary dilated cardiomyopathy. *Obstet Gynecol* 2002;99:928–30.

25. Bernstein PS, Magriples U. Cardiomyopathy in pregnancy: a retrospective study. *Am J Perinatol* 2001;18:163–8.

26. Elliott P, McKenna WJ. Hypertrophic cardiomyopathy. *Lancet* 2004;363:1881–91.

27. Thaman R, Varnava A, Hamid MS, Firoozi S, Sachdev B, Condon M, *et al.* Pregnancy related complications in women with hypertrophic cardiomyopathy. *Heart* 2003;89:752–6.

28. Autore C, Conte MR, Piccininno M, Bernabo P, Bonfiglio G, Bruzzi P, *et al.* Risk associated with pregnancy in hypertrophic cardiomyopathy. *J Am Coll Cardiol* 2002;40:1864–9.

29. Probst V, Langlard JM, Desnos M, Komajda M, Bouhour JB. Familial hypertrophic cardiomyopathy. French study of the duration and outcome of pregnancy. *Arch Mal Coeur Vaiss* 2002;95:81–6.

Chapter 17
Ischaemic heart disease

Jolien W Roos-Hesselink

Introduction

The prevalence of coronary artery disease in women is increasing owing to changing patterns of lifestyle, including cigarette smoking, diabetes and stress. Up to 10% of women with myocardial infarction are currently under the age of 35 years.[1] Because women are delaying childbearing until an older age, in the future the occurrence of acute myocardial infarction during pregnancy will be encountered more frequently. When infarction occurs in pregnancy, it constitutes a particular problem for the woman and the treating physician because the selection of diagnostic and therapeutic approaches is greatly influenced not only by maternal but also by fetal safety. In the literature the risk of a myocardial infarction in women during pregnancy is estimated as 1 per 10 000.[2-4] Myocardial infarction can occur at all stages of the pregnancy but the peak incidence is in the third trimester, in parous women older than 33 years.[5]

In normal pregnancy, the circulatory changes not only ensure the adequate supply of nutrients and oxygen to the developing fetus but also change the load on the cardiac muscle. Blood volume and cardiac output increase by 30–50%. This increase reaches a peak at around the 24th to 28th week of gestation and stays high or slowly decreases until term. Furthermore, there is an increase in heart rate of 10–20 beats per minute. Gestational hormones and circulating prostaglandins, in combination with the low vascular resistance of the placenta and the uterus, decrease the peripheral vascular resistance and blood pressure. Additionally, labour and its uterine contractions result in a further increase in blood pressure and cardiac output. Finally, after delivery, there is a significant increase in cardiac preload as a result of decompression of the inferior vena cava and the return of uterine and placental blood into the circulation. The reabsorption of extracellular fluids into the circulation in the postpartum period also results in an increase in intravascular volume. Most haemodynamic adaptations resolve within 2–6 weeks postpartum.[6]

During pregnancy there is a higher risk of thrombotic events owing to hyper-coagulability induced by hormone changes. The changed cardiac and haemodynamic situation and especially the hypercoagulability during pregnancy and the postpartum period possibly contribute to the spectrum of causes of myocardial infarction. In a series of women who underwent coronary angiography during pregnancy,[5] coronary atherosclerosis (with or without thrombus) was found in 43% and thrombus without signs of atherosclerosis was present in 21% of the women. Coronary dissection was found in 16% and was the primary cause of infarction in the postpartum period, while normal coronary arteries were reported in 20% of the women. The role of coronary spasm as a causative factor remains unclear.

The estimated mortality in pregnancy during acute myocardial infarction before the current practice of primary percutaneous transluminal coronary angioplasty (PTCA) was 20–37% for the mother and 17% for the baby.[7,8] The diagnosis is often missed because women may report chest pain during normal pregnancy, and also because the physician does not expect to diagnose myocardial infarction. The differential diagnosis of ischaemic chest pain includes haemorrhage, sickle cell crises, pre-eclampsia, acute pulmonary embolism and aortic dissection.[9] The diagnosis is confirmed by the characteristic electrocardiographic changes and the increase in cardiac enzyme levels.

In the acute phase, the treatment options for an acute myocardial infarction are percutaneous intervention, thrombolysis or coronary artery bypass grafting (CABG). At present, the primary choice of treatment in the general population is PTCA with stenting. However, the selection of diagnostic and therapeutic approaches during pregnancy is influenced by considerations of fetal as well as maternal safety.

Treatment of an acute coronary syndrome

Treatment in pregnancy is not based on randomised trials but on limited data from case reports (success tends to be reported), observational studies and individual clinical experience. During cardiac catheterisation, less than 20% of the radiation exposure reaches the fetus because of tissue attenuation. Radiation exposure to the fetus is kept to a minimum if PTCA is performed through the radial artery. Furthermore, shielding the gravid uterus from direct radiation, shortening of fluoroscopic time, delaying the procedure until at least the completion of the period of major organogenesis (more than 15 weeks after the last menstrual period) will minimise the radiation exposure. The amount of fetal exposure to radiation during chest radiography in PTCA results in a mean exposure of 0.02 mSv and a maximum of 0.1 mSv in difficult PTCA procedures (Table 17.1).[10] Therefore, PTCA should probably be considered acceptably safe but should still only be used during pregnancy when absolutely necessary because of the possible detrimental effects on the fetus (Table 17.2). The 8th to 15th week of gestation is the most radiation-sensitive period as far as the fetus is concerned.

Equally, as with PTCA, there is little experience with thrombolytic therapy during myocardial infarction. Streptokinase and low-dose recombinant tissue plasminogen activator (rtPA, or alteplase) do not cross the placenta in non-human animals. There is very little information available regarding humans, but streptokinase does not appear to cross the human placenta during late pregnancy.[11,12] It is not known whether rtPA crosses the human placenta but, in one case where it was used, intracranial haemorrhage was reported in the newborn infant.[13] The few available reports do not mention any teratogenic effect.

Most experience with thrombolytic therapy during pregnancy had been with streptokinase in women with pulmonary embolism, deep venous thrombosis or cardiac valve thrombosis. Complications that have been reported include maternal haemorrhage, uterine haemorrhage at emergency caesarean section, preterm delivery, fetal loss, fatal placental abruption, postpartum haemorrhage and spontaneous miscarriage. Haemorrhagic risks increase if thrombolytic therapy is given at the time of delivery.

Therefore, during pregnancy PTCA seems to be the first-line therapy, not only because of the relatively low fetal risks but also because other causes, for example coronary artery dissection, can be detected and treated. The use of stenting during

Table 17.1. Fetal radiation doses from X-ray investigations

Investigation	Fetal dose (mSv)	
	Mean	Maximum
Abdomen	1.4	4.2
Colon	6.8	24
Thorax	< 0.01	< 0.01
CT thorax	0.06	0.96
CT abdominal	8	49
CT pelvis	25	79
PTCA	0.02	0.1

CT = computed tomography; PTCA = percutaneous transluminal coronary angioplasty

PTCA implies the use of platelet aggregation inhibitors in the post–PTCA period. No information is available on the effects of clopidogrel on the fetus, although animal experiments have not shown a teratogenic effect.[14] Therefore, in these women balloon dilatation without stenting may be an alternative.

Because of the hypercoagulability state of pregnant women, thrombus formation can be a cause of myocardial infarction. Treatment with low molecular weight heparin is generally safe during pregnancy. More recently, 2b3a-receptor inhibitors have been introduced. However, there are no clinical or experimental data available on the fetal effects of this drug and therefore they are not currently recommended for use during pregnancy.

Morphine, which is used to treat the pain of myocardial infarction, does not cause teratogenic anomalies but crosses the placenta and can cause respiratory depression if given shortly before delivery.[15] Specific information on the safety of nitrates and sodium nitroprusside is lacking. Intravenous as well as oral nitrates have been used in a few women for the treatment of hypertension, myocardial ischaemia and heart failure; however, case reports of fetal heart decelerations associated with their use have been reported (most likely from decreased placental perfusion associated with hypotension).[16,17]

Table 17.2. Effects of radiation on the fetus

Period of exposure	Effect	Incidence (%)	Comments
Until 8 days	Spontaneous abortion	50–75	Rejection, all or nothing
9 days to 8 weeks	Deformation of organs	6	Small change – a relatively, high dose is needed
8–15 weeks	Mental retardation	0.5	500–1000 mSv: brain damage, from lower IQ to severe incomplete development
After 15 weeks	Childhood cancer	0.1	500 mSv: delayed growth, mental retardation (3 IQ points per 100 mSv)

After the acute phase of myocardial infarction, several drugs can be used to reduce the risk of recurrence or to reduce the progression of atherosclerosis. In general, beta blockers and digoxin are relatively safe. The calcium antagonist diltiazem should be avoided because of its suggested teratogenic effect.[18] Aspirin in low doses (less than 150 mg/day) is considered safe. High doses can cause premature closure of the ductus arteriosus, fetal congenital abnormalities and fetal and maternal haemorrhage.[19–22] Angiotensin-converting enzyme (ACE) inhibitors should be withdrawn during pregnancy because of their feto-toxic effects. Reported complications include fetal and neonatal renal failure, oligohydramnios, intrauterine growth restriction and hypoplasia of the skull bones (especially in the second and third trimester).[23]

There are no data available on the use of angiotensin II receptor antagonists in pregnancy, but their actions are similar to those of ACE inhibitors and so most consider them contraindicated.[24] Treatment options in myocardial infarction with cardiac failure are diuretics (furosemide and spironolactone)) and hydralazine, which are considered safe. Thiazides are not recommended because of reports of neonatal thrombocytopenia, jaundice, hyponatraemia and bradycardia.[25,26] Statins are contraindicated owing to feto-toxic effects.[14]

Cardiac surgery

Open-heart surgery can be performed during pregnancy with the same risk to the mother as outside pregnancy but with a high incidence (20–33%) of fetal death. The best period to perform it is early in the second trimester because in the first trimester surgery may cause miscarriage, and in the third trimester premature labour. The poor fetal outcome is due to the non–pulsatile blood flow and hypotension associated with cardiopulmonary bypass that adversely affect placental blood flow. Cardiopulmonary bypass in pregnancy should if possible be performed at high flow, high pressure, without hypothermia, and with the shortest possible cross-clamping time.

Delivery

Delivery does not need to be expedited because it is optimal to wait at least 2 or 3 weeks after the myocardial infarction to allow adequate healing. The mode of delivery should be determined by obstetric reasons and the clinical status of the mother. No convincing data showing an advantage to either vaginal delivery or caesarean section have been reported.[2]

Previous myocardial infarction

In addition to the acute coronary syndrome, women with previous myocardial infarction may also request counselling about a desired pregnancy. Impaired left ventricular function is one of the main determinants of maternal and neonatal outcome. No reviews are available that indicate a cut-off value for left ventricular ejection fraction below which pregnancy is contraindicated. An echocardiographic ejection fraction (EF) above 40% with a good rise of systemic arterial pressure on an exercise test suggests a good pregnancy outcome although complications can still occur. If the EF is below 40% with an increased left ventricular dimension, pregnancy should be discouraged.[27]

Pregnant women with heart disease and their close relatives should receive general advice before conception. Recommendations should include stopping smoking and avoiding excessive alcohol intake and any unnecessary medications. The use of any medication in pregnancy and during lactation requires consideration of the safety and tolerability for the fetus and infant, the physiological maternal changes and the risk–benefit ratio. In women who are already taking cardiovascular medication, the discontinuation of potentially harmful medication or a switch to a 'safer' drug should be discussed before conception. When ACE inhibitors and/or angiotensin II inhibitors are being used, stopping this medication and performing an echo-cardiographic and exercise test after 3 months is advised before making any recom-mendations about the wisdom of going ahead with a pregnancy.

Advice during pregnancy should include limiting physical activity (up to complete bed rest in cases where heart failure develops) and salt and fluid restriction. Self-weighing should be encouraged and in the event of sudden unexpected weight gain the woman should contact the physician in case pre-eclampsia is developing. Serial echocardiogram evaluation should be performed.

Particular attention should be focused on the recognition of ventricular arrhythmias during pregnancy and after delivery. Pregnancy increases the incidence of arrhythmias. Most antiarrhythmic drugs can be prescribed safely in pregnancy but every effort should be made to diagnose a correctable cause before starting therapy. All antiarrhythmic drugs cross the placental barrier and their potentially toxic effect on the fetus should be taken into consideration, particularly during the first weeks of pregnancy.[28]

Conclusion

The diagnosis of an acute myocardial infarction is often missed in pregnant women. Prompt diagnosis and therapy are necessary for reduction of the high mortality of child and mother. Atherosclerosis is one of the causes of myocardial infarction during pregnancy but other causes such as dissection and thrombus have also been found to be relatively frequent. Thrombolytic therapy can be given but serious adverse effects have been reported. Radiation exposure of the fetus during angiography and angioplasty appears to be acceptable, but is preferably postponed until after the 15th week of pregnancy. Finally, it is recommended that pregnant women with angina or myocardial infarction should be treated in a centre with facilities for interventional cardiology.

References

1.   Croft P, Hannaford PC. Risk factors for acute myocardial infarction in women: evidence from the Royal College of General Practitioners oral contraceptive study. *BMJ* 1989;298:165–8.

2.   Cohen WR, Steinman T, Patsner B, Snyder D, Satwicz P, Monroy P. Acute myocardial infarction in a pregnant woman at term. *JAMA* 1983;250:2179–81.

3.   Ginz B. Myocardial infarction in pregnancy. *J Obstet Gynaecol Br Commonw* 1970;77:610–15.

4.   Petitti DB, Sidney S, Quesenberry C Jr, Bernstein A. Incidence of stroke and myocardial infarction in women of reproductive age. *Stroke* 1997;28:280–3.

5.   Roth A, Elkayam U. Acute myocardial infarction associated with pregnancy. *Ann Intern Med* 1996;9:751–62.

6.   Hunter S, Robson SC. Adaptations of the maternal heart in pregnancy. *Br Heart J* 1992;68:540–3.

7 Ascarelli MH, Grider AR, Hsu HW. Acute myocardial infarction during pregnancy managed with immediate percutaneous transluminal coronary angioplasty. *Obstet Gynecol* 1996;88:655–7.

8. Badui E, Enciso R. Acute myocardial infarction during pregnancy and puerperium: a review. *Angiology* 1996;47:739–56.

9. Ray P, Murphy GJ, Shutt LE. Recognition and management of maternal cardiac disease in pregnancy. *Br J Anaesth* 2004;93:428–39.

10. Teunen D. The European Directive on health protection of individuals against the dangers of ionising radiation in realtion to medical exposures. *J Radiol Prot* 1998;18:133–7.

11 Turrentine MA, Braems G, Ramirez MM. Use of thrombolytics for the treatment of tromboembolic disease during pregnancy. *Obstet Gynecol Surv* 1995;50:534–41.

12. Pfeifer GW. The use of thrombolytic therapy in obstetrics and gynaecology. *Australas Ann Med* 1970;19(Suppl 1):28–31.

13. Baudo F, Caima TM, Redaelli R, Nosari AM, Mauri M, Leonardi G, et al. Emergency treatment with recombinant tissue plasminigen activator of pulmonary embolism in a pregnant woman with antithrombin 3 deficiency. *Am J Obstet Gynecol* 1990;163(4 Pt 1):1274–5.

14. *Farmacotherapeutisch Kompas.* Amstelveen: College voor Zorgverzekeraars; 2003, 2004.

15. Heinonen OP, Slone D, Shapiro S. *Birth Defects and Drugs in Pregnancy.* Littleton: Publishing Sci; 1977. p. 434.

16. Sheikh AU. Harper MA. Myocardial infarction during pregnancy: management and outcome of two pregnancies. *Am J Obstet Gynecol* 1993;169(2 Pt 1):279–84.

17. Shalev Y, Ben-Hur H, Hagay Z, Blickstein I, Epstein M, Ayzenberg O, et al. Successful delivery following myocardial ischaemia during the second trimester of pregnancy. *Clin Cardiol* 1993;16:754–6.

18. Briggs GG, Freeman RK, Yaffe SJ, editors. *Drugs in Pregnancy and Lactation: A Reference Guide to Fetal and Neonatal Risk.* 4th ed. Baltimore: Williams & Wilkins; 1994. p. 287–8.

19. Stuart MJ, Gross SJ, Elrad H, Graeber JE. Effects of acetylsalicylic-acid ingestion on maternal and neonatal haemostasis. *N Engl J Med* 1982;307:909–12.

20. Zierler S, Rothman KJ. Congenital heart disease in relation to maternal use of Bendectin and other drugs in early pregnancy. *N Engl J Med* 1985;313:347–52.

21. Viinikka L, Hartikainen-Sorri AL, Lumme R, Hiilesmaa V, Ylikorkala O. Low dose aspirin in hypertensive pregnant women: effect on pregnancy outcome and Prostacyclin–thromboxane balance in mother and newborn. *Br J Obstet Gynaecol* 1993;100:809–15.

22. CLASP (Collaborative Low-dose Aspirin Study in Pregnancy) Collaborative Group. CLASP: a randomised trial of low-dose aspirin for the prevention and treatment of pre-eclampsia among 9364 pregnant women. *Lancet* 1994;343:619–29.

23. Buttar HS. An overview of the influence of ACE inhibitors on fetal–placental circulation and perinatal development. *Mol Cell Biochem* 1997;176:61–71.

24. Hanssens M, Keirse MJ, Vankelecom F, Van Assche FA. Fetal and neonatal effects of treatment with angiotensin converting enzyme inhibitors in pregnancy. *Obstet Gynecol* 1991;78:128–35

25. Elkayam U. Pregnancy and cardiovascular disease. In: Braunwald E, editor. *Heart Disease. A Textbook of Cardiovascular Medicine.* 5th ed. Philadelphia: W.B. Saunders Company; 1997. p. 1843–64.

26. Opasich C, Russo A, Colombo E, Aldrovandi M, Addis A, Tavazzi L. Your cardiac patient wants to become a mother. Risk considerations and advice. Part II – Your cardiac patient is pregnant. *Ital Heart J* 2000;1:667–73.

27. Oakley C, Child A, Lung B, Presbitero P, Tornos P, Klein W, *et al.* Expert consensus document on management of cardiovascular diseases during pregnancy: The Task Force on Management of Cardiovascular Diseases During Pregnancy of the European Society of Cardiology. *Eur Heart J* 2003;24:761–81.

28. Gowda RM, Khan IA, Mehta NJ, Vasavada BC, Sacchi TJ. Cardiac arrhythmias in pregnancy: clinical and therapeutic considerations. *Int J Cardiol* 2003;88:129–33.

Chapter 18
Maternal cardiac arrhythmias

Koichiro Niwa and Shigeru Tateno

Arrhythmias without underlying cardiac disease

Incidence of arrhythmias in women of childbearing age

From published cardiac screening studies,[1,2] the incidence of arrhythmias in female students in junior high school, university students and women aged 35–40 years is reported to be 1.9–3.6%. Extrasystoles, I–II atrioventricular block (AVB) and right bundle branch block (RBBB) are all common in women of childbearing age.[3] Complex arrhythmias are rare.[1-3]

Incidence of arrhythmias during pregnancy

New onset or increased frequency of pre-existing arrhythmia is seen during the course of pregnancy in otherwise healthy women because of maternal neural, hormonal and physiological changes.[4] However, most of these arrhythmias are benign and asymptomatic, and without clinical significance.[4-6] Arrhythmias seen during pregnancy include premature supraventricular or ventricular extrasystoles, supraventricular tachyarrhythmia (SVT) such as paroxysmal supraventricular tachycardia (PSVT), atrial fibrillation (AF), atrial flutter (AFL), ventricular tachycardia (VT), conduction disturbances and Wolff–Parkinson–White (WPW) syndrome. The exact incidence of each arrhythmia during pregnancy is unknown but arrhythmias other than monofocal or multifocal extrasystoles, or couplets/triplets of supraventricular extrasystole, are rare. From a recent study based on Holter monitoring analysis in volunteers during pregnancy, 95% of the women showed supraventricular and/or ventricular extrasystoles but none showed complex arrhythmias.[7] Ventricular extrasystole is observed in up to 60% of pregnant women.[4]

The incidence of pre-excitation arrhythmias such as WPW syndrome varies from 0.1 to 3.7 per 1000 population.[8] Most adults with a pre-excitation syndrome have a normal heart. The incidence of PSVT increases during pregnancy in women with WPW.[9] However, pregnancy does not appear to predispose otherwise healthy hearts to AFL/AF.[3] AFL/AF are usually only observed during pregnancy in women with heart disease.

VT is rare in the general population. Idiopathic VT with a right ventricular focus has been observed during pregnancy,[10] but in a study of 50 healthy pregnant women who underwent Holter monitoring, only one episode of three-beat VT was recorded.[3]

In one study of long QT syndrome,[11] arrhythmic events such as syncope or cardiac arrest were observed more frequently postpartum compared with during pregnancy. Beta blockers produce a significant reduction of arrhythmic events and are thus useful in the management of pregnant women with long QT syndrome.

The incidence of bradyarrhythmias is lower than that of tachyarrhythmias during pregnancy. Most such arrhythmias are asymptomatic and have no clinical importance.[10] The incidence of sinus node dysfunction during pregnancy is unknown but clinically relevant cases are rare. Complete AVB has been observed during pregnancy but it is not clear whether a woman with congenital complete AVB would benefit from elective implantation of a permanent pacemaker.[12] If there is no associated heart disease and the woman remains asymptomatic with a good escape mechanism, a pacemaker is not necessary.

Bundle branch block (BBB) appearing *de novo* in pregnancy has not been reported, but pregnant women may present with fascicular blocks, isolated or in combination with right BBB. Left BBB is very rare in women of childbearing age and, when seen, is usually associated with significant heart disease.

Arrhythmia in women with CHD during pregnancy

In recent years, increasing numbers of women with repaired congenital heart disease (CHD) have been reaching childbearing age. The prevalence of arrhythmia in repaired CHD rises with age, as a result of surgical scars, the underlying lesion specific to each patient (some lesions have intrinsic conduction abnormalities), and ageing. In spite of improvements in the antiarrhythmic treatments available, some of these arrhythmias have a significant negative impact on life expectancy.[13,14]

Arrhythmias in women with CHD during pregnancy may be attributable not only to dramatic changes in haemodynamics, hormones, catecholamine levels and autonomic nervous system activity during pregnancy[4] but also to the underlying specific haemodynamics of CHD and the presence in the heart of surgical scars. The intravascular volume increases during pregnancy, especially in preload, and can unveil an arrhythmogenic focus in atrial or ventricular tissue, which is augmented by the underlying haemodynamic abnormalities. Poor functional status and a history of pre-existing decompensated cardiac failure are additional risk factors for arrhythmias.[15,16] During pregnancy there is typically an increase in the heart rate, which may promote arrhythmia by modifying the effective refractory period, the velocity of conduction and the spatial dispersion of refractoriness.[17] Rapid heart rate is induced by increased sympathetic or impaired parasympathetic nerve activity[18,19] and can be accompanied by significant SVT or VT during pregnancy. Volume overload with neurohormonal activation and imbalance between sympathetic and parasympathetic systems secondary to inhibited autonomic nerve function may also play a contributory role. The mechanism of VT in women with CHD is typically re-entry, involving a disparity in conduction between normal and diseased myocardium or operative scar. In contrast, the most common mechanism of VT in pregnancy may be increased catecholamine sensitivity.[20] This hypothesis is supported by the observation that increased rest during pregnancy decreases the incidence of SVT or VT. In one study,[21] a blunted heart-rate response during exercise in pregnancy in women with CHD after repair (especially in tetralogy of Fallot) was reported.[22]

Arrhythmias, especially SVT, VT and high-degree AVB, during pregnancy in women with CHD can cause significant haemodynamic compromise to both the mother and fetus.[23] Prompt and accurate diagnosis and treatment of these arrhythmias is likely to reduce maternal and fetal morbidity and mortality. In one report,[7] no maternal deaths were observed in women with repaired CHD and arrhythmias during pregnancy. However, it should be remembered that pharmacological agents used for the arrhythmia control during pregnancy may have adverse effects on the mother and fetus.[24]

Tachyarrhythmias

Of the various reviews of pregnancy in women with CHD,[15,16,25–28] none have focused specifically on arrhythmia during pregnancy. However, in one study of 233 pregnancies in women with CHD,[16] 20 with arrhythmias (including two women with AFs and four with PSVTs) were reported. In another study of 132 pregnancies there was one case of VT and four of SVTs,[15] and in a multicentre study of 445 pregnancies two women with VTs and 14 with SVTs were reported.[25] Finally, in another study of 309 pregnancies there was only one woman reported to have an arrhythmia.[28] In the most recent reported series,[7] the incidence of significant arrhythmias during pregnancy in women with CHD was 6.9%, with SVT being more frequent than VT.

SVTs may be associated with atrial dilatation, for example secondary to atrio-ventricular valve regurgitation, atrial septal defect or Fontan procedure. Pregnancy may cause an increased incidence of paroxysmal AF in women with CHD. VT has been observed in women with repaired tetralogy of Fallot, with free pulmonary regurgitation and right ventricular dilatation, and it can induce right ventricular failure and sudden death.[14] VT is reported to be an unusual event in pregnancy[20] and is relatively rare even in women with CHD. However, sustained VT needs urgent treatment when it does occur.

The precise incidence of the new onset of sick sinus syndrome during pregnancy is unknown[5,6,29] but pregnancy does not appear to predispose women to develop II–III degree AVB.[12] Complete AVB or sick sinus syndrome is sometimes seen as a surgical complication but in a recent cohort of women with CHD requiring surgery it was rare even in this context.[30]

Arrhythmia management during pregnancy

Data on the effects of antiarrhythmic medications on the fetus are very limited.[5,6,24,31,32] Most such drugs are in the US Food and Drug Administration (FDA) category C ('animal studies have shown an adverse effect and there are no adequate and well-controlled studies in pregnant women' or 'no animal studies have been conducted and there are no adequate and well-controlled studies in pregnant women'; www.perinatology.com/exposures/Drugs/FDACategories.htm). Especially during the first trimester, administration of drugs is probably best avoided owing to the possibility of unknown unfavourable effects on the fetus.[31,32] Most drugs have not been thoroughly tested in pregnancy and, as far as is currently known, all antiarrhythmic drugs can cross the placenta.[31,32] Most of them also transmit from mother to baby through breastfeeding.[32] The altered risk–benefit ratio of antiarrhythmic therapy during pregnancy in women with CHD affects the traditional concepts of manage-ment. Most SVTs and VTs of short duration (non-sustained) are benign and are not usually associated with any symptoms other than palpitations. Treatment of arrhythmia may be more harmful than the arrhythmia itself in this situation. However, some episodes of tachyarrhythmia can be associated with severe or even life-threatening symptoms in women with CHD. In considering therapy for cardiac arrhythmias, and sometimes for subsequent cardiac failure, the altered haemodynamics of pregnancy need to be taken into account. Immediate medical attention is warranted, especially for persistent SVT or sustained VT or severe bradyarrhythmias. These can affect the mother and fetus adversely, resulting in haemodynamic compromise that jeopardises not only the mother's but also the fetus's wellbeing (by decreasing uterine blood flow). In this situation, antiarrhythmic medication must be initiated as soon as possible after the appropriate diagnosis has been made.

Ventricular tachycardia

Ventricular tachycardia can occur in structurally normal hearts but it is more commonly associated with structurally abnormal hearts as in women with CHD. In one study,[4] non-sustained VT was observed in three of 26 women with CHD. One woman with a repaired tetralogy of Fallot developed VT during delivery and was successfully treated with intravenous mexiletine. In the series reported by Brodsky *et al.*,[20] two of 40 women with VT during pregnancy died. The risk of death is further increased when concomitant ventricular dysfunction is present. Thus, in women with symptomatic VT, urgent therapy is indicated. Lidocaine, mexiletine or procainamide can be administered safely and effectively in sustained VT with stable haemodynamics.[33] Beta blockers can also be effective for VT originating from the right ventricular outflow tract.[2]

Supraventricular tachyarrhythmia

Supraventricular tachyarrhythmia is observed more frequently than VT, and two-thirds of SVT cases will need treatment with antiarrhythmic medication (Table 18.1).[7] When SVT is observed in women with low functional class (lower than NYHA II (New York Heart Association)) or pre-existing cardiac failure, meticulous care should be taken and antiarrhythmic therapy should be initiated as soon as the diagnosis has been made. In women with a history of persistent SVT before pregnancy, the recurrence rate of SVT during pregnancy is high (36%)[15] and thus catheter ablation should be considered before pregnancy, if appropriate. In cases with sustained VT or persistent SVT and unstable haemodynamics, prompt direct current (DC) synchronised cardioversion is necessary.[33,34]

Supraventricular tachyarrhythmia includes a number of different types of tachycardia with varying features and clinical mechanisms, such as PSVT (sinus nodal re-entry tachycardia (SNRT), intra-atrial re-entrant tachycardia (IART), atrioventricular nodal re-entrant tachycardia (AVNRT), atrioventricular reciprocating tachycardia (AVRT)), automatic atrial tachycardia (AAT), multiple atrial tachycardia (MAT), AF and AFL. Intravenous adenosine infusion is effective in most cases of PSVT.[35,36] Beta blockers and/or digoxin are safe and effective for prevention of PSVT for long-term use.[37] A selective beta 1 blocker, for example metoprolol, is safer than a non-specific beta blocker, especially in the first trimester.[37] In cases of drug-resistant incessant PSVT, catheter ablation can be performed in the third trimester.[38] Pre-excitation may be associated with Ebstein anomaly of the tricuspid valve and left ventricular non-compaction. (The latter is a cardiomyopathy characterized by numerous excessive trabeculations and deep intertrabecular recesses with a high manifestation of SVT.) AF with pre-excitation carries the potential risk of rapid conduction over accessory pathways, permitting an extremely rapid ventricular response that can lead to ventricular fibrillation. Meticulous care should be taken in

Table 18.1. Drugs for supraventricular tachyarrhythmia; data from *Drug Facts and Comparisons*[72]

Treatment	Recommendation[a]	FDA class[b]
Termination		
Vagal manoeuvres	I	None
Adenosine	I	C
DC cardioversion	I	None
Metoprolol, propranolol	IIa	C
Verapamil	IIb	C
Prophylaxis		
Digoxin	I	C
Metoprolol	I	C
Propranolol	IIa	B
Sotalol, flecainide	IIa	C
Quinidine, propafenone, verapamil	IIb	C
Procainamide	IIb	C
Catheter ablation	IIb	None
Atenolol	III	D
Amiodarone	III	D

[a] Recommendation classes:I = recommended; IIa = relative recommendation; IIb = not recommended; III = avoid
[b] See www.perinatology.com/exposures/Drugs/FDACategories.htm for descriptions of the FDA classes

the use of digoxin and verapamil since both may increase transmission of impulses through the accessory pathway to the ventricle.[5]

Atrioventricular nodal re-entry tachycardia

Short runs of AVNRT and AVRT require no treatment. However, prolonged episodes of these can occur in women with CHD, producing haemodynamic compromise requiring medication or even cardioversion. Adenosine has been shown to terminate more than 90% of SVTs involving the atrioventricular node as part of the re-entry circuit, and it has been shown to be safe and useful during pregnancy.[35,36] Intravenous verapamil may be used, but the safety of verapamil during pregnancy is not fully established.[32,39] For AVRT, procainamide to slow the conduction of the bypass tract can also terminate the arrhythmia.[31] For women with severe symptoms, a combination of digoxin and a beta blocker appears to be safe and effective during pregnancy.[5] In women with AVNRT, digoxin or a beta blocker can be useful.[5] For severely symptomatic women who become refractory to medication, radiofrequency ablation of the bypass tract or slow pathway has been successfully performed during pregnancy.[38]

Sinus nodal re-entry tachycardia and intra-atrial re-entrant tachycardia

Sinus nodal re-entry tachycardia and IART can be managed by blocking either atrioventricular nodal conduction or the recurrent re-entry circuit. Digoxin or a beta blocker are safe and effective. Type Ia drugs can be used to terminate re-entrant circuits. Flecainide has been reported to be useful for the termination of atrial tachycardia during pregnancy.[40]

Atrial flutter

Chronic AFL is usually associated with significant heart disease. It may occur as a result of increased atrial pressure, atrial dilatation, post-surgical scarring or unusual haemodynamics such as more than moderate atrioventricular valve regurgitation or Fontan circuit. The approach to AFL in pregnant women depends on the degree of haemodynamic compromise. The mechanism of AFL often involves atrial macro re-entry or, rarely, focal ectopic origin due to enhanced automaticity.[5] In typical AFL, the atrial depolarisation is usually seen as negative deflections in the inferior leads (II, III, AVF) of the electrocardiogram (ECG).

In a haemodynamically stable woman, the ventricular rate can be controlled with intravenous digoxin. Beta blockers and/or digoxin are also safe and are usually effective for rate control. In resistant cases, calcium channel blockers can be used. Alternatively, class I antiarrhythmic agents such as procainamide can be used to convert AFL to sinus rhythm. In women with more severe CHD, and haemodynamic compromise, urgent synchronised cardioversion should be used.[34,41] The need for continuing medication for sinus rhythm maintenance will depend on the severity and frequency of the symptoms.

Atrial fibrillation

In women with CHD, pregnancy can cause an increased incidence of AF. The increased morbidity and mortality in such cases can be explained by the haemo-dynamic changes and the increased risk of thromboembolism, especially in the third trimester with its hypercoagulable state. Haemodynamically, AF is poorly tolerated in women with inflow stenosis (mitral stenosis, tricuspid stenosis, increased ventricular end–diastolic pressure). Atrial emptying is severely impaired because of the shortened diastolic filling time. This results in a rise in atrial and pulmonary venous pressure, as well as pulmonary oedema and decreased cardiac output. The risk of systemic embolisation in AF during pregnancy is probably due to circulatory stasis in the atrium and left atrial appendage, and the hyperviscosity and hypercoagulable state of pregnancy with subsequent thrombus formation.

The aetiology of AF is associated with postoperative scarring and increased atrial pressure. The most common cardiac conditions associated with this arrhythmia during pregnancy are mitral or tricuspid stenosis, more than moderate CHD after repair such as tetralogy of Fallot, complete transposition of the great arteries after atrial switch repair, systemic inflow and outflow stenosis of the ventricle, pulmonary venous high flow such as atrial septal defect, atrioventricular valve regurgitation and special haemodynamics such as Fontan. Electrophysiologically, AF is due to the simultaneous discharge of multiple atrial foci, resulting in a high atrial rate and no apparent p waves in the ECG. The ventricular rate depends on atrioventricular nodal refractoriness.

The management of AF is similar to that of AFL. In haemodynamically stable women, the ventricular rate should be controlled by digoxin, a beta blocker or a calcium channel blocker, or a combination of these. As alternative to rate control, drugs such as procainamide may be useful for conversion to sinus rhythm. Synchro-nised cardioversion can be used to convert AF to sinus rhythm in women with compromised haemodynamics. In an elective situation, procainamide should be started and a therapeutic level achieved before cardioversion to prevent relapse. In emergency cases, cardioversion should be performed, so long as there is no evidence of atrial thrombus, assessed by transoesophageal echocardiography.

DC cardioversion

An electric shock, by depolarising all excitable myocardium and possibly by prolonging refractoriness, interrupts re-entry circuits, discharges foci and establishes the electrical homogeneity that terminates re-entry. DC cardioversion will terminate most tachycardias effectively, whether SVT or VT, at any stage of pregnancy.[5,6,36,42,43] Reported fetal complications from DC cardioversion are few but include the occurrence of a transient fetal bradycardia that resolved spontaneously.[5] It is good practice to scan the fetal heart immediately after successful DC cardioversion of the mother, and this should be encouraged.

Implantable cardioverter defibrillators

The outcome of pregnancy in women with implanted permanent cardioverter defibrillators has been assessed and no increased risk of major complications during pregnancy has been reported.[44]

Electrophysiological study and catheter ablation

Both electrophysiological evaluation and radiofrequency ablation require the use of ionising radiation and are thus better avoided during pregnancy. However, electrophysiological study (EPS) can be performed during pregnancy using echocardiographic guidance for the evaluation of pre-syncope, syncope or VT,[45] as can catheter ablation[46] (see Chapter 8).

Bradyarrhythmias

Most bradyarrhythmias and conduction abnormalities during pregnancy in women with repaired CHD are a residual effect of surgery.

Sinus node dysfunction

The incidence of sinus node dysfunction during pregnancy is unknown. A pacemaker (temporary or permanent) is necessary in surgically induced sick sinus syndrome.[47,48]

Second or complete atrioventricular block

Although pregnancy does not appear to predispose woman to develop second- or third-degree AVB[12], several reports of pregnancy with complete AVB have been published.[5] Common cardiac conditions associated with high-degree AVB are corrected transposition of the great arteries, ventricular septal defect and tetralogy of Fallot. In women with CHD and post-surgical complete AVB, permanent pacemaker implantation is indicated. In those with post-surgical high-grade AVB, pacemaker insertion before pregnancy is advisable.

Intraventricular conduction block

QRS duration can be prolonged during pregnancy secondary to ventricular dilatation associated with the high cardiac output. The potential clinical implications of this QRS prolongation have, however, not been documented even among women with repaired tetralogy of Fallot (where QRS prolongation represents a risk factor for VT and sudden cardiac death). Left BBB is usually associated with structural heart disease or surgical complications.

Pacemaker implantation

Permanent pacemaker implantation is indicated in women with sick sinus syndrome or AVB during pregnancy. Pacemaker implantation can be performed safely after 12 weeks of gestation,[5,10] but it is probably better performed before pregnancy to avoid fetal radiation exposure. Women who already have an implanted pacemaker prior to conception tolerate pregnancy well.[49]

Specific considerations of antiarrhythmic drugs

Procainamide has a long record of safety during pregnancy (Table 18.2).[50] Lidocaine has also been widely used and it also appears to be relatively safe and not teratogenic. It is classified as category B by the FDA ('animal studies have revealed no evidence of harm to the fetus, however, there are no adequate and well-controlled studies in pregnant women').[51] Bradycardia and adverse effects on the central nervous system have been observed only rarely.[12,23] Although there is less experience with flecainide, particularly during the early stages of fetal development, it appears to be relatively well tolerated during pregnancy.[23,40,51] No adverse effects have been reported for propafenone, but experience during pregnancy is very limited. There has been extensive experience with beta blockers since these have been used in various situations such as arrhythmias, hypertension and aortic dilatation.[52,53] They appear to be relatively safe although growth restriction, bradycardia and hypoglycaemia in the fetus have occasionally been reported for propranolol.[23,51] Cardioselective beta blockers seem to be preferable. Sotalol appear to be well tolerated but experience with its use during pregnancy is very limited.[40] Amiodarone may be teratogenic as an increase in the rate of congenital abnormalities has been observed with its use.[32] In addition, an association of amiodarone with fetal hypothyroidism is quite common (approximately 9%), and growth restriction and preterm birth have also been reported.[54,55] It is thus classified as FDA category D ('adequate well-controlled or observational studies in pregnant women have demonstrated a risk to the fetus. However, the benefits of therapy may outweigh the potential risk. For example, the drug may be acceptable if needed in a life-threatening situation or serious disease for which safer drugs cannot be used or are ineffective') and should be avoided during pregnancy unless considered essential.[23,51] Calcium channel blockers are considered relatively safe, but bradycardia, heart block and hypotension have been encountered with the use of verapamil.[23,50,51] Generally, beta blockers, digoxin and adenosine are preferred over calcium antagonists. There has been more experience with digoxin and it is probably the safest drug to use during pregnancy, although an increased incidence of low birthweight infants has been reported as an adverse effect.[23,50] Adenosine also appears to be safe, but there is only limited experience during early pregnancy.[36]

Arrhythmia during pregnancy in specific categories of CHD

In one report concerning tetralogy of Fallot, two of 72 pregnant women developed SVT.[56] From another report[57] on Ebstein anomaly of the tricuspid valve and pregnancy, although 14% of the women had one or more accessory conduction pathways at the

Table 18.2. Antiarrhythmic drugs during pregnancy; data from *Drug Facts and Comparisons*[72] and American Academy of Pediatrics Committee on Drugs[73]

Drug	Vaughan Williams class[a]	FDA class[b]	Indication	Adverse effects	Teratogenic	Lactation
Quinidine	IA	C	Various arrhythmias	Thrombocytopenia	No	Compatible
Procainamide	IA	C	Various arrhythmias	Lupus-like syndrome	No	Compatible
Disopyramide	IA	C	Various arrhythmias	Uterine contraction	No	Compatible
Lidocaine	IB	B	VT	Bradycardia, CNS adverse effects	No	Compatible
Mexiletine	IB	C	VT	Bradycardia, CNS adverse effects, LBWI	No	Compatible
Phenytoin	IB	D	Digoxin toxicity	Fetal hydantoin syndrome	Yes	Compatible
Flecainide	IC	C	VT, SVT	None	No	Compatible
Propafenone	IC	C	VT, SVT	None	No	Unknown
Propranolol	II	C	SVT, VT, AF	IUGR, bradycardia, hypoglycaemia	No	Compatible
Atenolol	II	C	SVT, VT, AF	None	No	Caution
Amiodarone	III	D	VT	Hypothyroidism, IUGR anomaly	Yes	Avoid
Sotalol	III	B	VT, SVT	Bradycardia	No	Compatible
Verapamil	IV	C	SVT, VT, AF	Hypotension, bradycardia	No	Compatible
Adenosine	N/A	C	SVT	None	No	Unknown
Digoxin	N/A	C	SVT, AF	LBWI	No	Compatible

[a] See Vaughan Williams[74]

[b] See www.perinatology.com/exposures/Drugs/FDACategories.htm for descriptions of the FDA classes

AF = atrial fibrillation; CNS = central nervous system; IUGR = intrauterine growth restriction; LBWI = low birthweight infant; SVT = supraventricular tachyarrhythmia; VT = ventricular tachycardia; N/A = not available

time of pregnancy, there were no episodes of clinical arrhythmia requiring hospital admission. Similarly, there was no sustained arrhythmia requiring hospital admission in 29 pregnancies among women with corrected transposition of the great arteries.[58] In another survey,[7] however, two women with the same congenital heart defect had episodes of SVT and AFL and needed antiarrhythmic medication. A recent paper has detailed the course of 48 pregnancies in 34 pregnant women with complete transposition of the great arteries and a Mustard procedure: only one episode of AFL was reported in a woman with relevant previous history.[59–61] In another study of women with systemic right ventricles,[7] one woman with complete transposition of the great arteries and a Mustard procedure required pacemaker implantation during pregnancy owing to sick sinus syndrome. Both AFL and PSVT have been reported in one of 14 pregnancies among Fontan patients.[62]

Influence of arrhythmia on the mother and fetus

Arrhythmia management in women with CHD is basically the same as in those without cardiac disease. However, the underlying haemodynamic conditions unique to each syndrome must be taken into account. In cases of repaired CHD with residual abnormalities and/or ventricular dysfunction and tachyarrhythmia during pregnancy, morbidity in the mother and fetus is high.[7,16,25] Attention should be focused on whether the arrhythmia has significant clinical effects, such as causing deterioration of the underlying cardiac condition, and the adverse effects of antiarrhythmic medication. During the 12 year period from 1979 to 1990, there were no reports of maternal deaths from primary tachyarrhythmia in the UK, although some deaths involved tachyarrhythmia in association with structural heart disease.[63] In recent reports from Canada and Japan, reported arrhythmias in pregnant women with CHD did not result in maternal death.[7,25]

In women with cyanosis and CHD, the incidence of low birthweight infants, stillbirth or miscarriage has been found to be high.[64] The rate of successful pregnancies has been reported to improve when cyanotic patients became acyanotic following surgical repair, with babies subsequently having normal intrauterine growth.[15,16,26,27] In a survey on pregnancy in women with CHD and arrhythmias,[7] the incidence of low birthweight infants (24%) and miscarriage or stillbirth (11%) was higher than in previous reports on pregnancy in women with repaired CHD.

Counselling of pregnancy and fetal cardiac screening in women with arrhythmias

The cardiologist's role is to give the woman an estimate of both maternal and fetal risk so as to allow her to make an informed decision about pregnancy, and to provide appropriate antenatal care.[42,65] In women with a history of arrhythmia, it is recommended to evaluate the type and nature of arrhythmia, the haemodynamics of the underlying CHD, cardiac function and the type of antiarrhythmic medication prior to conception. In women with risk factors for arrhythmias during pregnancy, such as those with cardiac failure or poor functional class or significant atrio-ventricular valve regurgitation, meticulous care must be taken both during and after pregnancy. Ideally, catheter ablation should be performed before pregnancy, when appropriate. Prepregnancy exercise ECG testing can be helpful to predict new onset or recurrence of arrhythmias or cardiac failure during pregnancy.[65]

Contraception in women with arrhythmias

In high-risk conditions, such as pulmonary arterial hypertension, severe obstructive lesions or Marfan syndrome with a large aorta, women should be advised against pregnancy because of the underlying lesion itself. If pregnancy occurs, termination should be considered.[42] However, arrhythmia is not in itself an indication for such advice or action.[5,6] For detailed comments on contraception, see Chapter 2.

Maternal follow-up during pregnancy

There is no consensus at present on the most appropriate follow-up interval during pregnancy for women with CHD (with or without arrhythmia).[42,66] Intervals should be shorter for women with moderate cardiovascular disease and arrhythmias than in those with uncomplicated mild cardiovascular disease. In women with arrhythmias, ECG and Holter monitoring can be easily performed before, during and after pregnancy. Arrhythmias are prone to develop in women with cardiac failure and thus serial evaluation of cardiac function by echocardiography, brain natriuretic peptides

(BNP) and atrial natriuretic peptides (ANP) levels may assist management. Hospitalisation and urgent treatment are necessary in women with incessant tachyarrhythmia that may result in acute deterioration of their cardiac condition.

Management and anaesthesia of women with arrhythmias during delivery

Significant haemodynamic changes due to the effects of uterine contractions, increased catecholamine levels, significant blood loss (average 300–800 ml) during delivery and a massive increase in venous return immediately after delivery are important cardiac challenges that can induce arrhythmias in women with CHD.[67] Close monitoring of heart rate, rhythm and blood pressure is thus mandatory during delivery and the postpartum period.

A normal vaginal delivery with good analgesia and a low threshold for assisted delivery is the safest mode of delivery for a woman with CHD and arrhythmias, since it is associated with less blood loss and less rapid haemodynamic changes than caesarean section.[42,43,68] Effective analgesia is necessary for women with CHD during delivery because their condition can easily deteriorate owing to the acute haemodynamic changes of birth and delivery-related stress.[67,69]

Multidisciplinary team approach during pregnancy and delivery

In pregnant women with CHD, timely management of complications such as cardiac failure, arrhythmias, thrombosis and hypertension is essential.[25,42] Close monitoring of haemodynamic changes during pregnancy and delivery in women with CHD is also mandatory. Clearly, therefore, appropriate levels of evaluation and management of the cardiac condition by cardiologists throughout the pregnancy are necessary. Anaesthetists who are used to caring for women with heart disease are essential for safe and effective analgesia. The incidence of premature and/or low birthweight infants is high in women with CHD and arrhythmias, and thus the support of neonatologists is sometimes necessary.[65–69] A multidisciplinary team that consists of obstetricians, cardiologists, anaesthetists, neonatologists, cardiac surgeons, geneticists and other specialised consultants is a key feature of caring for women with CHD and arrhythmias during pregnancy and delivery.[67] Pregnant women with moderate to complex CHD are best managed in specialist tertiary care facilities.[66,70]

Postpartum management of women with arrhythmias

Cardiac failure or new onset or increased frequency of significant arrhythmia can occur after delivery. Close follow-up of these women after delivery is thus essential.

Lactation

All antiarrhythmiac drugs are excreted into breast milk but concentrations are generally low.[31,71] Amiodarone should be avoided since it appears at high levels in breast milk. Beta blockers, digoxin, lidocaine, calcium antagonists, sotalol and flecainide may be compatible with breastfeeding, but experience is particularly limited with the last three.[50] They should therefore be used with caution.

Conclusions

Arrhythmias are probably the most frequent complication of pregnancy in women with CHD. However, many of them are benign. Nevertheless, new onset or increased frequency of pre-existing arrhythmias can occur during pregnancy, which in turn may cause significant haemodynamic compromise to both the mother and fetus. DC cardioversion is safe during pregnancy. Drug therapy requires careful consideration of the risk–benefit ratio for both the mother and fetus. A multidisciplinary approach with close monitoring of the woman and with timely arrhythmia therapy, when needed, are required to optimise maternal and neonatal outcomes.

References

1. Niwa K, Warita N, Sunami Y, Shimura A, Tateno S, Sugita K. Prevalence of arrhythmias and conduction disturbances in large population-based samples of children. *Cardiol Young* 2004;14:68–74.
2. Tsuda J, Niimura I, Matsuo M. Statistics of arrhythmias in school age. Health guidance of heart disease in childhood. *Nihon-Ijishinpo* 1982;3035:43–8.
3. Sobotka PA, Mayer JH, Bauernfeind RA, Kanakis C Jr, Rosen KM. Arrhythmias documented by 24-hour continuous ambulatory electrocardiographic monitoring in young women without apparent heart disease. *Am Heart J* 1981;101:753–9.
4. Shotan A, Ostrzega E, Mehra A, Johonson JV, Elkayam U. Incidence of arrhythmias in normal pregnancy and relation to palpitations, dizziness, and syncope. *Am J Cardiol* 1997;79:1061–4.
5. Leung CY, Broadsky MA. Cardiac arrhythmias and pregnancy. In: Elkayam U, Gleicher N, editors. *Cardiac Problems in Pregnancy*, 3rd edn. New York: Wiley-Liss; 1998. p. 155–74.
6. Anderson MH. Rhythm disorders. In: Oakley C, editor. *Heart Disease in Pregnancy*. London: British Medical Journal Publishing Group; 1997. p. 248–81.
7. Tateno S, Niwa K, Nakazawa M, Akagi T, Shinohara T, Yasuda T. Arrhythmia and conduction disturbances in patients with congenital heart disease during pregnancy: multicenter study. *Circ J* 2003;67: 992–7.
8. Wellens HJ. Wolff–Parkinson–White syndrome: diagnosis, arrhythmias and identification of the high risk patient. *Mod Concepts Cardiovasc Dis* 1983;52:53–9.
9. Widerhorn J, Widerhorn AL, Rahimtoola SH, Elkayam U. WPW syndrome during pregnancy: increased incidence of supraventricular arrhythmias. *Am Heart J* 1992;123:796–8.
10. Page RL, Hamdan MH, Joglar JA. Arrhythmias occurring during pregnancy. *Cardiac Electrophysiol Rev* 2002;6:136–9.
11. Rashba EJ, Zareba W, Moss AJ, Hall WJ, Robinson J, Locati EH, et al. Influence of pregnancy on the risk for cardiac events in patients with hereditary long QT syndrome. *Circulation* 1998;97:451–6.
12. Dalvi BV, Chaudhuri A, Kulkazrni HL, Kale PA. Therapeutic guidelines for congenital complete heart block presenting in pregnancy. *Obstet Gynecol* 1992;79:802–4.
13. Silka M, Hardy B, Menashe V, Morris CD. A population-based prospective evaluation of risk of sudden cardiac death after operation fro common congenital heart defects. *J Am Coll Cardiol* 1998;32:245–51.
14. Gatzoulis MA, Balaji S, Webber SA, Siu SC, Hokanson JS, Poile C, et al. Risk factors for arrhythmia and sudden cardiac death late after repair of tetralogy of Fallot: a multicentre study. *Lancet* 2000;356:975–81.

15. Siu SC, Sermer M, Harrison DA, Grigoriadis E, Liu G, Sorensen S, *et al.* Risk and predictors for pregnancy-related complications in women with heart disease. *Circulation* 1997;96:2789–94.

16. Whittemore R, Hobbins JC, Engle MA. Pregnancy and its outcome in women with and without surgical treatment of congenital heart disease. *Am J Cardiol* 1982;50:641–51.

17. Schwarz PJ, Priori SG. Symptomatic nervous system and cardiac arrhythmias. In: Zipes PD, Jalife J, editors. *Cardiac Electrophysiology: from Cell to Bedside.* Philadelphia: World Bank Saunders; 1990. p. 330–43.

18. Barron WM, Mujais SK, Zinaman M, Bravo EL, Lindheimer MD. Plasma catecholamine responses to physiologic stimuli in normal human pregnancy. *Am J Obstet Gynecol* 1986;154:80–4.

19. Zimmermann M, Maisonblanche P, Cauchemez B, Leclercq JF, Coumel P. Determinants *of* the spontaneous ectopic activity in repetitive monomorphic idiopathic ventricular tachycardia. *J Am Coll Cardiol* 1986;7:1219–27.

20. Brodsky M, Doria R, Allen B, Sato D, Thomas G, Sada M. New-onset ventricular tachycardia during pregnancy. *Am Heart J* 1992;123:933–41.

21. Niwa K, Tateno S, Akagi T, Nakazawa M. Incidence of arrhythmias and heart rate response during pregnancy in CHD after repair: Holter monitoring analysis. *J Cardiol* 2003;42 Suppl I:228.

22. Ohuchi H, Ohashi H, Park J, Hayashi J, Miyazaki A, Echigo S. Abnormal post exercise cardiovascular recovery and its determinants in patients after right ventricular outflow tract reconstruction. *Circulation* 2002;106:2819–26.

23. Mendelsohn CL. Disorders of the heart beat during pregnancy. *Am J Obstet Gynecol* 1956;72:1268–301.

24. Joglar JA, Page RL. Antiarrhythmic drugs in pregnancy. *Curr Opin Cardiol* 2001;16:40–5.

25. Siu SC, Sermer M, Colman JM, Alvaletz N, Mercier LA, Morton BC, *et al.* Prospective multicenter study of pregnancy outcomes in women with heart disease. *Circulation* 2001;104:515–21.

26. Shime J, Mocarski E, Hastings D, Webb GD, McLaughlin PR. Congenital heart disease in pregnancy: short- and long-term implications. *Am J Obstet Gynecol* 1987;156:313–22.

27. McFaul P, Dornan J, Lamki H, Boyle D. Pregnancy complicated by maternal heart disease: a review of 519 women. *Br J Obstet Gynaecol* 1988;95:861–7.

28. Zuber M, Gautschi N, Oechslin E, Widmer V, Kiowski W, Jenni R. Outcome of pregnancy in women with congenital shunt lesions. *Heart* 1999;81:271–5.

29. Eddy W, Frankenfeld R. Congenital complete heart block in pregnancy. *Am J Obstet Gynecol* 1977;128:223–35.

30. Weindling SN, Saul JP, Gamble WJ, Mayer JE, Wessel D, Walsh EP. Duration of complete atrioventricular block after congenital heart surgery. *Am J Cardiol* 1998;82:525–7.

31. Page RL. Treatment of arrhythmias during pregnancy. *Am Heart J* 1995;130:871–6.

32. Briggs GG, Freeman RK, Yaffe SJ. *Drugs in Pregnancy and Lactation,* 7th edn. Philadelphia: Lippincott Williams and Willkins; 2005.

33. Cox JL, Gardner MJ. Treatment of cardiac arrhythmias during pregnancy. *Prog Cardiovasc Dis* 1993;36:137–78.

34. Schroeder JS, Harrison DC. Repeated cardioversion during pregnancy: treatment of refractory paroxysmal atrial tachycardia during three successive pregnancies. *Am J Cardiol* 1971;27:445–6.

35. Mason BA, Ricci-Goodman J, Koos BJ. Adenosine in the treatment of maternal paroxysmal supraventricular tachycardia. *Obstet Gynecol* 1992;80:478–80.

36. Elkayam U, Goodwin TM.. Adenosine therapy for supraventricular tachycardia during pregnancy. *Am J Cardiol* 1995;75:521–3.

37. Blomstrom-Lundqvist C, Scheinman MM, Aliot EM, Alpert JS, Calkins H, Camm AJ, *et al.*; European Society of Cardiology Committee, NASPE-Heart Rhythm Society. ACC/AHA/ESC guidelines for the management of patients with supraventricular arrhythmias – Executive summary. *J Am Coll Cardiol* 2003;42:1493–531.

38. Dominguez A, Iturralde P, Hermosillo AG, Colin L, Kershenovich S, Garrido LM. Successful radiofrequency ablation of an accessory pathway during pregnancy. *Pacing Clin Electrophysiol* 1999;22:131–4.

39. Magee LA, Schick B, Donnenfeld AE, Sage SR, Conover B, Cook L, *et al.* The safety of calcium channel blockers in human pregnancy: a prospective, multicenter cohort study. *Am J Obstet Gynecol* 1996;174:823–8.

40. Wagner X, Jouglard J, Moulin M, Miller AM, Petitjean J, Pisapia A. Coadministration of flecainide acetate and sotalol during pregnancy: lack of teratogenic effects, passage across the placenta, and excretion in human breast milk. *Am Heart J* 1990;119:700–2.

41. Gowda RM, Khan IA, Mehta NJ, Vasavada BC, Sacchi TJ. Cardiac arrhythmias in pregnancy: clinical and therapeutic considerations. *Int J Cardiol* 2003;88:129–33.

42. Oakley C, Child A, Jung B, Task Force on the Management of Cardiovascular Diseases During Pregnancy of the European Society of Cardiology. Expert consensus document on management of cardiovascular disease during pregnancy. The Task Force on the Management of Cardiovascular Disease During Pregnancy of the European Society of Cardiology. *Euro Heart J* 2003;24:761–81.

43. Connolly HM, Warnes CA. Pregnancy and contraception. In: Gatzoulis MA, Webb GD, Daubeney PEF, editors. *Diagnosis and Management of Adult Congenital Heart Disease.* Edinburgh: Churchill Livingstone; 2003. p. 135–44.

44. Natale A, Davidson T, Geiger MJ, Newby K. Implantable cardioverter-defibrillators and pregnancy: a safe combination? *Circulation* 1997;96:2808–12.

45. Lee MS, Evans SJ, Blumberg S, Bodenheimer MM, Roth SL. Echocardiographically guided electrophysiologic testing in pregnancy. *J Am Soc Echocardiogr* 1994;7:182–6.

46. Gras D, Mabo P, Kermarrec A, Bazin P, Varin C, Daubert C. Radiofrequency ablation of atrioventricular conduction during the 5th month of pregnancy. *Arch Mal Coeur Vaiss* 1992;85:1873–7.

47. Schatz JW, Fischer JA, Lee RF, Lampe RM. Pacemaker therapy in pregnancy for management of sinus bradycardia-junctional tachycardia syndrome. *Chest* 1974;65:461–3.

48. Abramovici H, Faktor JH, Gonen Y, Brandes JM, Amikan S. Maternal permanent bradycardia: pregnancy and delivery. *Obstet Gynecol* 1984;63:381–3.

49. Jaffe R, Gruber A, Fejgin M, Altaras M, Ben-Aderet N. Pregnancy with an artificial pacemaker. *Obstet Gynecol Surv* 1987;42:137–9.

50. Baumgartner H. Reproductive issues in adults with congenital heart disease: arrhythmias during pregnancy: importance, diagnosis and therapy. *Thorac Cardiov Surg* 2001;49:94–7.

51. Chow TH, Galvin J, McGovern B. Antiarrhythmiac drug therapy in pregnancy and lactation. *Am J Cardiol* 1998;82:581–621.

52. Frishman WH, Chesner M. Beta-adrenergic blockers in pregnancy. *Am Heart J* 1988;115:147–52.

53. Lip GYH, Beevers M, Churchill D, Shaffer LM, Beevers DG. Effect of atenolol on birth weight. *Am J Cardiol* 1997;79:1436–8.

54. Ovadia M, Brito M, Hoyer GL, Marcus FI. Human experience with amiodarone in the embryonic period. *Am J Cardiol* 1994;73:316–17.

55. Widerhorn J, Bhanadari AK, Bughi S, Rahimtoola SH, Elkayam U. Fetal and neonatal adverse effects profile of amiodarone treatment during pregnancy. *Am Heart J* 1991;22:1162–5.

56. Veldman GR, Connolly HM, Grogan M, Ammash NM, Warnes CA. Outcomes of pregnancy in women with tetralogy of Fallot. *J Am Coll Cardiol* 2004;44:174–80.

57. Connolly HM, Warnes CA. Ebstein's anomaly: outcome of pregnancy. *J Am Coll Cardiol* 1994;23:1194–8.

58. Connolly HM, Grogan M, Warnes CA. Pregnancy among women with congenitally corrected transposition of great arteries. *J Am Coll Cardiol* 1999;6:1692–5.

59. Genoni M, Jenni R, Hoerstrup SP, Vogt P, Turina M. Pregnancy after atrial repair for transposition of the great arteries. *Heart* 1999;81:276–7.

60. Lao TT, Sermer M, Colman JM. Pregnancy following surgical correction for transposition of the great arteries. *Obstet Gynecol* 1994;83:665–8.

61. Clarkson PM, Wilson NJ, Neutze JM, North RA, Calder AL, Barratt-Boyes BG. Outcome of pregnancy after the Mustard operation for transposition of the great arteries with intact ventricular septum. *J Am Coll Cardiol* 1994;24:190–3.

62. Canobbio MM, Mair DD, van der Velde M, Koos BJ. Pregnancy outcomes after the Fontan repair. *J Am Coll Cardiol* 1996;28:763–7.

63. *Reports On Confidential Enquiries into Maternal Deaths in England and Wales.* 1979–1981, 1982–1984, 1985–1987, 1988–1990. London: HMSO.

64. Presbitero P, Somerville J, Stone S, Aryta E, Spiegelhalter D, Rabajoli F. Pregnancy in cyanotic congenital heart disease. Outcome of mother and fetus. *Circulation* 1994;89:2673–6.

65. Thorne SA. Pregnancy in heart disease. Congenital heart disease. *Heart* 2004;90:450–6.

66. Therrien J, Gatzoulis M, Graham T, Bink-Boelkens M, Connelly M, Niwa K, *et al.* Canadian Cardiovascular Society Consensus Conference 2001 update: Recommendations for the Management of Adults with Congenital Heart Disease – Part II. *Can J Cardiol* 2001;17:1029–50.

67. Perloff JK. Pregnancy and congenital heart disease. *J Am Coll Cardiol* 1991;18:340–2.

68. Warnes C, Elkayam U. Congenital heart disease and pregnancy. In: Elkayam U, Gleicher N editors: *Cardiac Problems in Pregnancy*, 3rd edn. New York: Wiley-Liss; 1998. p. 39–53.

69. Ramanathan J, D'Alessio JG, Geller E, Rudick V, Niv D. Analgesia and anesthesia during pregnancy. In: Elkayam U, Gleicher N, editors. *Cardiac Problems in Pregnancy*, 3rd edn. New York: Wiley-Liss; 1998. p. 285–313.

70. Niwa K, Perloff JK, Webb GD, Murphy D, Liberthson R, Warnes C, *et al.* Survey of specialized tertiary care facilities for adults with congenital heart disease. *Int J Cardiol* 2004;96:211–16.

71. American Academy of Pediatrics Committee on Drugs. Transfer of drugs and other chemicals into human milk. *Pediatrics* 2001;108:776–89.

72. *Drug Facts and Comparisons.* St Louis: Facts and Comparisons; 1997.

73. American Academy of Pediatrics Committee on Drugs. The transfer of drugs and other chemicals into human milk. *Pediatrics* 1994;93:137–50.

74. Vaughan Williams EM. A Classification of antiarrhythmic actions after a decade of new drugs. *J Clin Pharmacol* 1984;24:129–47.

Chapter 19
Maternal endocarditis

Graham Stuart

Introduction

Endocarditis in pregnancy is rare. However, when it does occur it can result in serious morbidity or death to both mother and fetus. The aim of this chapter is to examine the incidence of endocarditis in pregnancy and to assess the predisposing risk factors and the efficacy of preventative measures. Finally, a protocol for prevention, diagnosis and treatment of endocarditis in pregnancy is proposed.

Definition

Infective endocarditis is one of the most serious complications of heart disease. It is usually defined as a bacterial or fungal infection within the heart. A precise definition of infective endocarditis confines it to infection of the heart valves, septal defects and endocardium, but the clinical spectrum includes infection that occurs on arterial shunts, arteriovenous malformations and coarctation of the aorta – 'infective endarteritis'. In the past, endocarditis was classified as acute or subacute. This was based on the clinical course of the disease before the advent of antimicrobial therapy. Acute endocarditis was an overwhelming infection that occurred in association with a coexisting debilitating illness such as tuberculosis or immunodeficiency. Subacute endocarditis had a more prolonged course, with multiple physical signs including embolic phenomena, new cardiac murmurs, splenomegaly and fever. In most early studies, the infecting organism identified was *Streptococcus viridans* and there was often an underlying structural cardiac abnormality.[1] Modern classifications of infective endocarditis are based on the infecting organism and underlying cardiac anatomy. This has enabled the development of targeted therapy and a rational approach to individual management.

Incidence of endocarditis

Despite apparent improvements in preventative strategies, the overall incidence of endocarditis has changed very little over the past 20 years. The incidence in Europe and North America is 1.7–6.2 per 100 000 person-years, with a 1 year mortality of almost 40%.[2] The typical textbook presentation has been modified by a decline in rheumatic heart disease, increased prevalence of implanted devices and prosthetic valves and the rise in intravenous drug abuse. At the same time there has been a rise in the prevalence of staphylococcal infections and the development of infective organisms that may be multi-drug resistant or difficult to culture in the laboratory.[3,4]

Endocarditis in pregnancy

It has been suggested for many years that women are at a higher risk of endocarditis when they are pregnant.[5] However, the incidence of endocarditis in pregnancy is low, and few accurate data on incidence are available. In a 1986 literature review, Seaworth and Durack[6] calculated an incidence of 0.03–0.14 per 1000 deliveries. This was based on 124 cases of endocarditis reported in the preceding 40 years. In a similar review in 2003, Campuzano et al.[7] found only 68 cases recorded in the previous 38 years, with maternal and fetal mortality rates of 22.1.% and 14.7%, respectively. In this study the valve-specific maternal mortality was 42.1%, 21.7% and 9.5% for the aortic, mitral and tricuspid valves, respectively. The valve-specific perinatal mortality was 15.8%, 8.7% and 9.5%, respectively. The most common infecting organism was S. viridans. A summary of published cases of infectious endocarditis in pregnancy from 1965 to 2005 is shown in Table 19.1.

Any assessment of the incidence of endocarditis in pregnancy is limited by the lack of prospective studies. The only recent large study from an unselected cohort is from Saudi Arabia[8] and may not accurately reflect the situation in the UK or Europe. A summary of recent pregnancy outcome studies is shown in Table 19.2. This includes both unselected reviews and studies in women with heart disease published between 1986 and 2005. Only 15 cases of endocarditis were reported, with a case series mortality ranging from 0% to 100%. It is likely that many cases of endocarditis were not reported and the true incidence and outcome are unknown.

Table 19.1. Literature review of reported cases of endocarditis in pregnancy, 1965–2005; modified and updated from Campuzano et al.[7]

Organism	Aorta	Mitral valve	Tricuspid/ pulmonary valve	No valve specified
Streptococcus viridans	3	9	1	2
Group B streptococcus	2	3	4	0
Other streptococcus	5	6	1	1
Staphylococcus aureus	1	1	5	3
Other staphylococcus	2	0	3	0
Neisseria	2	1	1	0
Other	3	1	3	5
No organism reported	3	2	5	2
Total	**21**	**23**	**23**	**13**
Maternal mortality	8 (38%)	5 (22%)	2 (7%)	1 (8%)
Perinatal Mortality	4 (19%)	2 (9%)	2 (9%)	2 (15%)
References	59,61–77	12,75,78–90	7,12,75,91–102	32,33,65,81,87,97,103–105

Table 19.2. Incidence of endocarditis during pregnancy

Study	Population	Number of women in study		Women with endocarditis		Mortality	Comment
		Total	Women with cardiac disease	Normal heart before pregnancy	Known cardiac disease		
Asghar[103]	Pakistani study, unselected population	5100	50	1 (0.002%)	1 (2%)	0%	28% CHD, 66% RHD; no endocarditis in normal hearts; antibiotic policy not recorded
Rahman[8]	Arabic women with heart disease	38 166	229	2 (0.005%)	2 (0.9%)	0%	1982–98, 18% CHD, 76% RHD; antibiotics given in all at delivery
Faiz[106]	Arabic women with heart disease	33 200	166	0	0	N/A	1993–97; antibiotics given in 83%; data for women with valve disease only
Avila[33]	Brazilian study	1000	1000	N/A	5 (0.5%)	0%	1989–99; 19% CHD, 56% RHD, 25% other cardiac disease; one woman required aortic valve replacement but survived
Kaemmerer[92]	Multicentre study	106	106	0	1 (0.9%)	0%	All women in the study group had CHD; cardiac problems occurred in 11%; endocarditis occurred postpartum despite antibiotics
Sadler[107]	Women with prosthetic valves	79 women, 147 pregnancies	79	N/A	0 (0%)	0%	1972–92; all women had a prosthetic valve (homografts/ mechanical or bioprosthetic valves)
Presbitero[108]	Cyanotic women	44 women, 96 pregnancies	44	N/A	1 (1%)	100%	Two-centre study
McFaul[109]	Women with known heart disease	519	519	N/A	0	N/A	1970–83; prophylactic antibiotics not used
Shime[110]	Single centre, women with CHD	144	144	N/A	2	0%	One woman required aortic valve replacement after delivery
Ben Ismael[111]	Women with prosthetic valves	51 women, 76 pregnancies	51	N/A	2 (2.6%)	100%	
Hall[112]	Women with prosthetic valves	38 women, 59 pregnancies	38	N/A	4 (6.8%)	5%	1989–96; one women with endocarditis required valve replacement in pregnancy and survived
Siu[34]	13 Canadian centres	562 women, 599 pregnancies	562	N/A	0	0%	1994–99; prospective multicentre study
Total		**79 009**	**2988**	**3**	**18**		

CHD = congenital heart disease; RHD = rheumatic heart disease; N/A = not applicable

In the 1997–99 report of the Confidential Enquiries into Maternal Deaths in the United Kingdom it was estimated that 10% of maternal cardiac deaths are due to endocarditis.[9] Relevant data from recent Confidential Enquiries into Maternal Deaths in the United Kingdom data are shown in Table 19.3. Although these data do not give the incidence of the condition, they clearly demonstrate that endocarditis is an important and continuing cause of maternal death in the UK.

Pathogenesis of endocarditis

A detailed discussion of the clinical features of endocarditis is beyond the scope of this chapter but is covered elsewhere.[10] In brief, endocarditis occurs owing to a complex interaction between the host vascular endothelium, haemostatic response and transient bacteraemia. Normal endothelium is non-thrombogenic and poorly receptive to adhesion by most bacteria. When an endothelial surface is damaged, the denuded surface exposes sub-endothelial factors (for example, thromboplastin and extracellular matrix proteins) that promote adherence of platelets and fibrin. The resulting thrombus provides a receptive surface for bacteria during episodes of bacteraemia. When bacteria bind to the thrombus, there is a cascade reaction leading to monocyte activation with production of cytokines and tissue factors. This causes the vegetation to enlarge and may result in abscess formation, septic emboli and systemic vasculitis. It is not known whether the coagulation changes of pregnancy influence this process.[11]

Only certain bacteria cause endocarditis. In 1988, Cox et al.[12] found the most common infecting organism to be streptococcus (60%), with an increasing number of infections due to staphylococcus (18%) and a small number of other organisms, including fungi (2%), multiple bacteria (4%) and other less common bacteria (6%). Cultures were negative in 5%. In several reports, Staphylococcus aureus has been identified as a leading cause of endocarditis in the non-pregnant population.[2,13,14]

In patients with congenital heart disease, endothelial damage usually occurs as a result of a 'jet' lesion. For example, in someone with a ventricular septal defect (VSD), vegetations are often found in the right ventricular outflow tract where the VSD jet has damaged the endocardium. In those who do not have an underlying cardiac defect, inflammation can induce expression of $beta_1$ integrins by endothelial cells. This facilitates adhesion by certain bacteria that carry fibronectin-binding proteins on their surface (e.g. S. aureus). In drug addicts, endocarditis is usually related to intravenous drug abuse and affects the right side of the heart.[15] In developing countries, gynae-cological events, puerperal sepsis and septic abortion are the most common cause of isolated right-sided endocarditis.[16–18]

Diagnosis

The diagnosis of endocarditis during pregnancy requires a high degree of suspicion. In particular, endocarditis should be considered in any pregnant woman with unexplained fever and a heart murmur.[19] Occasionally, endocarditis in pregnancy is associated with an atypical presentation (Table 19.4). Both the European Society of Cardiology (ESC) and American Heart Association (AHA) have recently published guidelines for the diagnosis and treatment of endocarditis.[3,20] The diagnostic criteria for endocarditis are identical in the pregnant and non-pregnant state.

In theory, the precise diagnosis of endocarditis requires both persistent bacteraemia and anatomical lesions on the valves or endocardium. In practice, blood cultures are

Table 19.3. Endocarditis data from the Confidential Enquiries into Maternal Deaths in the United Kingdom

Era	Endocarditis (n)	Normal heart (n)	Substandard care (n)	Co-factors	Cardiac deaths		Comment
					n	% endocarditis	
1985–87, 1988–90, 1991–93	9	N/A	N/A	N/A	78	N/A	Data unavailable.
1994–96	2[a]	1	1	Diabetes in one	39	5.1%	Patient 1: aortic valve disease/IDD; was admitted at 29 weeks of gestation with collapse; died following emergency aortic valve surgery Patient 2: developed endocarditis on structurally normal aortic valve; repeated admissions with a headache and positive blood cultures (Gram-positive cocci) 2 weeks pre-admission; new murmur 2 days post delivery; echocardiogram showed aortic valve vegetations; sudden collapse. Patient 3: a third woman with SLE died while having a non-viable pregnancy terminated; non-specifically unwell, autopsy showed Libman–Sacks endocarditis.[a]
1997–99	3	1	–	Psychiatric history in one	35	8.6%	Patient 1: known prosthetic aortic valve; developed LVF; died post CS. Patient 2: known coarctation of aorta (post surgery); died after mitral and aortic valve replacements and CS. Patient 3: no known cardiac anomaly; pyrexia of unknown origin; repeated self-discharge; died 4 weeks post CS; autopsy diagnosids.
2000–02	1	1	–	GBS colonisation	44	2.3%	Patient infected with GBS; aortic valve previously normal.
Total	**14**	**3**	**1**[b]		**152**	**9.2%**	

[a] Libman–Sacks endocarditis is found in approximately 50% of patients with SLE and is characterised by sterile vegetations on the heart valves; secondary infective endocarditis was not found in this woman; this case has a different aetiology from infective endocarditis

[b] Full data not available for each triennium

CS = caesarean section; GBS = group B streptococcus; IDD = Insulin-dependent diabetes; LVF = left ventricular failure; SLE = systemic lupus erythematosus; N/A = not available

Table 19.4.   Unusual features of endocarditis in pregnancy

Study	Feature	Comment
Siva[113]	Splenic infarction	Presented left upper quadrant pain
Kang[114]	Acute respiratory distress syndrome	Libman–Sacks endocarditis with obstructive sterile vegetations
Pantanowitz[115]	Arthritis and septicaemia	Following threatened termination and gonococcaemia
Oohara[80]	Stroke	Secondary to mycotic aneurysm
Downs[116]	Massive haemoptysis	Due to bronchial artery haemorrhage
Caraballo[117]	Myocardial infarction	Due to coronary artery septic embolism
Collins[118]	Breathlessness	Pneumothorax
Henry[119]	Septic renal embolus	Haematuria and flank pain

negative in around 10% of cases.[21] Criteria for the diagnosis of endocarditis were proposed in 1994 and modified in 2000 to take into account negative blood cultures.[22,23] These criteria have been validated in several studies and provide a useful aid to diagnosis in difficult cases. An outline of the modified Duke criteria is shown in Figure 19.1. Culture-independent molecular techniques can be used to improve the diagnostic yield of standard bacterial culture techniques.[24]

Predisposing factors

The frequency of bacteraemia with obstetric and gynaecological procedures is shown in Table 19.5. These data have to be interpreted with caution. Bacteraemia is found in 3% of blood cultures after simple tooth brushing.[25] Moreover, a case report described endocarditis following removal of an intrauterine device despite another study of 100 women that found 0% post-procedure bacteraemia and concluded that antibiotic prophylaxis is unnecessary.[26,27] It is likely that sustained bacteraemia with an appropriate bacterium is necessary for endocarditis to develop. Sustained bacteraemia is more likely if there is localised infection. The incidence of bacteraemia during urethral catheterisation thus increases if there is bacteruria.[28,29]

Additional predisposing factors for developing endocarditis are likely to be important and include the existence of a structural cardiac abnormality, intravenous drug abuse, periodontal disease and local infection. Several workers have shown that endocarditis can occur following both normal delivery and septic miscarriage.[30,31]

Depending on the population studied, a pre-existing cardiac defect may be present in up to 75% of women who develop endocarditis in pregnancy.[30,32] However, endocarditis is rare even in women with structural heart abnormalities. Thus, in two large prospective studies of women with heart disease, the incidence of endocarditis was less than 0.5%.[33,34] All cardiac patients do not have the same risk of endocarditis. High- and low-risk groups can be identified on the basis of underlying cardiac disease.[35] (Figure 19.2). Paradoxically, certain low-risk conditions may carry a higher risk of endocarditis after medical intervention. This includes some conditions requiring pacemaker implantation, and trans-catheter occlusion of an atrial septal defect.[36–38] In addition, intravenous drug abuse is emerging as a major cause of endocarditis in patients with normal cardiac anatomy.[12,21,39] A previous history of endocarditis is an important additional risk factor for the development of a second infection.[15]

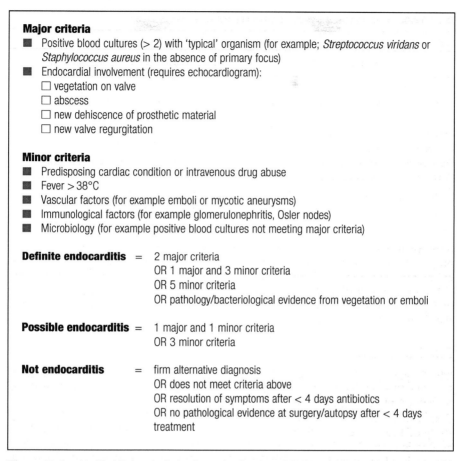

Major criteria
- Positive blood cultures (> 2) with 'typical' organism (for example; *Streptococcus viridans* or *Staphylococcus aureus* in the absence of primary focus)
- Endocardial involvement (requires echocardiogram):
  - ☐ vegetation on valve
  - ☐ abscess
  - ☐ new dehiscence of prosthetic material
  - ☐ new valve regurgitation

Minor criteria
- Predisposing cardiac condition or intravenous drug abuse
- Fever > 38°C
- Vascular factors (for example emboli or mycotic aneurysms)
- Immunological factors (for example glomerulonephritis, Osler nodes)
- Microbiology (for example positive blood cultures not meeting major criteria)

Definite endocarditis	=	2 major criteria
		OR 1 major and 3 minor criteria
		OR 5 minor criteria
		OR pathology/bacteriological evidence from vegetation or emboli
Possible endocarditis	=	1 major and 1 minor criteria
		OR 3 minor criteria
Not endocarditis	=	firm alternative diagnosis
		OR does not meet criteria above
		OR resolution of symptoms after < 4 days antibiotics
		OR no pathological evidence at surgery/autopsy after < 4 days treatment

Figure 19.1.   Modified Duke criteria for diagnosis of endocarditis; adapted from Li *et al.*[22] and Durack *et al.*[23]

Preventative measures

It is not known whether antibiotic prophylaxis can prevent endocarditis.[40,41] Most cases of endocarditis are not attributable to an invasive procedure and recommendations for the use of prophylactic antibiotics vary considerably in different countries.[42–44] Although some authorities do not recommend antibiotic prophylaxis for normal vaginal delivery,[45] many specialists feel that the theoretical benefit, together with the severe consequences of endocarditis in a high-risk woman, make antibiotic administration a prudent, if not an evidence-based, strategy.[44,46,47] Thus, Iserin[48] recommends prophylactic ampicillin at the start of labour and for the subsequent 48 hours. This view has been reinforced in a recent publication from the Royal College of Physicians of London and the British Cardiac Society.[35] Conversely, the American College of Obstetricians and Gynecologists guidelines[49] on the administration of prophylactic antibiotics in labour and delivery suggest that women with high-risk

Table 19.5. Bacteraemia and pregnancy-related events and procedures

Event/procedure	% bacteraemia	Comment
Termination of pregnancy	Unknown	Endocarditis reported but rare[6,30,120,121]
Vaginal delivery	0–5%	Endocarditis reported[30,122]
Caesarean section	14%	0% bacteraemia unless in labour; risk increased if preterm, low birthweight, positive chorioamnionic culture or intrauterine monitoring[123]
Dilatation and curettage	5%	No reports of endocarditis[124]
Insertion/removal of intrauterine device	0%	Endocarditis reported[26,27,125]
Sterilisation procedures	Unknown	No reports of endocarditis
Cervical smear	Unknown	Endocarditis reported[126]
Endometrial biopsy	8%	No reports of endocarditis[25]
Oocyte retrieval	Unknown	Endocarditis reported[127]
Urethral catheterisation	18–33%	Endocarditis reported[28,29]

cardiac conditions should only be given antibiotic prophylaxis if there is intra-amniotic infection. This report suggests antibiotic prophylaxis should be optional for cardiac patients (high and low risk) in uncomplicated delivery. Curiously, prophylactic antibiotics are recommended for all high-risk cardiac patients if caesarean section is required, although this may be based on the established ability of such prophylaxis to reduce substantially postoperative sepsis (that might subsequently act as a focus producing bacteraemia). The authors recognise that these recommendations are made on the basis of professional consensus rather than strong scientific evidence. Antibiotic prophylaxis is thought to be most effective when given perioperatively in doses adequate to ensure therapeutic serum levels and most authorities recommend that they are continued for 6–8 hours only.[44]

There is evidence that maternal periodontal disease is a risk factor for endo-carditis.[50] To prevent an oral inflammatory process evolving into a full-blown form of periodontitis with recurrent bacteraemia, mothers should receive regular professional oral hygiene care throughout pregnancy.[51] Similarly, preterm rupture of membranes is associated with bacteraemia and administration of antibiotics reduces maternal and fetal infectious morbidity.[52] A recent Cochrane review suggested that prophylactic antibiotics in the second or third trimester of pregnancy can reduce the risk of postpartum endometritis, although possibly at the cost of increasing neonatal sepsis.[53] Although this review was not designed to assess the effect on maternal endocarditis, it did suggest a benefit in reducing puerperal sepsis and this may represent an appropriate intervention in very high-risk women, for example in the context of a previous history of endocarditis in conjunction with a high-risk cardiac lesion. Similarly, serious non-cardiac infection (for example pyelonephritis) can result in septicaemia.[54] The possibility of endocarditis should always be considered in a woman who is refractory to standard treatment of non-cardiac infection.

- Prosthetic heart valves[a]
- Complex congenital heart disease[a]
- Surgically constructed pulmonary or systemic conduits[a]
- Previous infective endocarditis[a]
- Acquired heart valve disease
- Mitral valve prolapse with valvular regurgitation or severe leaflet dysplasia
- Non-cyanotic congenital heart disease (except unoperated secundum atrial septal defect)
- Hypertrophic cardiomyopathy
- Implanted intracardiac device (e.g. pacemaker, intravascular stent or occlusion device)[b]

[a] High-risk group
[b] Potential risk – discuss with cardiologist

Figure 19.2. Cardiac conditions at risk of endocarditis; modified from Horstkotte *et al*.[15]

Protocol for prevention, diagnosis and treatment of endocarditis in pregnancy

A protocol for prevention, diagnosis and treatment is described below. Intravenous drug abusers should be treated similarly to 'high-risk' cardiac patients.

Prevention

The prevention of endocarditis in pregnancy in women with structural heart disease should begin with education. Many patients and their families have a poor understanding of the risks of endocarditis.[55] Endocarditis risk should be discussed repeatedly during childhood and should be rediscussed on transfer to adult cardiology follow-up. There is considerable evidence that 'at risk' women benefit from being given regular, repeated and written advice concerning measures that will minimise the risk of endocarditis.[56] This should include the need for good dental hygiene, avoidance of intravenous drug abuse and early treatment of skin sepsis. Women should receive professional oral hygiene care throughout pregnancy. Moreover, all women should be issued with an endocarditis prophylaxis card giving details of their cardiac defect and cardiology centre contact.

There is no evidence that prophylactic administration of antibiotics will prevent endocarditis following uncomplicated vaginal delivery. However, despite the lack of prospective trial data, there is a strong case for the administration of prophylactic antibiotics to every high-risk woman undergoing a procedure that will lead to significant or prolonged bacteraemia (see Table 19.5). For women with pre-existing cardiac disease deemed to be at low risk, the administration of antibiotics is optional but there should be a low threshold if there is any suspicion of chorioamnionitis or other persistent local infection. Although this policy will lead to many women with cardiac disease receiving antibiotics at delivery, it is likely to reduce the small but very important group who suffer the catastrophic consequences of endocarditis with associated mortality and morbidity.

Diagnosis

A high index of suspicion in 'at risk' women is particularly important. The diagnosis of endocarditis in pregnancy should be made using the modified Duke criteria (Figure 19.1). If endocarditis is suspected, at least three blood culture sets should be taken using optimal antiseptic skin preparation. Both aerobic and anaerobic cultures should be taken and appropriately modified culture medium should be used if antibiotics have been given. There is no rationale for waiting until pyrexia before taking blood cultures.[57] Positive blood cultures in a febrile or unwell woman should never be ignored. Similarly, new cardiac murmurs in the context of a febrile woman should not be assumed to be innocent. If endocarditis is suspected, early cardiology assessment should be sought and echocardiography carried out.

Treatment

The effective treatment of infective endocarditis in pregnancy requires multidisciplinary cooperation between the fetal and obstetric team and specialists in infectious disease, cardiology and cardiac surgery. The mainstay of therapy is the administration of bactericidal antibiotics. The choice of antibiotic will depend on the nature of the cultured organism and antibiotic susceptibility testing.[21] Long-term parenteral therapy should usually be recommended. Treatment guidelines should predominantly follow those currently used for non-pregnant patients.[58] The precise treatment of culture-negative endocarditis is difficult and will depend on the likely source of infection and local antibiotic sensitivities. The need for cardiac surgery should be discussed with a surgeon at an early stage. If cardiac surgery is necessary, the risk to the mother is similar to that for non-pregnant female patients (3%) but fetal mortality remains high (19%).[59,60] During the third trimester, delivery of the child immediately before commencing cardiopulmonary bypass may be the safest option.

Conclusion

Endocarditis in pregnancy is a life-threatening disease. Despite improvements in outcome, significant morbidity and mortality still occur. Primary prevention is very important and should include early recognition of risk factors and use of strategies to minimise bacteraemia. Effective diagnosis and treatment involves a multidisciplinary approach and may include cardiac surgery and early delivery. Early detection, accurate diagnosis and aggressive appropriate treatment may significantly improve outcome

References

1. Herrmann GR. Bacterial endocarditis or valvulitis. In: Herrmann GR, editor. *Synopsis of Diseases of the Heart and Arteries*. St Louis: CV Mosby; 1941. p. 283–290.

2. Cabell CH, Jollis JG, Peterson GE, Corey GR, Anderson DJ, Sexton DJ, *et al.* Changing patient characteristics and the effect on mortality in endocarditis. *Arch Intern Med* 2002;162:90–4.

3. Baddour LM, Wilson WR, Bayer AS, Fowler VG Jr, Bolger AF, Levison ME, *et al.* Infective endocarditis: diagnosis, antimicrobial therapy, and management of complications: a statement for healthcare professionals from the Committee on Rheumatic Fever, Endocarditis, and Kawasaki Disease, Council on Cardiovascular Disease in the Young, and the Councils on Clinical Cardiology, Stroke, and

Cardiovascular Surgery and Anesthesia, American Heart Association – executive summary: endorsed by the Infectious Diseases Society of America. *Circulation* 2005;111:3167–84.

4. Prendergast BD. The changing face of infective endocarditis. *Heart* 2004;90:611–13.
5. Anonymous. Heart disease in pregnancy. *Lancet* 1941;237:82.
6. Seaworth BJ, Durack DT. Infective endocarditis in obstetric and gynecologic practice. *Am J Obstet Gynecol* 1986;154:180–8.
7. Campuzano K, Roque H, Bolnick A, Leo MV, Campbell WA. Bacterial endocarditis complicating pregnancy: case report and systematic review of the literature. *Arch Gynecol Obstet* 2003;268:251–5.
8. Rahman J, Rahman MS, Al Suleiman SA, Al Jama FE. Pregnancy complicated by maternal cardiac disease: a review of 274 patients. *J Obstet Gynaecol* 2000;20:242–5.
9. Cardiac disease. In: Lewis G, editor. *Why Mothers Die 1997–1999. The 5th Report of the Confidential Enquiries into Maternal Deaths in the United Kingdom.* London: RCOG Press; 2001. p.153–64.
10. Mylonakis E, Calderwood SB. Infective endocarditis in adults. *N Engl J Med* 2001;345:1318–30.
11. Brenner B. Haemostatic changes in pregnancy. *Thromb Res* 2004;114:409–14.
12. Cox SM, Hankins GD, Leveno KJ, Cunningham FG. Bacterial endocarditis. A serious pregnancy complication. *J Reprod Med* 1988;33:671–4.
13. Hoen B, Alla F, Selton-Suty C, Beguinot I, Bouvet A, Briancon S, et al. Changing profile of infective endocarditis: results of a 1-year survey in France. *JAMA* 2002;288:75–81.
14. Roder BL, Wandall DA, Frimodt-Moller N, Espersen F, Skinhoj P, Rosdahl VT. Clinical features of *Staphylococcus aureus* endocarditis: a 10-year experience in Denmark. *Arch Intern Med* 1999;159:462–9.
15. Horstkotte D, Follath F, Gutschik E, Lengyel M, Oto A, Pavie A, et al. Guidelines on prevention, diagnosis and treatment of infective endocarditis executive summary; the Task Force on Infective Endocarditis of the European Society of Cardiology. *Eur Heart J* 2004;25:267–76.
16. Grover A, Anand IS, Varma J, Choudhury R, Khattri HN, Sapru RP, et al. Profile of right-sided endocarditis: an Indian experience. *Int J Cardiol* 1991;33:83–8.
17. Swift PJ. *Staphylococcus aureus* tricuspid valve endocarditis in young women after gynaecological events. A report of 3 cases. *S Afr Med J* 1984;66:891–3.
18. Aslam AF, Aslam AK, Thakur AC, Vasavada BC, Khan IA. *Staphylococcus aureus* infective endocarditis and septic pulmonary embolism after septic abortion. *Int J Cardiol* 2005;105:233–5.
19. Montoya ME, Karnath BM, Ahmad M. Endocarditis during pregnancy. *South Med J* 2003;96:1156–7.
20. Horstkotte D, Follath F, Gutschik E, Lengyel M, Oto A, Pavie A, et al. [Guidelines on prevention, diagnosis and treatment of infective endocarditis. Executive summary]. *Rev Esp Cardiol* 2004;57:952–62.
21. Moreillon P, Que YA. Infective endocarditis. *Lancet* 2004;363:139–49.
22. Li JS, Sexton DJ, Mick N, Nettles R, Fowler VG Jr, Ryan T, et al. Proposed modifications to the Duke criteria for the diagnosis of infective endocarditis. *Clin Infect Dis* 2000;30:633–8.
23. Durack DT, Lukes AS, Bright DK. New criteria for diagnosis of infective endocarditis: utilization of specific echocardiographic findings. Duke Endocarditis Service. *Am J Med* 1994;96:200–9.
24. Breitkopf C, Hammel D, Scheld HH, Peters G, Becker K. Impact of a molecular

approach to improve the microbiological diagnosis of infective heart valve endocarditis. *Circulation* 2005;111:1415–21.

25. Livengood CH III, Land MR, Addison WA. Endometrial biopsy, bacteremia, and endocarditis risk. *Obstet Gynecol* 1985;65:678–81.

26. Wilson WR, Karchmer AW, Dajani AS, Taubert KA, Bayer A, Kaye D, *et al*. Antibiotic treatment of adults with infective endocarditis due to streptococci, enterococci, staphylococci, and HACEK microorganisms. American Heart Association. *JAMA* 1995;274:1706–13.

27. Everett ED, Reller LB, Droegemueller W, Greer BE. Absence of bacteremia after insertion or removal of intrauterine devices. *Obstet Gynecol* 1976;47:207–9.

28. Everett ED, Hirschmann JV. Transient bacteremia and endocarditis prophylaxis. A review. *Medicine (Baltimore)* 1977;56:61–77.

29. Sullivan NM, Sutter VL, Carter WT, Attebery HR, Finegold SM. Bacteremia after genitourinary tract manipulation: bacteriological aspects and evaluation of various blood culture systems. *Appl Microbiol* 1972;23:1101–16.

30. Nkoua JL, Kimbally-Kaky G, Ekoba J, Gombet T, Onkani AH, Oumba C, *et al*. [Infectious endocarditis of gyneco-obstetric origin. Apropos of 15 cases]. *J Gynecol Obstet Biol Reprod (Paris)* 1993;22:425–8.

31. Vaidya SS, Pandit S, Apte NV, Kelkar PN, Ramamoorthy K. Tricuspid valve endocarditis following septic abortion. *J Assoc Physicians India* 1986;34:157.

32. Cox SM, Leveno KJ. Pregnancy complicated by bacterial endocarditis. *Clin Obstet Gynecol* 1989;32:48–53.

33. Avila WS, Rossi EG, Ramires JA, Grinberg M, Bortolotto MR, Zugaib M, *et al*. Pregnancy in patients with heart disease: experience with 1,000 cases. *Clin Cardiol* 2003;26:135–42.

34. Siu SC, Sermer M, Colman JM, Alvarez AN, Mercier LA, Morton BC, *et al*. Prospective multicenter study of pregnancy outcomes in women with heart disease. *Circulation* 2001;104:515–21.

35. Ramsdale DR, Turner-Stokes L. Prophylaxis and treatment of infective endocarditis in adults: a concise guide. *Clin Med* 2004;4:545–50.

36. Erdinler I, Okmen E, Zor U, Zor A, Oguz E, Ketenci B, *et al*. Pacemaker related endocarditis: analysis of seven cases. *Jpn Heart J* 2002;43:475–85.

37. Balasundaram RP, Anandaraja S, Juneja R, Choudhary SK. Infective endocarditis following implantation of amplatzer atrial septal occluder. *Indian Heart J* 2005;57:167–9.

38. Calachanis M, Carrieri L, Grimaldi R, Veglio F, Orzan F. Infective endocarditis after transcatheter closure of a patent foramen ovale. *Catheter Cardiovasc Interv* 2004;63:351–4.

39. Pastorek JG, Plauche WC, Faro S. Acute bacterial endocarditis in pregnancy. A report of three cases. *J Reprod Med* 1983;28:611–14.

40. van der Meer JT, van Wijk W, Thompson J, Vandenbroucke JP, Valkenburg HA, Michel MF. Efficacy of antibiotic prophylaxis for prevention of native-valve endocarditis. *Lancet* 1992;339:135–9.

41. Chemoprophylaxis for infective endocarditis: faith, hope, and charity challenged. *Lancet* 1992;339:525–6.

42. de Jong J. [At which childbirth should endocarditis prophylaxis be given?]. *Ned Tijdschr Geneeskd* 1997;141:2134.

43. Danchin N, Duval X, Leport C. Prophylaxis of infective endocarditis: French recommendations 2002. *Heart* 2005;91:715–18.

44. Dajani AS, Taubert KA, Wilson W, Bolger AF, Bayer A, Ferrieri P, *et al*. Prevention of

bacterial endocarditis. Recommendations by the American Heart Association. *JAMA* 1997;277:1794–801.

45. Sugrue D, Blake S, Troy P, MacDonald D. Antibiotic prophylaxis against infective endocarditis after normal delivery – is it necessary? *Br Heart J* 1980;44:499–502.

46. Egdell RM, Reid S, Bending JJ, Cooke RP. Congenital heart lesions, childbirth, and antibiotic prophylaxis. *Lancet* 1992;340:1170–1.

47. Clark SL. Labor and delivery in the patient with structural cardiac disease. *Clin Perinatol* 1986;13:695–703.

48. Iserin L. Management of pregnancy in women with congenital heart disease. *Heart* 2001;85:493–4.

49. American College of Obstetricians and Gynecologists. ACOG practice bulletin Number 47, October 2003: Prophylactic Antibiotics in Labor and Delivery. *Obstet Gynecol* 2003;102:875–82.

50. Joshipura K, Ritchie C, Douglass C. Strength of evidence linking oral conditions and systemic disease. *Compend Contin Educ Dent Suppl* 2000;30:12–23.

51. Felice P, Pelliccioni GA, Checchi L. Periodontal disease as a risk factor in pregnancy. *Minerva Stomatol* 2005;54:255–64.

52. Mercer BM, Arheart KL. Antimicrobial therapy in expectant management of preterm premature rupture of the membranes. *Lancet* 1995;346:1271–9.

53. Thinkhamrop J, Hofmeyr GJ, Adetoro O, Lumbiganon P. Prophylactic antibiotic administration in pregnancy to prevent infectious morbidity and mortality. *Cochrane Database Syst Rev* 2002;(4):CD002250.

54. Hill JB, Sheffield JS, McIntire DD, Wendel GD Jr. Acute pyelonephritis in pregnancy. *Obstet Gynecol* 2005;105:18–23.

55. Bulat DC, Kantoch MJ. How much do parents know about their children's heart condition and prophylaxis against endocarditis? *Can J Cardiol* 2003;19:501–6.

56. Moons P, De Volder E, Budts W, De Geest S, Elen J, Waeytens K, *et al.* What do adult patients with congenital heart disease know about their disease, treatment, and prevention of complications? A call for structured patient education. *Heart* 2001;86:74–80.

57. Prendergast BD. Diagnostic criteria and problems in infective endocarditis. *Heart* 2004;90:611–13.

58. Fernandez-Perez ER, Salman S, Pendem S, Farmer JC. Sepsis during pregnancy. *Crit Care Med* 2005;33(10 Suppl):S286–93.

59. Westaby S, Parry AJ, Forfar JC. Reoperation for prosthetic valve endocarditis in the third trimester of pregnancy. *Ann Thorac Surg* 1992;53:263–5.

60. Parry AJ, Westaby S. Cardiopulmonary bypass during pregnancy. *Ann Thorac Surg* 1996;61:1865–9.

61. Takano Y, Matsuyama H, Fujita A, Kobayashi A, Kawamura M. [A case of urgent aortic valve replacement for infective endocarditis in pregnancy]. *Masui* 2003;52:1086–8.

62. Cavalieri RL, Watkins L Jr, Abraham RA, Berkay HS, Niebyl JR. Acute bacterial endocarditis with postpartum aortic valve replacement. *Obstet Gynecol* 1982;59:124–5.

63. Hanson GC, Phillips J. A fatal case of subacute bacterial endocarditis in pregnancy. A review of this condition in pregnancy including the incidence, diagnosis and treatment. *J Obstet Gynaecol Br Commonw* 1965;72:781–4.

64. Jeyamalar R, Sivanesaratnam V. Management of infective endocarditis in pregnancy. *Aust N Z J Obstet Gynaecol* 1991;31:123–4.

65. Sexton DJ, Rockson SG, Hempling RE, Cathey CW. Pregnancy-associated group B streptococcal endocarditis: a report of two fatal cases. *Obstet Gynecol* 1985;66(3 Suppl):44S–7S.

66. Hughes LO, McFadyen IR, Raftery EB. Acute bacterial endocarditis on a normal aortic valve following vaginal delivery. *Int J Cardiol* 1988;18:261–2.

67. Nazarian M, McCullough GH, Fielder DL. Bacterial endocarditis in pregnancy: successful surgical correction. *J Thorac Cardiovasc Surg* 1976;71:880–3.

68. O'Donnell D, Gillmer DJ, Mitha AS. Aortic and mitral valve replacement for bacterial endocarditis in pregnancy. A case report. *S Afr Med J* 1983;64:1074.

69. Holt S, Hicks DA, Charles RG, Coulshed N. Acute staphylococcal endocarditis in pregnancy. *Practitioner* 1978;220:619–22.

70. Burstein H, Sampson MB, Kohler JP, Levitsky S. Gonococcal endocarditis during pregnancy: simultaneous cesarean section and aortic valve surgery. *Obstet Gynecol* 1985;66(3 Suppl):48S–51S.

71. McComb JM, McNamee PT, Sinnamon DG, Adgey AA. Staphylococcal endocarditis presenting as meningitis in pregnancy. *Int J Cardiol* 1982;1:325–7.

72. Bataskov KL, Hariharan S, Horowitz MD, Neibart RM, Cox MM. Gonococcal endocarditis complicating pregnancy: a case report and literature review. *Obstet Gynecol* 1991;78(3 Pt 2):494–6.

73. Eilen B, Kaiser IH, Becker RM, Cohen MN. Aortic valve replacement in the third trimester of pregnancy: case report and review of the literature. *Obstet Gynecol* 1981;57:119–21.

74. Maeland A, Teieh AN, Arnesen H, Garborg I. Cardiobacterium hominis endocarditis. *Eur J Clin Microbiol* 1983;2:216–17.

75. Strasberg GD. Postpartum group B streptococcal endocarditis associated with mitral valve prolapse. *Obstet Gynecol* 1987;70(3 Pt 2):485–7.

76. van der Bel-Kahn JM, Watanakunakorn C, Menefee MG, Long HD, Dicter R. *Chlamydia trachomatis* endocarditis. *Am Heart J* 1978;95:627–36.

77. Hautman GD, Sherman SJ. Spontaneous bacterial endocarditis and aortic valve replacement complicating pregnancy. *Int J Gynaecol Obstet* 1996;54:173–4.

78. Castillo RA, Llado I, Adamsons K. Ruptured chordae tendineae complicating pregnancy. A case report. *J Reprod Med* 1987;32:137–9.

79. Hagay ZJ, Weissman A, Geva D, Snir E, Caspi A. Labor and delivery complicated by acute mitral regurgitation due to ruptured chordae tendineae. *Am J Perinatol* 1995;12:111–12.

80. Oohara K, Yamazaki T, Kanou H, Kobayashi A. Infective endocarditis complicated by mycotic cerebral aneurysm: two case reports of women in the peripartum period. *Eur J Cardiothorac Surg* 1998;14:533–5.

81. Ward H, Hickman RC. Bacterial endocarditis in pregnancy. *Aust N Z J Obstet Gynaecol* 1971;11:189–91.

82. Zimmerman J, Shotan A. Prosthetic valve endocarditis in pregnancy. *Acta Obstet Gynecol Scand* 1984;63:731–2.

83. Jemsek JG, Gentry LO, Greenberg SB. Malignant group B streptococcal endocarditis associated with saline-induced abortion. *Chest* 1979;76:695–7.

84. Saravolatz LD, Burch KH, Quinn EL, Cox F, Madhavan T, Fisher E. Polymicrobial infective endocarditis: an increasing clinical entity. *Am Heart J* 1978;95:163–8.

85. Bhoola RL, Rajmohamed SE. Acute bacterial endocarditis following criminal abortion. *S Afr Med J* 1979;56:85.

86. de Swiet M, de Louvois J, Hurley R. Letter: Failure of cephalosporins to prevent bacterial endocarditis during labour. *Lancet* 1975;2:186.

87. Dommisse J. Infective endocarditis in pregnancy. A report of 3 cases. *S Afr Med J* 1988;73:186–7.

88. Payne DG, Fishburne JI Jr, Rufty AJ, Johnston FR. Bacterial endocarditis in pregnancy. *Obstet Gynecol* 1982;60:247–50.

89.   Rosenberg K. Subacute bacterial endocarditis complicating pregnancy. *Proc Rudolf Virchow Med Soc City NY* 1965;24:132–5.

90.   Yacoub M, Pennacchio L, Ross D, McDonald L. Replacement of mitral valve in active infective endocarditis. *Br Heart J* 1972;34:758–60.

91.   Crespo A, Retter AS, Lorber B. Group B streptococcal endocarditis in obstetric and gynecologic practice. *Infect Dis Obstet Gynecol* 2003;11:109–15.

92.   Kaemmerer H, Bauer U, Stein JI, Lemp S, Bartmus D, Hoffmann A, *et al.* Pregnancy in congenital cardiac disease: an increasing challenge for cardiologists and obstetricians – a prospective multicenter study. *Z Kardiol* 2003;92:16–23.

93.   Vartian CV, Septimus EJ. Tricuspid valve group B streptococcal endocarditis following elective abortion. *Rev Infect Dis* 1991;13:997–8.

94.   Handa R, Aggarwal P, Biswas A, Wali JP. Right-sided endocarditis following abortion – underdiagnosed condition case report. *Indian J Med Sci* 1997;51:430–1.

95.   Murata T, Fujino M, Sasaki J, Takii M, Arakawa K. Right atrial vegetation in left ventricular-right atrial communication. *Clin Cardiol* 1987;10:61–2.

96.   Norro G, Pothuizen LM, Roos JP. Isolated tricuspid endocarditis. *Acta Cardiol* 1974;29:157–63.

97.   Pastorek JG, Plauche WC, Faro S. Acute bacterial endocarditis in pregnancy. A report of three cases. *J Reprod Med* 1983;28:611–14.

98.   Calleja F, Eguaras MG, Chacon A, Vivancos R, Montero A, Concha M. Pulmonary valve endocarditis during puerperal sepsis. *J Cardiovasc Surg (Torino)* 1992;33:292–4.

99.   Kennedy JH, Sabga GA, Fisk AA, Sancetta SM. Isolated tricuspid valvular insufficiency due to subacute bacterial endocarditis. Report of a case with recovery following prosthetic replacement of the tricuspid valve. *J Thorac Cardiovasc Surg* 1966;51:498–506.

100. Deger R, Ludmir J. *Neisseria sicca* endocarditis complicating pregnancy. A case report. *J Reprod Med* 1992;37:473–5.

101. Schondelmeyer RW, Sunderrajan EV, Atay AE, Strickland JL, Walls JT. Successful tricuspid valvulectomy without replacement for endocarditis during pregnancy. *Am Heart J* 1986;112:859–61.

102. Kido T, Nakata Y, Aoki K, Hata N, Hazama S. Infective endocarditis of the tricuspid valve in a non-drug user. *Jpn J Med* 1991;30:154–6.

103. Asghar F, Kokab H. Evaluation and outcome of pregnancy complicated by heart disease. *J Pak Med Assoc* 2005;55:416–19.

104. Anand CM, Mackay AD, Evans JI. *Haemophilus* aphrophilus endocarditis in pregnancy. *J Clin Pathol* 1976;29:812–14.

105. Holshouser CA, Ansbacher R, McNitt T, Steele R. Bacterial endocarditis due to *Listeria monocytogenes* in a pregnant diabetic. *Obstet Gynecol* 1978;51(1 Suppl):9s–10s.

106. Faiz SA, Al Meshari AA, Sporrong BG. Pregnancy and valvular heart disease. *Saudi Med J* 2003;24:1098–101.

107. Sadler L, McCowan L, White H, Stewart A, Bracken M, North R. Pregnancy outcomes and cardiac complications in women with mechanical, bioprosthetic and homograft valves. *Br J Obstet Gynaecol* 2000;107:245–53.

108. Presbitero P, Somerville J, Stone S, Aruta E, Spiegelhalter D, Rabajoli F. Pregnancy in cyanotic congenital heart disease. Outcome of mother and fetus. *Circulation* 1994;89:2673–6.

109. McFaul PB, Dornan JC, Lamki H, Boyle D. Pregnancy complicated by maternal heart disease. A review of 519 women. *Br J Obstet Gynaecol* 1988;95:861–7.

110. Shime J, Mocarski EJ, Hastings D, Webb GD, McLaughlin PR. Congenital heart disease in pregnancy: short- and long-term implications. *Am J Obstet Gynecol* 1987;156:313–22.

111. Ben Ismail M, Abid F, Trabelsi S, Taktak M, Fekih M. Cardiac valve prostheses, anticoagulation, and pregnancy. *Br Heart J* 1986;55:101–5.

112. Hall DR, Olivier J, Rossouw GJ, Grove D, Doubell AF. Pregnancy outcome in women with prosthetic heart valves. *J Obstet Gynaecol* 2001;21:149–53.

113. Siva S, Smoleniec J. Splenic infarction in pregnancy. *Aust N Z J Obstet Gynaecol* 1999;39:252–4.

114. Kang AH, Graves CR. Libman–Sacks endocarditis in a pregnant woman with acute respiratory distress syndrome. *Obstet Gynecol* 1999;93(5 Pt 2):819–21.

115. Pantanowitz L, Hodkinson J, Zeelie R, Jones N. Gonococcal endocarditis after a threatened abortion. A case report. *J Reprod Med* 1998;43:1043–5.

116. Downs TW, Chao CR. Massive hemoptysis in pregnancy treated with bronchial artery embolisation. *Am J Perinatol* 1997;14:51–3.

117. Caraballo V. Fatal myocardial infarction resulting from coronary artery septic embolism after abortion: unusual cause and complication of endocarditis. *Ann Emerg Med* 1997;29:175–7.

118. Collins JH Jr, Gomes G, Brown JW III, Muller R. Infective endocarditis presenting with a pneumothorax in a patient 32 weeks pregnant. *J La State Med Soc* 1985;137:60–3.

119. Henry DM, Cotton DB. Bacterial endocarditis in pregnancy associated with septic renal embolization. *South Med J* 1985;78:355–6.

120. Panigrahi NK, Panda RS, Panda S. Tricuspid valve endocarditis following elective abortion. *Indian J Chest Dis Allied Sci* 1998;40:69–72.

121. Kangavari S, Collins J, Cercek B, Atar S, Siegel R. Tricuspid valve group B streptococcal endocarditis after an elective termination of pregnancy. *Clin Cardiol* 2000;23:301–3.

122. Redleaf PD, Fadell EJ. Bacteremia during parturition; prevention of subacute bacterial endocarditis. *J Am Med Assoc* 1959;169:1284–5.

123. Boggess KA, Watts DH, Hillier SL, Krohn MA, Benedetti TJ, Eschenbach DA. Bacteremia shortly after placental separation during cesarean delivery. *Obstet Gynecol* 1996;87(5 Pt 1):779–84.

124. Sacks PC, Tchabo JG. Incidence of bacteremia at dilation and curettage. *J Reprod Med* 1992;37:331–4.

125. de Swiet M, Ramsay ID, Rees GM. Bacterial endocarditis after insertion of intrauterine contraceptive device. *Br Med J* 1975;3:76–7.

126. Mong K, Taylor D, Muzyka T, Freed D, Koshal A. Tricuspid endocarditis following a Papanicolaou smear: case report. *Can J Cardiol* 1997;13:895–6.

127. Bilavsky E, Bilavsky HY, Zeidman A. Infective tricuspid valve endocarditis following fertility treatments. *Eur J Intern Med* 2005;16:618.

Section 5

Intrapartum care

Chapter 20
Pregnancy and cardiac disease – peripartum aspects

Jacqueline Durbridge, Martin Dresner, Kate R Harding
and Steve M Yentis

Introduction

Pregnancy is in itself a cardiovascular stress and during the peripartum period the stress is even greater. Central to the optimum peripartum management of women with cardiac disease is careful planning and preparation for any complications that might occur.

Obstetric issues

Mode of delivery

During labour, cardiac output as measured by Doppler and cross-sectional echo-cardiography at the pulmonary valve, increases from a prelabour mean of 7.0–7.9 l/minute. This increase is predominantly as a result of increased stroke volume, although the heart rate also increases. In the absence of anaesthesia, stroke volume and heart rate increase further during contractions, raising the cardiac output to a mean of 10.6 l/minute. Heart rate returns to normal by 1 hour post delivery, although stroke volume, cardiac output and systolic blood pressure may take 24 hours to return to prelabour values.[1] It is thought that these cardiovascular changes in labour, and the associated increase in oxygen consumption, are largely related to uncontrolled pain and without effective analgesia/anaesthesia (see below) they may be poorly tolerated by women with cardiac disease. There is a similar though less marked increase in cardiac output during caesarean section.

The mode of delivery will generally be determined by obstetric rather than cardiac indications, with caesarean section rates varying between 21% and 51%.[2-4] Caesarean section is associated with increased risks of haemorrhage, postpartum infection, puerperal fluid shifts and metabolic demands.[5] In a large prospective study in Canada of 566 women,[6] there was no association between the type of delivery and the rate of peripartum cardiac events (3% versus 4% for vaginal versus caesarean delivery ($P = 0.46$)). However, studies in women with pulmonary vascular disease or a previous history of myocardial ischaemia suggest a doubling of maternal mortality in association with caesarean section.[7] In a systematic 18 year overview from 1978 to

1996, Weiss *et al.*[8] found a 2.5-fold (95% CI 1.1–5.2) increase in maternal mortality in women with pulmonary vascular disease undergoing caesarean section.

Traditionally, labour is conducted with the woman sitting upright (or in the lateral decubitus position) to avoid aortocaval compression. Effective analgesia (see below) reduces the cardiac stress induced by painful contractions. Some women with cardiac disease (for example those with cyanotic heart disease or those with a fixed or reduced cardiac output) have an increased risk of poor uteroplacental perfusion, and for these women continuous fetal heart-rate monitoring is particularly important.

Vaginal delivery is best performed with the woman sitting upright and her feet supported on foot rests or on reversed lithotomy poles. If the woman needs to lie on her back it is important to use a wedge to minimise aortocaval compression (which decreases venous return from the lower limbs) and to minimise elevation of her legs (which may increase venous return) – the aim is to maintain cardiovascular stability. Active pushing should be limited since this can cause considerable haemodynamic instability in some women. In women with severe cardiac disease (such as critical mitral stenosis) it may be considered necessary to avoid an active second stage. In such cases effective regional analgesia is extremely helpful in allowing the fetal head to descend to the perineum without active pushing and then a ventouse or forceps delivery can be performed. In a study in Malaysia of 143 women with acyanotic heart disease in 1998 there was a significantly greater operative delivery rate (35.7% versus 5.7%) when compared with 19 151 controls, although this was obviously not a randomised study.[9]

Timing of delivery

Women with moderate to severe cardiac disease may require delivery at a time and in a place that will ensure that the intrapartum team (see below) is readily available (although ideally, as women may go into labour at any time, a tertiary referral centre should be able to provide care all day, every day). For a woman who lives some distance from the maternity centre, this may entail her spending time in hospital at the end of the third trimester to avoid the possibility of going into labour distant from the hospital in which she is planning to deliver. In these women and in those who live locally but in whom the timing of the delivery is thought to be of importance, induction may be considered for 'timing' rather than obstetric or cardiac indications, although it is important to balance the risks of failed induction and caesarean section against the risks of awaiting spontaneous labour. A study in Israel between 1995 and 2001 looked at 121 consecutive pregnancies complicated by cardiac disease.[4] Forty-seven women (39%) had labour induced (68% of these were to optimise the timing of delivery). Of those who were induced, only 21% required a caesarean section compared with 19% among normal controls, suggesting that generally the risk of failed induction is small. Delivery was achieved during 'normal working hours' (8 a.m. to 4 p.m.) in 55% of women.

The provision of on-site or nearby 'hotel facilities' may avoid the need for induction or even operative delivery for 'logistical', rather than clinical, indications (for example timing of anticoagulation therapy, availability of staff, etc.). Women (and their families) can get very fed up with their having to stay in a hospital bed when it is not absolutely necessary and this is a wasteful use of limited resources. If tertiary centres can provide a convenient place for the woman and her family to stay, and from where she can easily attend the maternity unit for regular check-ups and access the delivery suite, induction may be prevented and the likelihood of vaginal delivery enhanced.

If the woman's condition worsens during pregnancy, early delivery should be considered. In such cases, the benefit to the woman needs to be balanced with the risk to the neonate from prematurity. In the most extreme cases (such as pulmonary hypertension), too early a delivery may risk a disabled baby with limited benefit to the mother (if her risk of dying is high whatever the gestation), and the father may be left with a disabled child to care for on his own. Steroids should be given if delivery is planned before 34 weeks of gestation although in cases of severe cardiac function impairment the associated fluid retention can precipitate cardiac failure and the use of prophylactic diuretics should be considered.

Both induction of labour and stimulation of slow progress in labour should be performed with care. Prostaglandin E_2 can be used for induction, as can intravenous oxytocin. There is about a 1% risk of uterine hyperstimulation with prostaglandins, and the use of beta sympathomimetics to counter it can lead to cardiac problems including tachycardia and arrhythmia. Additionally, acute fetal hypoxia can be precipitated by the hyperstimulation, necessitating urgent delivery with its attendant risks. On the other hand, with oxytocin, special care needs to be taken with regard to the volume of intravenous fluid given during labour, as oxytocin can cause water retention owing to its antidiuretic effects. Oxytocin should be given via a syringe driver in a small volume of saline, for example 10 iu in 50 ml starting at 0.6 ml/hour (2 miu/minute).

Third stage management

During the third stage of labour there are two counterbalancing effects on cardio-vascular physiology. As the placenta delivers and the uterus contracts (either spontaneously or in response to uterotonics), there is an increase in intravascular volume of approximately 500 ml. At around the same time, there is haemorrhage associated with delivery, which averages 500 ml. Measurements of cardiac output following caesarean section show a peak increase (from pre-delivery) at 15 and 30 minutes post delivery of around 30% and 20%, respectively, returning to preoperative levels by 60 minutes.[10] In some situations, judicious use of furosemide may be required to prevent pulmonary oedema.

In healthy women, oxytocin causes a small reduction in arterial blood pressure 30 seconds after a 10 iu intravenous bolus, followed by an increase in cardiac output (60 seconds after 5–10 iu and 120 seconds after 5 iu).[11] The initial change is due to peripheral vasodilatation with the increase in cardiac output secondary to autotransfusion as described above. Oxytocin also has a direct effect on the heart, causing decreased cardiac contractility and heart rate.[12] These effects may be catastrophic in women with cardiac disease.[13] If oxytocin is to be used, it should be given by very slow intravenous infusion. In contrast, the alternative oxytocic commonly used in normal women, ergometrine, causes peripheral vascular constriction and coronary vasospasm and should therefore also be avoided in women with hypertension or myocardial ischaemia. Carboprost (prostaglandin $F_{2\alpha}$) and misoprostol are both potent synthetic prostaglandins that are effective in causing tonic uterine contractions. Carboprost given intravascularly can cause bronchospasm and both carboprost and misoprostol are contraindicated in myocardial ischaemia. Misoprostol is not currently licensed for use in the third stage of labour and there are some concerns about its adverse effects of shivering (frequent) and hyperpyrexia (rare but serious) in women with cardiac disease; it should therefore only be used where it is considered that the benefit outweighs the risks. Further studies to clarify its risk–benefit ratio are justified. Some obstetricians have used mechanical manoeuvres to reduce postpartum haemorrhage, such as bimanual compression (in the short term), uterine compression sutures and intrauterine balloons, rather than using pharmacological oxytocics; this approach also warrants further study.

Postpartum haemorrhage is not uncommon in women with cardiac disease, both because the use of uterotonics is often avoided for the reasons described above and for haematological reasons such as the use of heparin thromboprophylaxis, and/or platelet dysfunction in the presence of mechanical heart valves. Such women often tolerate hypovolaemia poorly and it is of the utmost importance that attention be given to haemostasis both at caesarean section and for any perineal trauma.

Regional anaesthesia/analgesia

The term 'regional anaesthesia' describes dense neural blockade such as that required for a pain-free operative delivery. As well as producing sensory and motor blockade, epidural and spinal anaesthesia cause autonomic paralysis. This can lead to profound vasodilatation and hypotension in normal individuals, let alone those affected by cardiac disease. 'Regional analgesia', on the other hand, describes pain relief rather than complete neural blockade. Effective relief of labour pain can be achieved with minimal haemodynamic effect[14] by using weaker drug combinations than those used for anaesthesia. While analgesia and anaesthesia merge in a continuous spectrum, the two are not synonymous.

Regional anaesthesia

Regional anaesthesia is now the default technique for caesarean section in the UK.[15] It is considered safer than general anaesthesia in most cases, because failed intubation and aspiration of stomach contents, traditionally the main causes of anaesthetic maternal deaths, are avoided.[16] Regional anaesthesia also confers important advantages related to aesthetics and the quality of the birth experience for the mother and her family, such as:

- the presence of the woman's birth partner at delivery
- immediate intimate contact between mother and baby
- improved postoperative analgesia
- improved maternal satisfaction with the anaesthetic and birth experience.

Women with cardiac disease should not be denied these benefits without good reason.

The usual contraindications for regional anaesthesia still apply, such as refusal by the woman, bacteraemia or skin infection. There are also some contraindications specifically related to cardiac disease, such as anticoagulation (for example for prosthetic valves or thromboprophylaxis), anxiety so extreme as to increase the risk of arrhythmia, and a severely limited and fixed cardiac output.

Although regional anaesthesia is generally preferred to general anaesthesia, uncontrolled regional anaesthesia is extremely hazardous in the presence of cardiac disease. A rapid-onset, high-level spinal block can drastically reduce cardiac output both by reducing venous return through peripheral vasodilatation and by blocking the cardiac sympathetic supply. The safe use of regional anaesthesia depends on three technical considerations:

1. Incremental induction of regional blockade – this may be achieved using epidural anaesthesia alone, by combined spinal–epidural anaesthesia (in which a small intrathecal dose is followed by incremental epidural doses to extend the block), or by intrathecal catheter techniques. There is no evidence base to determine the best technique for particular cardiac lesions but there are many case reports of the successful use of each in a variety of clinical circumstances.

2. Control of peripheral vasodilatation with appropriate agents – in most cases a pure alpha agonist such as phenylephrine to avoid tachycardia.

3. Judicious intravenous fluid therapy, since excessive fluid preloading given to reduce the severity of hypotension may precipitate cardiac failure as the regional blockade dissipates.

The relative importance of each will vary from case to case. It is important to note that the appropriate bedside manner and technical skills necessary to deliver incremental, cardiostable regional anaesthesia in a safe and confident manner are not generic qualities possessed by all anaesthetists. Therefore, women whose cases are complicated by cardiac disease should be managed by specific consultant anaesthetists who form part of the multidisciplinary team charged with their care.

Regional analgesia

The increased risks associated with caesarean section (anaesthesia-related problems, bleeding, infection, deep vein thrombosis, etc.) compared with vaginal delivery, together with the ability to obtund the considerable cardiac stresses of pain and the efforts of pushing that effective regional analgesia can offer, have led to a move away from the traditional choice of caesarean section for all women with cardiac disease. In a UK series of over 250 cardiac cases reported to a voluntary registry, 49% of mothers had a vaginal delivery and 73% of these had some form of regional analgesia.[2]

Regional analgesia for pain relief in labour follows the same principles as regional anaesthesia but intrinsically carries less risk because of the lower local anaesthetic doses required compared with anaesthesia for obstetric surgery. However, haemodynamic monitoring remains essential, the level of which can only be determined on a case-by-case basis. If operative delivery is required, the epidural can be topped up to provide anaesthesia if time allows.[17]

The combination of regional anaesthesia/analgesia and aortocaval compression can produce profound haemodynamic compromise. Attention to detail in this regard is most important. The same is true for the use of oxytocin by intravenous bolus injection during caesarean section.[11] This can be effectively and safely substituted with uterine massage with or without a slow intravenous infusion of oxytocin.

General anaesthesia

Certain aspects of general anaesthesia are particularly relevant to women with cardiac disease, in whom general anaesthesia may have a number of advantages and disadvantages.

Advantages of general anaesthesia

Women with severe cardiac disease may be particularly anxious about the risks of delivery and the associated increase in sympathetic drive may threaten the balance between cardiac oxygen supply and demand. Although increased sympathetic tone may persist during and beyond induction of general anaesthesia, this technique avoids the situation of an awake and frightened mother undergoing caesarean section and possibly requiring sedation, especially if surgery is complicated. Similarly, if regional anaesthesia is sub-optimal, this too may have undesirable cardiovascular effects and may necessitate intravenous analgesia/sedation, and possibly the need to convert to general anaesthesia intraoperatively in a less controlled manner. A well-controlled, smooth 'cardiac'-style anaesthetic, conversely, may provide extremely stable cardio-vascular parameters and avoid both the adverse effects of anxiety/pain and the hypotension that may typically occur with regional anaesthesia.

General anaesthesia allows a number of therapeutic options more easily during surgery, such as direct current (DC) cardioversion in women suffering from or at risk of arrhythmias, or administration of 100% oxygen, whose pulmonary vasodilatory effect may be useful in women with pulmonary hypertension. It also allows post-operative ventilation if this is felt appropriate, without the need for any extra intervention at the end of the operation.

For women already receiving anticoagulant drugs, or for those in whom the risk of thromboembolism is considered high (many if not most women with cardiac disease fall into one of these groups), general anaesthesia allows standard anticoagulant therapies to be used without the need to manipulate their timing because of fears over spinal haematoma.[18] The risk of spinal haematoma, and of 'breakthrough' thromboembolism when treatment is stopped to allow regional anaesthesia, can thus be minimised.

Disadvantages of general anaesthesia

The main risks from general anaesthesia in obstetric cases are difficult/failed tracheal intubation and aspiration/regurgitation of gastric contents.[16] Unless the mother has an associated abnormality affecting the airway, this risk should be no greater because of the presence of cardiac disease than in anyone else. However, the consequences of such complications in a woman with cardiac disease may be catastrophic.

Although a 'cardiac' anaesthetic may be cardiostable, the use of large doses of opioids as part of the technique may lead to significant neonatal respiratory depression (although the newer, ultra-short-acting opioid remifentanil may solve this problem[19]). In addition, even a 'cardiac' anaesthetic cannot guarantee cardiovascular stability: there may be hypotension on induction of anaesthesia because of the cardiodepressant effects of the induction agent, hypertension/tachycardia on tracheal intubation (and extubation) and hypotension due to maintenance of anaesthesia intraoperatively. If anaesthesia is too light because of concerns over the cardiovascular effects of excessive dosage, this may risk maternal awareness. In pulmonary hypertension, light anaesthesia, instrumentation of the airway and coughing or bucking on the tracheal tube/ventilator may lead to acute increases in pulmonary pressures.

Blood loss is generally greater during caesarean section under general anaesthesia than under regional anaesthesia, largely because of effects on the distribution of blood volume (although high concentrations of volatile anaesthetic agents may cause uterine relaxation, this is minimal at the usual doses at caesarean section). In women with actual or potential right-to-left shunts, there is a risk of systemic air embolism, and if nitrous oxide is used as part of the anaesthetic technique this risk is increased since the gas tends to expand air-filled cavities and bubbles because of differences between its solubility and that of nitrogen.[20]

Women under general anaesthesia are unable to see or bond with their baby and in general it is inadvisable for her partner to be present. In addition, even with routine, non-'cardiac' anaesthetics, the neonate may be affected by the maternal anaesthetic drugs. Finally, postoperative pain, nausea and vomiting, respiratory depression and deep vein thrombosis are all thought to be more likely after general anaesthesia than regional anaesthesia.

Choice of anaesthetic

The overall choice of anaesthetic technique will depend on the relative importance of the above factors in each particular case, the preference of the anaesthetist and the wishes of the woman. Traditionally, general anaesthesia has been the preferred method although recent opinion is that regional anaesthesia is suitable in many – if not most – cases. However, the choice for women with severe disease remains more controversial.[21,22] In a UK series of over 250 cardiac cases reported to a voluntary registry, 39% of caesarean sections were under general anaesthesia, over three times the background proportion.[2] It should be noted that whatever the method of anaesthesia, intravenous oxytocin may cause disastrous haemodynamic instability, especially if given by rapid bolus (see above).[13]

Maternal monitoring

Basic non-invasive monitoring

Monitoring starts with the continuous clinical observation by a trained attendant, usually a midwife, in the peripartum period. The need for further haemodynamic monitoring should be adapted to each individual woman's needs. It will depend on the severity of the cardiac condition and the type of planned delivery, as well as the available technical expertise, cost–benefit analysis and individual preference. A minimum level can be preplanned but may need to be changed depending on the clinical condition of the woman.

The basic minimum of intermittent non-invasive blood pressure recording, continuous electrocardiography (ECG) and pulse oximetry should be used for all except the most minor conditions.[23] The limitations of the measurements must be kept in mind: for instance, the pulse oximeter is not a monitor of ventilation, such that a low arterial saturation 'cured' by administration of oxygen may reassure staff despite impending respiratory failure.[24] Attention should be paid to fluid balance with accurate recording of input and output.

Invasive monitoring

An arterial line is a relatively simple addition to basic monitoring that provides beat-to-beat measurements of blood pressure and heart rate.[25] It may also give an indication of fluid status and provides access for blood sampling. It will also continue to provide reliable information during hypotension, when automated external blood pressure monitors and even pulse oximeters may fail to give an accurate reading.

The decision to insert a central venous catheter must balance the potential benefits of monitoring and assessing the trend of the woman's fluid status against the knowledge that these measurements actually often correspond poorly to true volume status and to the functioning of the left side of the heart.[25] Furthermore, insertion carries the risk of vascular damage, pneumothorax, endocarditis and paradoxical embolus.

A pulmonary artery catheter allows semi-continuous measurement of cardiac output, pressure in the right atrium and pulmonary artery, and mixed venous oxygen saturation.[25] It also allows assessment of right ventricular volume and ejection fraction. The benefit of these measurements to guide therapy must be considered against the risks of placement, as with those of central venous access discussed above, plus the provocation of arrhythmias, pulmonary infarction or artery rupture; in general, these militate against its use. The potential benefits may outweigh the risks in severe valvular disease. The use of a pulmonary artery catheter in critical care remains controversial and its use has been associated with serious maternal and fetal complications.[26] If the risk of insertion is accepted, then it is clearly essential that the information gained be taken fully into account in any management decisions for the benefits to be realised.

Non-invasive cardiac output monitoring

Oesophageal ultrasound Doppler monitoring of cardiac function is relatively non-invasive but is too uncomfortable for routine use in awake women. It gives rapid beat-to-beat estimation of stroke volume and cardiac output and has been used in a number of critically ill obstetric patients with good effect.[27] However, one study found that it consistently underestimated cardiac output in pre-eclamptic women;[28] further evaluation is clearly required.

Pulse contour analysis provides continuous cardiac output monitoring by analysis of the pulse wave. In non-obstetric patients it appears to correlate well with measurements made using a pulmonary artery catheter, but its use in pregnancy remains unvalidated. Other non-invasive monitors are being developed but have not been widely used or proven to be accurate even in non-obstetric patients.[29]

Resources

Staff

For the best management of delivery in women with cardiac disease, a dedicated named multidisciplinary team is essential, including obstetrician, cardiologist and/or obstetric physician, and anaesthetist (with access to both obstetric and cardiac anaesthetic expertise), with input from an intensivist in high-risk cases, each with a named back-up for occasions when they are unavailable. Involvement of a neonatologist will also be appropriate if the birth is preterm or the baby is otherwise at risk. A team of midwives with a special interest and training in high-dependency care is also required (in some countries, this will be a team of specially trained maternity nurses). All members of the team should understand the effects of labour and delivery on the mother's cardiovascular status and the effect of her cardiac disease on placental perfusion, and ideally all should have become familiar with the woman and her partner during pregnancy, and vice versa. Maintaining vigilance is vital as women with cardiac disease do not have low-risk deliveries, and one of the biggest challenges is ensuring that everyone who comes into contact with them appreciates this. A multidisciplinary clinic is a very useful place to review these women and plan their care individually. Communication between the team members is crucial. It may occasionally be necessary to induce labour to ensure that the optimal team is present, although as labour can be unpredictable, it is important that in tertiary centres properly trained staff are available on-call 24 hours a day, 365 days per year.

The attitude of the team is also important. Deliveries of mothers with cardiac disease can become very 'medicalised', to the detriment of the mother's birth experience, and a relaxed and positive team approach can minimise the impact of this and produce as satisfying an experience as possible for the woman and her partner.

Training and resuscitation

All staff caring for mothers with cardiac disease should be adequately trained in recognising when the woman is acutely sick, in the management of obstetric emergencies, and in the resuscitation of adults and neonates. There are a variety of courses run nationally that may be helpful in achieving this, including Managing Obstetric Emergencies and Trauma,[30] Acute Life-threatening Events – Recognition and Treatment,[31] Immediate Life Support,[32] Advanced Life Support[33] and Newborn Life Support.[34] Cardiac arrest in mothers with cardiac disease is more likely than in those without cardiac disease, and obstetric emergencies such as haemorrhage are no less common. The management of cardiac arrest should be in accordance with national guidelines,[35] and the principles of basic and advanced life support are the same as for non-pregnant patients. Early involvement of medical emergency teams or hospital outreach teams in the assessment of acutely unwell women is emphasised in these latest guidelines for the prevention of cardiac arrest. In an emergency, the ABCDE approach should be used (Figure 20.1).

Attention to the prevention or relief of aortocaval compression is vital. The immediate summoning of expert obstetric, anaesthetic and neonatal help is necessary for the effective resuscitation of mother and fetus. Early tracheal intubation is desirable to prevent aspiration of gastric contents but may be more difficult in a pregnant woman. Defibrillation should be used in standard energy doses but the placement of the apical paddle may be more difficult owing to left lateral tilt and large breasts. Adhesive defibrillator pads may overcome this. If initial resuscitation attempts are unsuccessful, urgent caesarean delivery of the fetus may improve the chances of successful maternal and fetal resuscitation. The best survival rates are likely when delivery of the fetus is within 5 minutes of maternal cardiac arrest. Regular training drills for a variety of obstetric emergencies including cardiopulmonary resuscitation is recommended in all maternity units in the latest report of the Confidential Enquiries into Maternal and Child Health (CEMACH).[16]

A	**Airway and cervical spine control**
B	**Breathing and oxygenation**
C	**Circulation and haemorrhage control**
D	**Dysfunction and disability of the central nervous system**
E	**Exposure and environmental control**

Figure 20.1.   The ABCDE approach to emergency care

Equipment and environment

Twenty-four hour dedicated obstetric and anaesthetic services are essential. Access to an area on or near the labour ward where invasive monitoring can be accommodated is vital, and on-site critical care support and facilities are also important. If cardiac critical care or surgical facilities are not on-site, a very clearly defined referral policy needs to be in place.

Monitors that allow continuous monitoring of both non-invasive and invasive parameters are obviously a prerequisite. Staff must be familiar with all monitors used in the area and understand their limitations and problems. Access to a 12-lead ECG machine and blood gas monitor is important. Access to all the usual resuscitation equipment and obstetric haemorrhage management devices is also essential.

Most deliveries will be performed in the maternity suite but in some circumstances it may be preferable to operate in cardiac or main theatres. If there is a particularly high risk of a woman requiring cardiac bypass or cardiac support systems, the cardiac team should be readily available. The location of the critical care unit should also be considered since if such care is predicted and the unit is adjacent to the main or cardiac theatres, it may be safer to move the mother there for delivery rather than transfer her postpartum. Equipment to provide pulmonary vasodilatation may be deemed necessary and consideration of this should be made when planning the place of delivery. Disadvantages of performing operative deliveries outside the maternity unit include the lack of familiarity of the maternity team with their surroundings, the distance from the neonatal unit, the difficulty of having the partner present for the delivery, and possibly an increased risk of hospital-acquired infection.

Conclusions

- Vaginal delivery is optimal unless there is a fetal or obstetric indication for caesarean section.
- Care needs to be taken in the third stage to avoid postpartum haemorrhage, hypotension and pulmonary oedema.
- Communication between all members of the intrapartum team and the woman is of paramount importance to ensure a satisfactory outcome.

References

1. Robson SC, Dunlop W, Boys RJ, Hunter S. Cardiac output in labour. *BMJ* 1987;295:1169–72.
2. Dob DP, Yentis SM. UK Registry of High-risk Obstetric Anaesthesia: report on cardiorespiratory disease. *Int J Obstet Anesth* 2001;10:267–72.
3. Avila WS, Rossi EG, Ramires JA, Grinberg M, Bortolotto MR, Zugaib M, et al. Pregnancy in patients with heart disease: experience of 1,000 cases. *Clin Cardiol* 2003;26:135–42.
4. Oron G, Hirsch R, Ben-Haroush A, Hod M, Gilboa Y, Davidi O, et al. Pregnancy outcome in women with heart disease undergoing induction of labour. *BJOG* 2004;111:669–75.
5. Van Mook WN, Peeters L. Severe cardiac disease in pregnancy, Part II: impact of congenital and acquired cardiac diseases during pregnancy. *Curr Opin Crit Care* 2005;11:435–48.
6. Siu SC, Sermer M, Colman JM, Alvarez AN, Mercier LA, Morton BC, et al.

Prospective multicentre study of pregnancy outcomes in women with heart disease. *Circulation* 2001;104:515–21.

7. Gei AF, Hankins GDV. Cardiac disease and pregnancy. *Obstet Gynecol Clin N Am* 2001;28:465–511.

8. Weiss BM, Zemp L, Seifert B, Hess OM. Outcome of pulmonary vascular disease in pregnancy: A systematic overview from 1978–1986. *J Am Coll Cardiol* 1998;31:1650–7.

9. Chia S, Raman S, Tham SW. The pregnancy outcome of acyanotic heart disease. *J Obstet Gynaecol Res* 1998;24:267–73.

10. James CF, Banner T, Caton D. Cardiac output in women undergoing caesarean section with epidural or general anesthesia; *Am J Obstet Gynecol* 1989;160:1178–84.

11. Pinder AJ, Dresner M, Calow C, Shorten GD, O'Riordan J, Johnson R. Haemodynamic changes caused by oxytocin during caesarean section under spinal anaesthesia. *Int J Obstet Anesth* 2002;11:156–9.

12. Mukaddam-Daher S, Yin YL, Roy J, Gutkowska J, Cardinal R. Negative inotropic and chronotropic effects of oxytocin. *Hypertension* 2001;38:292–6.

1. Lewis G, editor. *Why Mothers Die 1997–1999. The Fifth Report of the Confidential Enquiries into Maternal Deaths in the United Kingdom.* London: RCOG Press; 2001.

14. Hawthorne L, Slaymaker A, Bamber J, Dresner M. Effect of fluid preload on maternal haemodynamics for low-dose epidural analgesia in labour. *Int J Obstet Anesth* 2001;10:312–15.

15. *NHS Maternity Statistics, England: 1998–99 to 2000–01.* London: Department of Health; 2002.

16. Lewis G, editor. *Why Mothers Die 2000–2002: The Sixth Report of Confidential Enquiries into Maternal Deaths in the United Kingdom.* London: RCOG Press; 2004.

17. Suntharalingam G, Dob D, Yentis SM. Obstetric epidural analgesia in aortic stenosis: a low-dose technique for labour and instrumental delivery. *Int J Obstet Anesth* 2001;10:129–34.

18. Horlocker TT, Wedel DJ, Benzon H, Brown DL, Enneking FK, Heit JA, *et al.* Regional anesthesia in the anticoagulated patient: defining the risks (the Second ASRA Consensus Conference on Neuraxial Anesthesia and Anticoagulation). *Reg Anesth Pain Med* 2003;28:172–97.

19. Orme RM, Grange CS, Ainsworth QP, Grebenik CR. General anaesthesia using remifentanil for caesarean section in parturients with critical aortic stenosis: a series of four cases. *Int J Obstet Anesth* 2004;13:183–7.

20. Grocott HP, Sato Y, Homi HM, Smith BE. The influence of xenon, nitrous oxide and nitrogen on gas bubble expansion during cardiopulmonary bypass. *Eur J Anaesthesiol* 2005;22:353–8.

21. Whitfield A, Holdcroft A. Anaesthesia for caesarean section in patients with aortic stenosis: the case for general anaesthesia. *Anaesthesia* 1998;53:109–12.

22. Brighouse D. Anaesthesia for caesarean section in patients with aortic stenosis: the case for regional anaesthesia. *Anaesthesia* 1998;53:107–9.

23. Association of Anaesthetists of Great Britain and Ireland. *Recommendations for Standards of Monitoring During Anaesthesia and Recovery 3.* London: AAGBI; 2000.

24. Fu ES, Downs JB, Schweiger JW, Miguel RV, Smith RA. Supplemental oxygen impairs detection of hypoventilation by pulse oximetry. *Chest* 2004;126:1552–8.

25. Fujitani S, Baldisseri M. Hemodynamic assessment in a pregnant and peripartum patient. *Crit Care Med* 2005;33(10 Suppl):S354–61.

26. Crane-Elders AB, Nijhuis JG, van Dongen PW, vd Dries A. Severe maternal morbidity and fetal mortality caused by a diagnostic Swan–Ganz procedure: a case report. *Eur J Obstet Gynecol Reprod Biol* 1990;37:95–8.

27. Belfort MA, Rokey R, Saade GR, Moise KJ. Rapid echocardiographic assessment of left and right heart hemodynamics in critically ill obstetric patients. *Am J Obstet Gynecol* 1994;171:884–92.

28. Penny JA, Anthony J, Shennan AH, De Swiet M, Singer M. A comparison of hemodynamic data derived by pulmonary artery flotation catheter and the esophageal Doppler monitor in preeclampsia. *Am J Obstet Gynecol* 2000;183:658–61.

29. Rhodes A, Grounds RM. New technologies for measuring cardiac output: the future? *Curr Opin Crit Care* 2003;11:224–6.

30. Advanced Life Support Group. Managing Obstetric Emergencies and Trauma Course [www.ALSG.org.uk].

31. Smith GB, Osgood VM, Crane S. ALERT™ – A multiprofessional training course in the care of acutely ill adult patient. *Resuscitation* 2002;52:281–6.

32. Resuscitation Council (UK). Immediate Life Support Course [www.resus.org.uk/pages/ilsgen.htm].

33. Resuscitation Council (UK). Advanced Life Support Course [www.resus.org.uk/pages/alsgen.htm].

34. Resuscitation Council (UK). Newborn Life Support Course [www.resus.org.uk/pages/nlsgen.htm].

35. Resuscitation Council (UK). *Advanced Life Support*. 5th ed. London: Resuscitation Council (UK); 2005.

Section 6

Postpartum care

Chapter 21

Management of the puerperium in women with heart disease

Margaret Ramsay

Introduction

The puerperium is a dangerous time for women with heart disease, especially those with cardiomyopathy or pulmonary hypertension. This is the time of highest mortality and significant morbidity, when many changes occur that affect cardiac function. Some of these haemodynamic changes are predictable (e.g. 'autotransfusion' of blood into the systemic circulation as the uterus contracts) but others are unpredictable (e.g. a variable amount of blood loss from the genital tract around the time of delivery). Although it is possible to control what happens during delivery by planning either vaginal birth or caesarean section, the events of the puerperium are faced by every woman. Their cardiovascular challenges cannot be avoided.

Physiological changes occurring in the puerperium in healthy women

Haemodynamic changes

There have been a number of studies of the haemodynamic changes occurring during pregnancy and the puerperium. However, few of these have concentrated on events happening in the first 48 hours after delivery. Pregnancy is characterised by a volume-loaded state, with an increased cardiac output owing to an increased stroke volume and a higher heart rate, and increased preload, as demonstrated by enlarged ventricular end-diastolic dimensions.[1,2] Afterload is reduced, with reductions in both systemic and pulmonary vascular resistances.[3] Intrinsic myocardial contractility is increased in pregnancy.[2] Filling pressures on the left side of the heart (pulmonary capillary wedge pressure (PCWP)) and on the right side of the heart (central venous pressure (CVP)) are unchanged, as is pulmonary artery pressure.[3] Colloid osmotic pressure (COP) and the COP–PCWP gradient are low in late pregnancy, contributing to the vulnerability of women to pulmonary oedema around the time of delivery.[3,4]

During active labour without analgesia, cardiac output increases by 15–30% during contractions. This is associated with a 25–30% increase in stroke volume, an increase in blood pressure and a decrease in heart rate.[5,6] In the second stage of labour, cardiac output increases, reaching levels 40% higher than those recorded before labour, whereas in women with adequate regional anaesthesia, cardiac output hardly changes.[5]

Active bearing down ('pushing'), involving a repeated Valsalva manoeuvre, results in reduction of cardiac output, which overshoots as heart rate rises.[6] Pain and anxiety increase cardiac output.[6,7] Changing from the lateral to the supine posture usually diminishes cardiac output by 10–25%, with initially little change in heart rate and blood pressure, but then a progressive decrease in heart rate and an even more marked fall in cardiac output.[8]

Cardiac output increases very significantly immediately after delivery, typically 60% above prelabour values, regardless of the type of analgesia employed.[5] Not all of this rise in cardiac output can be explained by tachycardia. In one study,[5] 10 minutes after delivery of the baby, stroke volume was found to be 50% increased over prelabour values.

In another study,[9] at 1 and 2 hours post delivery, cardiac output was on average 22% higher and stroke volume 38% higher but heart rate lower than before the onset of labour. Serial CVP measurements in this study showed significantly increased values after delivery, and this was attributed to 'autotransfusion' of blood from the uteroplacental bed following delivery.

A high cardiac output is preserved for at least 48 hours, despite a reduction in heart rate at this time, while stroke volume increases.[1,10] There is an increase in left ventricular end-diastolic dimensions, suggesting an increased venous return due to an increased circulating volume.[10]

Cardiovascular parameters measured 2 weeks after delivery show a reduction in cardiac output, stroke volume and heart rate. Left ventricular end-diastolic dimensions, ejection fraction and circumferential shortening are also reduced, compared with values recorded in late pregnancy or the early puerperium.[10] These changes suggest not only that the circulating volume declines but also that there is reduction in myocardial contractility.[10]

By 6 weeks, some further reduction in cardiac output, stroke volume and heart rate has been reported, with increased systemic and pulmonary vascular resistance. Myocardial contractility is reduced further.[2] Left ventricular wall thickness decreases.[11] It is not clear when (or even whether) cardiovascular parameters reach a true 'non-pregnant' state. Robson et al.[11] followed a cohort of 15 women for 6 months from pregnancy, performing Doppler and M-mode echocardiography studies at 38 weeks of gestation, then at two, six, 12 and 24 weeks after delivery. Even at 24 weeks postpartum, there were many cardiovascular parameters significantly different from those found in an age-matched control group of women, none of whom were using hormonal contraception. In particular, postnatal women had higher left ventricular wall thickness, dilatation of aortic and pulmonary valve areas, higher stroke volume and reduced indices of left ventricular contractility.

Circulating volume changes

The concept of 'autotransfusion' of blood from the uteroplacental bed into the systemic circulation once the uterus contracts tonically after delivery of the placenta is an important one.[9] Studies have estimated the magnitude of these blood volume changes to be 300–500 ml.[6,7] Similar volumes of blood are squeezed from the uteroplacental bed during labour contractions, although these may be partly balanced by increases in the maternal intervillous blood volume as the venous outflow is occluded early in the contraction cycle. There is a rise in CVP measured during contractions and in the first 2 hours following delivery, consistent with these acute changes in circulating blood volume.[9] Post-delivery 'autotransfusion' is a significant haemodynamic phenomenon, if the blood losses during delivery have been average or less, although clearly this effect will be negated if there is above average postpartum haemorrhage.

There can also be increased venous return after delivery owing to relief of aortocaval compression by the uterus.[8,12]

Total blood volume may be diminished by blood loss at the time of delivery or during the following hours and days. It is not uncommon for brisk haemorrhage to arise from uterine atony, or for substantial losses to occur from vaginal, perineal or surgical trauma sustained during delivery. This will then represent an opposite cardiovascular stress to that associated with the 'autotransfusion' described above.

The increase in plasma volume noted during pregnancy diminishes over the weeks following delivery.[13] Most of the changes are likely to occur during the first 2 weeks, in parallel with the diminution of cardiac output.[11] The diuresis that occurs at this time is the response to the decreased activity of the renin–angiotensin–aldosterone axis following pregnancy.[14] Extravascular fluid is also mobilised, enters the circulation and is then lost from the body in the urine.

Effects of drugs and fluids

Many of the drugs used at the time of delivery have cardiovascular effects. Ergometrine causes vasoconstriction and transiently elevated blood pressure. Oxytocin given as an intravenous bolus can cause hypotension, while given as an intravenous infusion it has antidiuretic effects, leading to water retention and hyponatraemia.[15] In the early puerperium, there may also be residual effects from anaesthetic agents, particularly the sympathetic blockade created by regional anaesthesia. Intravenous fluids may also have been given during labour, as vehicles for drug administration, for hydration purposes, or in association with regional anaesthesia.

Haemostatic changes

The risk of thromboembolism is highest around the time of delivery, which stimulates maximal platelet activation and fibrin formation.[16,17] Additionally, by 3 hours post delivery, there is evidence of continuing enhanced clotting activity and also maximum fibrinolysis.[16] Physical factors such as immobility and impaired venous drainage contribute to the risk of venous thromboembolism; other factors such as pyrexia and dehydration may also be important.

Risks during the puerperium for women with heart disease

Healthy women mostly tolerate the dramatic haemodynamic changes of the puerperium without problems. However, women with underlying heart disease may be at risk of one or more of the following adverse events:

- pulmonary oedema
- systemic hypertension
- alterations in cardiac shunting of blood
- cyanosis
- thromboembolism
- rhythm disturbances

■ bacteraemia/sepsis
■ ventricular ischaemia.

The particular risks depend on the underlying cardiac condition but can also be influenced by intercurrent disease, particularly pre-eclampsia, thrombophilia, diabetes, haemorrhage and sepsis.

Pulmonary oedema

Fluid flow into the pulmonary interstitium depends on capillary permeability and the difference between hydrostatic and osmotic pressures within the capillaries. As discussed above, the COP–PCWP gradient is low in late pregnancy;[3] gradients of 4 mmHg or less are associated with pulmonary oedema.[4] Factors that increase PCWP, reduce COP or increase capillary permeability predispose to the development of pulmonary oedema. These may be inherent to cardiac disease (e.g. mitral stenosis causing increased PCWP) or consequent on other conditions (e.g. pre-eclampsia can be associated with increased PCWP, reduced COP and increased capillary permeability).[4]

Systemic hypertension

Fluid shifts occurring soon after delivery, as the uteroplacental circulation constricts, or later, as accumulated extracellular fluid is mobilised into the circulation, can give rise to systemic hypertension. High circulating catecholamine levels, due to anxiety or pain, result in elevated blood pressure and cardiac output.[6] Intercurrent pre-eclampsia is associated with labile and sometimes extremely elevated blood pressure, owing to increased vascular reactivity to circulating pressor agents.[18] Women with pre-eclampsia often have reduced plasma volumes in comparison with healthy women in late gestation; they thus often have much higher systemic vascular resistance than would be typical in pregnancy.[19]

Alterations in cardiac shunting of blood

Systemic vasoconstriction or vasodilatation, in response to blood loss or the sympathetic blockade of regional anaesthesia, alters the direction of blood flow through intracardiac shunts. This affects venous return, cardiac output and pulmonary blood flow. A sudden fall in ventricular output may cause cardiogenic shock.[20,21] There may be subtle changes in the balance of systemic and pulmonary vascular resistances following delivery owing to the loss of aortocaval compression, improvement of venous return to the heart and acute increase in plasma volume; these may be enough to affect the direction of shunt flow in women with pulmonary hypertension and a large intracardiac shunt.[21]

Cyanosis

Cyanosis can arise owing to an alteration in the direction of flow across an intracardiac shunt, such that blood flows right to left in the heart and does not enter the pulmonary circulation. Cyanosis can also be due to worsening pulmonary hypertension, as pulmonary vascular resistance increases gradually in the weeks after delivery or acutely in response to hypoxia, hypercarbia, acidosis, stress or pain.[22,23] Thrombosis in the small vessels of the pulmonary arterial system or multiple pulmonary emboli from a systemic venous thrombosis also increase pulmonary vascular resistance.[22,23]

Thromboembolism

When a deep vein thrombosis has formed, there may be pulmonary embolisation as an acute event, or multiple, recurrent events. In someone with an intracardiac shunt, there is the possibility of systemic embolisation, causing cerebral transient ischaemic attacks or infarction.[24,25] Clots may also develop in dilated or poorly contracting heart chambers, further compromising cardiac function.[26] Women with cyanotic heart disease are commonly polycythaemic and hence have increased blood viscosity, putting them at particular risk of thromboembolism.[21]

Rhythm disturbances

Effective ventricular filling and emptying depend on cardiac rate. Blood flow into the coronary arteries happens during diastole and can be impaired if there is a persistent tachycardia, especially when there is ventricular hypertrophy.[20] Acute rhythm disturbances are more likely when the cardiac chambers are dilated but may also be the consequence of re-entry phenomena, ischaemic heart disease or the long QT syndrome.[27]

Any acute or persistent tachyarrhythmia in the puerperium can impair cardiac output, cause syncope or angina or precipitate cardiac arrest.

Bacteraemia/sepsis

Caesarean delivery is associated with a higher incidence (approximately 3%) of bacteraemia than is vaginal delivery (0.1%).[28] The highest risks of bacteraemia are associated with prolonged rupture of the membranes, chorioamnionitis, pyelonephritis or endometritis, the latter particularly following caesarean delivery.[28] Most cases (approximately 80%) of severe sepsis in obstetric patients thus occur in the postpartum period. The risks for women with cardiac disease are those of general haemodynamic disturbances associated with a pyrexial illness (vasodilatation, tachycardia, etc.), increased risk for pelvic vein thromboembolism and risks of bacterial endocarditis in those with susceptible conditions (e.g. valvular disease, prosthetic valves, ventriculoseptal defects).[29]

Ventricular ischaemia

Myocardial infarction, although uncommon, is most likely to happen during labour or in the postpartum period.[30] The mechanism is most commonly coronary artery dissection, rather than atheromatous disease.[31] Haemodynamic changes around the time of delivery exert maximal sheer stresses in the aorta and coronary vessels, which may also have weakened collagen at this time.[31,32] The risks of dissection are greatest in women with a known connective tissue disorder, such as Marfan or Ehlers–Danlos syndrome. Ischaemia may also complicate the puerperium in women with ventricular outflow obstruction and ventricular wall hypertrophy, cardiac transplantation, coronary arteritis, collagen vascular diseases and those with known occlusive coronary artery disease.[31–33]

Timing of maternal deaths during the puerperium

Deaths from Eisenmenger syndrome, which has a 30–50% maternal mortality rate, usually occur within the first week after delivery.[21] Women with pulmonary hypertension, however, are as likely to die antenatally or in the late puerperium, as in the first weeks following delivery.[34] Cardiomyopathy-related deaths tend to happen many months after delivery and some occur even later.[35,36] The early puerperium is the most common time for deaths from myocardial infarction.[30,32]

Morbidity in the puerperium associated with specific cardiac conditions

Eisenmenger syndrome

Women with Eisenmenger syndrome have a poor tolerance of hypovolaemia, which leads to shunt reversal, reduced cardiac output and increased cyanosis. They are just as intolerant of an increased volume load because they have a fibrotic pulmonary vascular bed.[21] They are also vulnerable to thromboembolism into an already diseased pulmonary vascular bed.[21] Excitement, effort, anxiety and heat are known to provoke fainting and collapse in patients with this condition;[25] all these may be encountered during or soon after delivery.

Pulmonary hypertension

There may be both a fixed component to pulmonary hypertension, due to vascular remodelling, and a reactive component, due to vasoconstriction. The pulmonary vascular bed can be further compromised by emboli. Women with this condition experience haemodynamic instability during pregnancy. After delivery, an increase in blood volume easily provokes right ventricular failure. Any increase in pulmonary vascular resistance, such as may be provoked by hypercarbia, hypoxia, acidosis, stress and pain will further reduce effective gas exchange in the lungs.[34,37]

Cardiomyopathy

Women with pre-existing or peripartum cardiomyopathy exhibit symptoms and signs of left heart failure. They are intolerant of tachycardia, which impairs ventricular filling and emptying. They are also intolerant of the increased blood volume of the early puerperium (i.e. increased preload) and the changes in systemic vascular resistance and left ventricular contractility that happen over the following weeks and months.[35,36] Women with severe myocardial dysfunction due to peripartum cardiomyopathy may never regain normal cardiac function and they may become candidates for cardiac transplantation.[25,36]

Corrected tetralogy of Fallot

Unless they have pulmonary hypertension, left ventricular dysfunction or cyanosis, women with corrected tetralogy of Fallot do well in pregnancy and the puerperium. Their main vulnerability is to supraventricular tachycardia, pulmonary embolism or worsening right ventricular function.[38,39]

Fontan circulation

The Fontan procedure is palliative and usually involves creating a shunt between the right atrium and the pulmonary artery. There is no pump for the pulmonary circulation, so success depends on there being good left ventricular function. Women with this type of circulation are vulnerable to tachyarrhythmia and congestive cardiac failure. They have a limited ability to increase cardiac output and so may run into difficulties soon after delivery owing to increased blood volume and enhanced venous return.[40]

Valvular and aortic disease

The particular risks with valvular disease depend on its site and the associated pressure gradients. There is vulnerability to ventricular failure, causing peripheral or pulmonary oedema, with any increase in preload or tachyarrhythmia. Mechanical valve replacements are vulnerable to thrombosis and systemic emboli, particularly when there is the maximal haemostatic challenge around the time of delivery, or if thromboprophylaxis is inadequate.[41] Bioprosthetic valves, where there is no residual haemodynamic compromise, do not cause particular problems in the puerperium.[42] Sheer stress in the aortic root is greatest immediately postpartum, making women with aortic coarctation or dilated aortic root particularly vulnerable to aortic dissection at this time.[43]

Cardiac transplantation

The denervated transplanted heart is vulnerable to progressive occlusive coronary artery disease, causing ischaemia. There is no perception of ischaemic pain and the only symptom may be of dyspnoea. There is always the risk of organ rejection, causing deterioration in cardiac function. During and after delivery, the main maternal risks are due to an increased sensitivity of the denervated heart to vasoactive drugs and to hypovolaemia.[33] Hypertension and pre-eclampsia are more common in immuno-suppressed women with cardiac transplants. This brings an increased vulnerability to pulmonary oedema.[44]

Management of women with significant cardiac disease during the puerperium

Planning ahead with multidisciplinary input

It is important when making plans for safe delivery and care in the puerperium that there is as complete a cardiac diagnosis as possible. In someone with repaired congenital heart disease, it is important to have information from all previous hospital specialists involved in her care, and up-to-date echocardiography. This will enable the evolution of adverse features (e.g. pulmonary hypertension, left ventricular hypertrophy) to be appreciated, and knowledge as to whether there has been a good response previously to interventions, such as the administration of pulmonary vasodilators, is also useful. There can be serious unexpected cardiac problems even in cases where there was an apparently complete repair of a congenital lesion in childhood and there have been no recent symptoms.[45]

Discussions about the specific risks of the puerperium and its management options need to involve obstetricians, cardiologists, anaesthetists (including those with skills in obstetric and cardiac anaesthesia), intensive care medicine specialists and often haematologists. The issues can then be discussed in detail with the woman and her family, and an individual care plan can be formulated. The following areas need to be discussed:

■ What are the particular risks for this woman, given her cardiac condition and any other obstetric or medical problems?

■ What features should be monitored to determine stability of her cardiac condition? Should this include invasive haemodynamic monitoring and are there particular hazards in doing so?

■ How long will it be before the main dangers are past? For how long should monitoring in an intensive care or high-dependency care setting be maintained?

■ Plans for fluid management.

■ What thrombotic risks are there? What degree of thromboprophylaxis or anticoagulation should be used?

■ Plans for antibiotic prophylaxis.

■ What are the best options for analgesia?

■ Is there a particular requirement for cardiac rate or rhythm control and what agents should be used to achieve this?

■ Is any particular posture (e.g. sitting upright, lateral recumbence) likely to be beneficial?

Multidisciplinary care during the puerperium

For women with significant cardiac disease, care during the first few days of the puerperium needs to be based in an intensive care or high-dependency unit. Multidisciplinary input is required to attend to all needs and risks; good communication between the specialist teams is essential. It is important not to relax vigilance too quickly, bearing in mind that major changes in cardiac output and plasma volumes continue over at least the first 2 weeks following delivery.

Cardiovascular monitoring

Non-invasive monitoring of pulse rate, respiratory rate, blood pressure, transcutaneous oxygen saturation and fluid balance is a minimum requirement. For women at risk of arrhythmias, the electrocardiogram should also be monitored. Invasive monitoring can include just systemic arterial and central venous pressure monitoring, or full haemodynamic monitoring with insertion of a Swan–Ganz pulmonary artery catheter. This allows measurement of pulmonary artery pressure and PCWP, as well as cardiac output, using a thermodilution technique. From these measured variables, pulmonary and systemic vascular resistances, stroke volume and work, as well as the weight- and height-adjusted indices, can be calculated. Invasive haemodynamic monitoring carries risks of pneumothorax, ventricular arrhythmias, pulmonary artery rupture, local thrombosis, pulmonary infarction, damage to the heart valves and coiling up or knotting of the catheter within the heart chambers.[46]

Doppler echocardiography can also be used in obstetric critical care to measure indices of cardiac performance. Good correlation between invasive and echo techniques has been reported in several studies of critically ill obstetric patients.[47–49] Consistent underestimation of cardiac output was found with a transoesophageal Doppler technique in young women with pre-eclampsia, although the magnitude and direction of changes in cardiac output with time were documented accurately.[50] Importantly, these non-invasive echocardiographic techniques can provide crucial haemodynamic information when it is too hazardous to insert a pulmonary artery catheter.

Thromboprophylaxis and anticoagulation

Thromboprophylaxis is most conveniently achieved with low molecular weight heparin injections. The doses given can be adjusted with reference to assays for anti-Xa activity to ensure adequate prophylaxis or even full anticoagulation.[51] In some cases (e.g. mechanical heart valves or a recent episode of thromboembolism) intravenous unfractionated heparin may be the preferred means of anticoagulation, as the infusion rate can be adjusted to moderate the degree of anticoagulation on an hour-by-hour basis.

Pharmacological management of specific cardiac problems

Depending on the underlying cardiac pathology, intervention may be required in the puerperium to treat acute volume overload with diuretics, give inotropic support (e.g. angiotensin-converting enzyme (ACE) inhibitors, digoxin, dopamine, dobutamine), reduce preload (with venodilators or diuretics) or reduce afterload (with vasodilators).[52] Control of heart rate may require beta blockade; other arrhythmias should be managed according to their specific electrocardiographic features. In the puerperium, there is no longer any need to avoid valuable drugs that have adverse fetal side effects, although the passage of drugs into the breast milk must be taken into account in breastfeeding mothers (for example, some maternally administered beta blockers can cause neonatal bradycardia).

There may be a need to reduce pulmonary vascular resistance without also reducing systemic vascular resistance (so as to restore intracardiac shunt blood flow from left to right). Experience is increasing with the use of inhaled nitric oxide, inhaled or intravenous prostacyclin and inhaled iloprost for the treatment of pulmonary hypertension.[23,53–56] Nitric oxide donors (sildenafil and L-arginine) have also been used for the same purpose.[57]

Standard antibiotic regimens for the prevention of bacterial endocarditis should be followed where this is a particular risk.[52]

Pain relief, oxygen and posture

Breakthrough pain, with its associated anxiety and high circulating catecholamines, has adverse cardiac effects (as detailed earlier),[6] so adequate analgesia is still a priority even after delivery. Where regional analgesia has been used successfully during labour or operative delivery, then this can be continued. Opiates are often included in regional analgesic blocks and cause less systemic vasodilatation than local anaesthetic agents. Opiates may also be given orally or in patient-controlled infusions. Concurrent anticoagulation may preclude use of nonsteroidal analgesics.

Hypoxia increases pulmonary vascular resistance.[22,23] Supplemental oxygen should be given during the early puerperium to women with cyanosis, ventricular failure, pulmonary hypertension or intracardiac shunts.[34,37,58]

The effect of posture on cardiac function is often overlooked, other than to avoid the supine position before delivery. The left lateral position is the most favourable, as it avoids aortocaval compression.[12,59] It is the best posture to be adopted both for delivery and the first few hours thereafter in women vulnerable to sudden changes in preload. In women at risk from pulmonary oedema, a sitting-upright posture reduces left atrial pressures.[59]

Conclusions

It is important that multidisciplinary discussions about the care of women with serious cardiac problems do not just cover how they should be delivered. The early hours, days and weeks of the puerperium are equally, if not more, dangerous and need careful planning.

More women who have had surgical correction or palliation of congenital heart lesions are reaching childbearing age. Their safe care requires close liaison between specialists in congenital heart disease, adult cardiologists, intensive care specialists and obstetricians, sharing knowledge and ideas to solve their problems.

References

1. Spatling L, Fallenstein F, Huch A, Hich R, Rooth G. The variability of cardiopulmonary adaptation to pregnancy at rest and during exercise. *Br J Obstet Gynaecol* 1992;99 Suppl 8:18–20.

2. Gilson GJ, Samaan S, Crawford MH. Qualls CR, Curet LB. Changes in hemodynamics, ventricular remodelling, and ventricular contractility during normal pregnancy: a longitudinal study. *Obstet Gynecol* 1997;89:957–62.

3. Clark SL, Cotton DB, Lee W, Bishop C, Hill T, Southwick J, *et al*. Central hemodynamic assessment of normal term pregnancy. *Am J Obstet Gynecol* 1989;161:1439–42.

4. Zlatnik MG. Pulmonary edema: etiology and treatment. *Semin Perinatol* 1997;21:298–306.

5. Hansen JM, Ueland K. The influence of caudal analgesia on cardiovascular dynamics during normal labour and delivery. *Acta Anaesthesiol Scand Suppl* 1966;23:449–52.

6. Hendricks CH, Quilligan EJ. Cardiac output during labor. *Am J Obstet Gynecol* 1956;71:953–72.

7. Adams JQ, Alexander AM. Alterations in cardiovascular physiology during labor. *Obstet Gynecol* 1958;12:542–9.

8. Kerr MG. Cardiovascular dynamics in pregnancy and labour. *Br Med Bull* 1968;24:19–24.

9. Kjeldsen J. Hemodynamic investigations during labour and delivery. *Acta Obstet Gynecol Scand* 1979;58 Suppl 89:77–197.

10. Robson SC, Dunlop W, Hunter S. Haemodynamic changes during the early puerperium. *Br Med J* 1987;294:1065.

11. Robson SC, Hunter S, Moore M, Dunlop W. Haemodynamic changes during the puerperium: a Doppler and M-mode echocardiographic study. *Br J Obstet Gynaecol* 1987;94:1028–39.

12. Kerr MG, Scott DB, Samuel E. Studies of the inferior vena cava in late pregnancy. *Br Med J* 1964;1:532–3.

13. Hytten FE, Paintin DB. Increase in plasma volume during normal pregnancy. *J Obstet Gynaecol Br Emp* 1963;70:402–7.

14. August P. The renin angiotensin system in hypertensive pregnancy. In: Rubin PC, editor. *Handbook of Hypertension, Vol. 21: Hypertension in Pregnancy*. Amsterdam: Elsevier; 2000. p. 57–75.

15. Summaries of product characteristics for oxytocin and ergometrine. Multilex Drug Data File.

16. Gerbasi FR, Bottoms S, Farag A, Mammen EF. Changes in hemostasis activity during delivery and the immediate postpartum period. *Am J Obstet Gyncol* 1990;162:1158–63.

17. Reinthaller A, Musch-Edlmayr G, Tatra G. Thrombin-antithrombin III complex levels in normal pregnancy with hypertensive disorders and after delivery. *Br J Obstet Gynaecol* 1990;97:506–10.

18. Chesley LC. Vascular reactivity in normal and toxemic pregnancy. *Clin Obstet Gynecol* 1966;9:871–80.

19. Gallery EDM, Huntor SN, Györy AZ. Plasma volume contraction: a significant factor in both pregnancy-associated hypertension (pre-eclampsia) and chronic hypertension in pregnancy. *Q J Med* 1979;192:593–602.

20. Oakley C. Acyanotic heart disease. In: Oakley C, editor. *Heart Disease in Pregnancy*. London: BMJ Publishing Group; 1997. p. 63–82.

21. Gleicher N, Midwall J, Hochberger D, Jaffin H. Eisenmenger's syndrome and pregnancy. *Obstet Gynecol Surv* 1979;34:721–41.

22. Slomka F, Salmeron S, Zetlaoui P, Cohen H, Simonneau G, Samii K. Primary pulmonary hypertension and pregnancy: anaesthetic management for delivery. *Anesthesiology* 1988;69:959–61.

23. Rosenthal E, Nelson-Piercy C. Value of nitric oxide in Eisenmenger syndrome during pregnancy. *Am J Obstet Gynecol* 2000;183:781–2.

24. Harvey JR, Teague SM, Anderson JL, Voyles WF, Thadani V. Clinically silent atrial septal defects with evidence for cerebral embolisation. *Ann Intern Med* 1986;105:695–7.

25. Daliento L, Somerville J, Presbitero P, Menti L, Brach-Prever S, Rizzoli G, et al. Eisenmenger syndrome: factors relating to deterioration and death. *Eur Heart J* 1998;19:1845–55.

26. Oakley C. Peripartum cardiomyopathy and other heart muscle disorders. In: Oakley C, editor. *Heart Disease in Pregnancy*. London: BMJ Publishing Group; 1997. p. 210–25.

27. Anderson MH. Rhythm disorders. In: Oakley C, editor. *Heart Disease in Pregnancy*. London: BMJ Publishing Group; 1997. p. 248–81.

28. Gordon MC. Maternal sepsis. In: Foley MR, Strong TH, editors. *Obstetric Intensive Care: A Practical Manual*. Philadelphia: WB Saunders Company; 1997. p. 129–46.

29. Oakley C. Infective endocarditis. In: Oakley C, editor. *Heart Disease in Pregnancy*. London: BMJ Publishing Group; 1997. p. 147–52.

30. Hankins GDV, Wendel GD, Leveno KL, Stoneham J. Myocardial infarction during pregnancy: a review. *Obstet Gynecol* 1985;65:139–46.

31. Kearney P, Singh H, Hutter J, Khan S, Lee G, Lucey J. Spontaneous coronary artery dissection: a report of three cases and review of the literature. *Postgrad Med J* 1993;69:940–5.

32. Oakley C. Coronary artery disease. In: Oakley C, editor. *Heart Disease in Pregnancy*. London: BMJ Publishing Group; 1997. p. 237–47.

33. Kim K-M, Sukhani R, Slogoff S, Tomich PG. Central hemodynamic changes associated with pregnancy in a long-term cardiac transplant recipient. *Am J Obstet Gynecol* 1996;174:1651–3.

34. Bonnin M, Mercier FJ, Sitbon O, Roger-Christoph S, Jais X, Humbert M, et al. Severe pulmonary hypertension during pregnancy. *Anesthesiology* 2005;102:1133–7.

35. Heider AL, Kuller JA, Strauss RA, Wells SR. Peripartum cardiomyopathy: a review of the literature. *Obstet Gynecol Surv* 1999;54:526–31.

36. Witlin AG, Mabie WC, Sibai BM. Peripartum cardiomyopathy: a longitudinal echocardiographic study. *Am J Obstet Gynecol* 1997;177:1129–32.

37. Nelson DM, Main E, Crafford W, Ahumada GG. Peripartum heart failure due to primary pulmonary hypertension. *Obstet Gynecol* 1983;62 Suppl:58S–63S.

38. Singh H, Bolton PJ, Oakley CM. Pregnancy after surgical correction of tetralogy of Fallot. *Br Med J* 1982;285:168–70.

39. Veldtman GR, Connolly HM, Grogan M, Ammash NM, Warnes CA. Outcomes of pregnancy in women with tetralogy of Fallot. *J Am Coll Cardiol* 2004;44:174–80.

40. Cannobio MM, Mair DD, Van de Velde M, Koos BJ. Pregnancy outcomes after the Fontan repair. *J Am Coll Cardiol* 1996;28:763–7.

41. Chan WS, Anand S, Ginsberg JS. Anticoagulation of pregnant women with mechanical heart valves: a systematic review of the literature. *Arch Intern Med* 2000;160:191–6.

42. Avila WS, Rossi EG, Grinberg M. Influence of pregnancy after bioprosthetic valve replacement in young women: a prospective five-year study. *J Heart Valve Dis* 2002;11:864–9.

43. Head CEG, Thorne SA. Congenital heart disease in pregnancy. *Postgrad Med J* 2005;81:292–8.

44. Scott JR, Wagoner LE, Olsen SL, Taylor DO, Renlund DG. Pregnancy in heart transplant recipients: management and outcome. *Obstet Gynecol* 1993;82:324–7.

45. Jackson GM, Dildy GA, Varner MW, Clark SL. Severe pulmonary hypertension in pregnancy following successful repair of ventriculoseptal defect in childhood. *Obstet Gynecol* 1993;82:680–2.

46. Mabie WC. Basic hemodynamic monitoring for the obstetric care provider. In: Foley MR, Strong TH, editors. *Obstetric Intensive Care: A Practical Manual.* Philadelphia: WB Saunders Company; 1997. p. 1–19.

47. Belfort MA, Rokey R, Saade GR, Moise KJ. Rapid echocardiographic assessment of left and right heart hemodynamics in critically ill obstetric patients. *Am J Obstet Gynecol* 1994;171:884–92.

48. Rokey R. Belfort MA, Saade GR. Quantitative echocardiographic assessment of left ventricular function in critically ill obstetric patients: a comparative study. *Am J Obstet Gynecol* 1995;173:1148–52.

49. Lee W, Rokey R, Cotton DB. Noninvasive maternal stroke volume and cardiac output determination by pulsed Doppler echocardiography. *Am J Obstet Gynecol* 1988;158:505–10.

50. Penny JA, Anthony J, Shennan AH, De Swiet M, Singer M. A comparison of hemodynamic data derived by pulmonary artery flotation catheter and the oesophageal Doppler monitor in pre-eclampsia. *Am J Obstet Gynecol* 2000;183:658–61.

51. Greer I, Hunt BJ. Low molecular weight heparin in pregnancy: current issues. *Br J Haematol* 2005;128:593–601.

52. Koszalka MF. Cardiac disease in pregnancy. In: Foley MR, Strong TH, editors. *Obstetric Intensive Care: A Practical Manual.* Philadelphia: WB Saunders Company; 1997. p. 106–28.

53. Goodwin TM, Gherman RB, Hameed A, Elkayam U. Favorable response of Eisenmenger syndrome to inhaled nitric oxide during pregnancy. *Am J Obstet Gynecol* 1999;180:64–7.

54. Bildirici. 1, Shumway JB. Intravenous and inhaled epoprostenol for primary pulmonary hypertension during pregnancy and delivery. *Obstet Gynecol* 2004;103:1102–5.

55. Monnery L, Nanson J, Charlton G. Primary pulmonary hypertension in pregnancy: a role for novel vasodilators. *Br J Anaesth* 2001;87:295–8.

56. Easterling TR, Ralph DD, Schmucker BC. Pulmonary hypertension in pregnancy: treatment with pulmonary vasodilators. *Obstet Gynecol* 1999;93:494–8.

57. Lacassie HJ, Germain AM, Valdés G, Fernández MS, Allamand F, López H. Management of Eisenmenger syndrome in pregnancy with sildenafil and L-arginine. *Obstet Gynecol* 2004;103:1118–20.

58. Buckland R, Pickett JA. Pregnancy and the univentricular heart: case report and literature review. *Int J Obstet Anesth* 2000;9:55–63.

59.   Clark SL, Cotton DB, Pivarnik JM, Lee W, Hankins GDV, Benedetti TJ, *et al.* Position change and central hemodynamic profile during normal third-trimester pregnancy and postpartum. *Am J Obstet Gynecol* 1991;164:883–7.

Chapter 22

Impact of pregnancy on long-term outcomes in women with heart disease

Jack M Colman, Candice K Silversides and Samuel C Siu

Importance

Little is known about the impact of pregnancy on long-term outcomes in women with heart disease, even though it is such an important topic. In preconception counselling the possible effect of pregnancy on progression of disease, the potential need for earlier cardiac intervention and the likelihood of triggering other adverse effects on long-term prognosis are often among the first questions asked by the patient. There are data for women with heart disease on the risks during pregnancy and the puerperium of adverse cardiac, obstetrical, fetal and neonatal events but there is a paucity of information about late maternal prognosis.

A better understanding of the anticipated effects of pregnancy on maternal heart disease would allow better informed decisions regarding timing of interventions to be made. In order to allow a woman to enter pregnancy in the best possible state, the idea of a preconception cardiac surgical or interventional procedure to that end is intuitively attractive. However, in many heart conditions affecting adults, symptoms drive interventions and it is difficult to support a risk-associated intervention in an asymptomatic young woman intent on pregnancy without good data that overall risks to mother and child will be reduced.

There may be a role for pre-emptive institution of medical therapy intended as prophylaxis against progression of heart disease (for instance, systemic ventricular dysfunction) during pregnancy. However, there are inadequate data to establish the value of such interventions. Knowledge of the expected impact of pregnancy on long-term outcomes would provide the necessary basis for mounting trials of such therapeutic strategies.

Obstacles

There are a number of reasons why information is lacking on the long-term impact of pregnancy on women with heart disease. The late outcomes of many of the heart diseases under consideration are variable and not fully established, even in women who have never been pregnant. The number of women with any one specific lesion complicating pregnancy is low. It is difficult to identify the superimposed impact of pregnancy on conditions that are infrequent, non-homogeneous even within a single diagnostic category, and studied mainly through natural history studies and case series. In many cardiac conditions no studies whatsoever have been done of the long-term effects of pregnancy. Risk assessments have focused almost exclusively on antepartum and early postpartum outcomes. The measurable haemodynamic effects of pregnancy resolve rapidly postpartum in normal women such that the longest lasting pregnancy-induced changes have normalised by the 24th postpartum week.[1] It is not known if this is true in women with heart disease.

Randomised controlled trials of the effects of pregnancy on maternal heart diseases cannot be mounted. Descriptive attempts have been made to address such issues but, in conditions where events are expected independent of pregnancy and are age- and time-dependent, it is crucial to examine matched control groups, otherwise any conclusions are open to the challenge that the described findings are no more than what would be expected with the passage of time, independent of pregnancy.

Case series are clearly subject to reporting bias, triggered as they often are by a few adverse outcomes, and all retrospective studies are subject to ascertainment bias.

Historically, data collection in pregnancy has focused on maternal mortality. However, death rates related to pregnancy in the developed world are low, and death, while very important, is no longer the major outcome of interest. It is necessary also to understand the impact of pregnancy on long-term morbidity in women with heart disease but data on maternal morbidity are not widely collected in the same systematic fashion as are mortality data. Furthermore, the impact of pregnancy on late death and on morbidity in cardiac disease will be systematically underreported because it is likely that death or deterioration in status will be attributed to progression of the underlying heart disease and the role of pregnancy not explored. The likelihood of such an omission will increase as the time between the pregnancy and the change in status increases. It has long been recognised that there is a bias favouring reporting of pregnancy-related mortality and morbidity when pregnancy is the direct cause of the problem, whereas cases are underreported if pregnancy is an indirect cause, acting via adverse effects on the underlying disease.[2]

Current and future research

In women with underlying heart disease, more good data on the long-term impact of pregnancy on ventricular dysfunction, pulmonary vascular disease, structural changes in valves and conduits, function of mechanical valves, severity and frequency of cardiac arrhythmias, rate of progression of aortopathy, and development of chronic hypertension and late vascular disease are needed. On many of these subjects, the literature is silent. The European consensus document on management of heart disease in pregnancy[3] does not address long-term outcomes. The consensus statements on management of congenital heart disease from Canada,[4-6] the USA[7] and Europe[8] offer guidance only on acute risks and acute management of pregnancy. Neither the American College of Cardiology (ACC)/American Heart Association (AHA) guidelines for the management of patients with valvular heart disease[9] nor the ACC/AHA/European Society of Cardiology (ESC) guidelines for management of patients with supraventricular arrhythmias[10] discuss the long-term impact of pregnancy.

There is some published information for some lesions. In the aortopathy associated with Marfan syndrome, a recent review of 23 women undergoing pregnancy and 22 control women who did not become pregnant with mean aortic root size of 37 ± 5 mm, showed no difference in rate of aortic root expansion during a 6.4 year follow-up.[11]

In peripartum cardiomyopathy, the risk of recurrence and of worsening of left ventricular (LV) dysfunction in a subsequent pregnancy is high and death may ensue in women whose LV function has remained abnormal 6 months following the end of the index pregnancy. The risk of recurrence is lower and death is rare if LV function has normalised.[12]

It is recognised that bioprosthetic xenograft valves degenerate at an undesirably rapid rate in women of childbearing age but there is an emerging consensus supported by a number of studies that pregnancy itself may not hasten that process.[13,14]

There is some evidence that pre-eclampsia and gestational diabetes are associated with future development of acquired cardiovascular diseases such as hypertension, atherosclerosis and coronary artery disease, as well as diabetes mellitus and its complications.[15]

In an observational study,[16] a surprisingly frequent need for intervention for aortic stenosis at a mean of 4 years following pregnancy was noted. While there are data on rate of progression of aortic stenosis and its impact on prognosis,[9] there are no controlled data on whether pregnancy actually accelerates this rate.

A recent retrospective review[17] of 28 pregnancies in 16 women following the Mustard operation for classic transposition of the great arteries concluded that pregnancy imparts a risk of irreversible systemic right ventricular (RV) dysfunction. However, this study is limited because there were no matched controls and RV dysfunction was assessed only in a qualitative manner based on routine clinical transthoracic echocardiographic studies.

In future, studies are needed that incorporate matched control groups consisting of non-pregnant women of similar age with similar cardiac disease followed for similar periods of time. Ideally, such studies should be prospective. Most will need to be multicentre because of the low numbers of women in any one centre who have the pathology of interest. Until results from such studies are available, it will continue to be difficult to provide evidence-based guidance to women regarding the long-term impact of pregnancy on their heart disease.

References

1. Hunter S, Robson SC. Adaptation of the maternal heart in pregnancy. *Br Heart J* 1992;68:540–3.

2. Lewis G, editor. *Why Mothers Die 2000–2002: The Sixth Report of Confidential Enquiries into Maternal Deaths in the United Kingdom*. London: RCOG Press; 2004.

3. Task Force on the Management of Cardiovascular Diseases During Pregnancy of the European Society of Cardiology. Expert consensus document on management of cardiovascular diseases during pregnancy. *Eur Heart J* 2003;24:761–81.

4. Therrien J, Dore A, Gersony W, Iserin L, Liberthson R, Meijboom F, *et al.* Canadian Cardiovascular Society Consensus Conference. Update: recommendations for the management of adults with congenital heart disease. Part I. *Can J Cardiol* 2001;17:940–59.

5. Therrien J, Gatzoulis M, Graham T, Bink-Boelkens M, Connelly M, Niwa K, *et al.* Canadian Cardiovascular Society Consensus Conference. Update: recommendations for the management of adults with congenital heart disease. Part II. *Can J Cardiol* 2001;17:1029–50.

6. Therrien J, Warnes C, Daliento L, Hess J, Hoffmann A, Marelli A, *et al.* Canadian Cardiovascular Society Consensus Conference. Update: recommendations for the management of adults with congenital heart disease. Part III. *Can J Cardiol* 2001;17:1135–58.

7. Foster E, Graham TP Jr, Driscoll DJ, Reid GJ, Reiss JG, Russell IA, *et al.* Task force 2: special health care needs of adults with congenital heart disease. *J Am Coll Cardiol* 2001;37:1176–83.

8. Task Force on the Management of Grown Up Congenital Heart Disease of the European Society of Cardiology. Management of grown up congenital heart disease. *Eur Heart J* 2003;24:1035–84.

9. Task Force on Practice Guidelines (Committee on Management of Patients with Valvular Heart Disease). ACC/AHA guidelines for the management of patients with valvular heart disease. A report of the American College of Cardiology/American Heart Association. *J Am Coll Cardiol* 1998;32:1486–588.

10. Blomstrom-Lundqvist C, Scheinman MM, Aliot EM, Alpert JS, Calkins H, Camm AJ, *et al.* ACC/AHA/ESC guidelines for the management of patients with supraventricular arrhythmias – executive summary: a report of the American College of Cardiology/American Heart Association Task Force on Practice Guidelines and the European Society of Cardiology Committee for Practice Guidelines (Writing Committee to Develop Guidelines for the Management of Patients with Supraventricular Arrhythmias). *Circulation* 2003;108:1871–909.

11. Meijboom LJ, Vos FE, Timmermans J, Boers GH, Zwinderman AH, Mulder BJM. Pregnancy and aortic root growth in the Marfan syndrome: a prospective study. *Eur Heart J* 2005;26:914–20.

12. Elkayam U, Tummala PP, Rao K, Akhter MW, Karaalp IS, Wani O, *et al.* Maternal and fetal outcomes of subsequent pregnancies in women with peripartum cardiomyopathy. *N Engl J Med* 2001;344:1567–71.

13. Jamieson WR, Miller DC, Akins CW, Munro AI, Glower DD, Moore KA, *et al.* Pregnancy and bioprostheses: influence on structural valve deterioration. *Ann Thorac Surg* 1995;60(2 Suppl):S282–7.

14. Avila WS, Rossi EG, Grinberg M, Ramires JAF. Influence of pregnancy after prosthetic valve replacement in young women; a prospective 5 year study. *J Heart Valve Disease* 2002;11:864–9.

15. Williams D. Pregnancy: a stress test for life. *Curr Opin Obstet Gynecol* 2003;15:465–71.

16. Silversides CK, Colman JM, Sermer S, Farine D, Siu SC. Early and intermediate-term outcomes of pregnancy with congenital aortic stenosis. *Am J Cardiol* 2003;91:1386–9.

17. Guedes S, Mercier L-A, Leduc L, Berube L, Marcotte F, Dore A. Impact of pregnancy on the systemic right ventricle after a Mustard operation for transposition of the great arteries. *J Am Coll Cardiol* 2004;44:433–7.

Section 7

Consensus views

Chapter 23
Long-term outcome of pregnancy with heart disease

Carole A Warnes

Introduction

Very few data exist with regard to the long-term outcome for women with heart disease, even before the superimposed haemodynamic burden of pregnancy is considered. With the declining incidence of rheumatic heart disease in North America and Western Europe, most maternal cardiac disease is now congenital in origin. Because of the significant advances in surgical intervention, diagnostic imaging and treatment modalities, the last 50 years have seen dramatic changes in the lives of patients born with congenital heart disease. Adult survivors, both men and women, are burgeoning in their numbers and represent a fast-growing population. Issues of ventricular dysfunction, arrhythmias and valvular and vascular dysfunction are common and these patients require continuing care for their complex residua and sequelae. Patients with profoundly complex anatomy who would not have survived two or three decades ago are now presenting in cardiology clinics after having had innovative and complex surgical repairs. In many cases, the long-term outcomes are unknown, and there are no postoperative historical comparisons with which to compare. Women who had previously been physiologically ill-equipped to bear children or who would not, in all probability, have reached reproductive age, are now presenting for obstetric and cardiac care after earlier reparative surgery.

The interplay between the pregnancy-related adjustments in maternal circulatory and respiratory physiology and the growth of the fetus is complex and the factors relating to pregnancy outcomes are many and variable. Most of the published reports regarding pregnancy and maternal cardiac disease of any sort focus on whether the outcome of pregnancy was successful for the fetus and whether the mother experienced any complications during the pregnancy or shortly after. There are few if any data regarding the impact of pregnancy months or even years after delivery.

While normal pregnancy does not appear to have a deleterious effect on cardiac function in either the short or long term in women with normal cardiac anatomy, women with heart disease have less cardiac reserve and are thus more vulnerable. Although they often have a successful delivery and survive without major morbidity, there may be subtle changes in ventricular function or valve regurgitation, which do not return to normal after delivery. These, in turn, may cause a gradual deterioration in exercise capacity over the ensuing months. When symptoms eventually develop it is difficult, indeed impossible without proper comparative studies, to attribute the deterioration to the pregnancy rather than to the natural history of the cardiac problem. With the advances of non-invasive imaging in the last two decades, particularly two-dimensional echocardiography, it is now possible to serially follow changes in ventricular size and function, valvular abnormalities and aortic dimensions. This has facilitated the ability to determine the impact, positive or negative, of a therapeutic intervention, for example, or a haemodynamic burden such as pregnancy.

This review will focus on four cardiac problems where pregnancy has now been recognised as having a possible detrimental effect on maternal wellbeing and long-term outcome.

Ventricular dysfunction

Patients who have mild impairment of ventricular function frequently have at least mild atrioventricular (AV) valve regurgitation. The haemodynamic changes that take place during a normal pregnancy include a 40–50% increase in plasma volume, a heart rate increase of 10–20% and a fall in systemic and pulmonary vascular resistance.[1-6] The increased cardiac output necessary to sustain a pregnancy results in mild increases in cardiac chamber dimensions that have been documented by echocardiography.[7,8] These may affect the right-sided cardiac chambers slightly more than the left. Chamber enlargement can cause annular dilatation, and minor alterations in the geometry of the ventricles can impair effective coaptation of the AV valves. Once AV regurgitation occurs, this adds to the circulatory burden on the ventricles and tends to beget more AV valve regurgitation. These changes may be irreversible.

When the underlying cardiac anatomy is abnormal, not only are the baseline haemodynamics often impaired, but the changes imposed by pregnancy are likely to be more profound. This has been demonstrated in women whose systemic ventricles have right ventricular morphology, the so-called 'systemic right ventricle' (i.e. those with transposition of the great arteries after atrial switch procedures ? Mustard or Senning operations). Guedes et al.[9] reviewed 16 women who had 28 pregnancies and monitored their clinical status and echocardiographic parameters before, during and after pregnancy. All these women were in NYHA functional class I (n = 21) or II (n = 7) before pregnancy (see Appendix A for NYHA classifications). The functional class deteriorated in six women (38%) with no return to prepregnancy levels after delivery in two. Two of the 16 women required heart failure therapy during or soon after pregnancy. Echocardiographic parameters in relation to the right (systemic) ventricular dimensions, function and tricuspid regurgitation were reviewed before, during and after pregnancy. Data on right ventricular dimensions were available in 18 pregnancies: right ventricular dilatation was absent (n = 4), mild/moderate (n = 12) or severe (n = 2) and progressed in five women (31%) with no recovery in any of the women in a follow-up period of 24 months. Data on right ventricular function were available in 21 pregnancies: before pregnancy dysfunction was absent (n = 16), mild/moderate (n = 4) or severe (n = 1). Systolic dysfunction progressed in four women (25%) with no recovery in three cases. Tricuspid regurgitation was absent (n = 8), mild (n = 9) or moderate (n = 3) before pregnancy and deteriorated in eight women (50%) with no recovery in three women.

This study underscores the progression and deterioration of haemodynamic changes during pregnancy in these women with complex anatomy. While it is possible that they could be attributable to the natural history of the anomaly, the short time frame involved makes that explanation unlikely.

This is one of the very few studies that have evaluated serial echocardiographic parameters before and during pregnancy and for several months after delivery. It is certainly possible that such changes in ventricular dimensions, function and secondary AV valve regurgitation might be seen in other maternal cardiac disease, particularly when ventricular function is borderline or mildly reduced prepregnancy. Whether any form of stress testing prepregnancy might delineate impaired cardiac reserve remains to be determined.

Peripartum cardiomyopathy

Many women who have had an episode of peripartum cardiomyopathy subsequently normalise their ventricular function, and a common question is whether or not it is advisable for them to have another pregnancy.[10-12] The evidence suggests that a subsequent pregnancy may be associated with recurrent left ventricular dysfunction, which is sometimes persistent and associated with symptomatic heart failure. Rarely, profound clinical deterioration and even death may occur. It has been suggested that the haemodynamic changes of pregnancy unmask subclinical myocardial dysfunction, or perhaps there is a reactivation of the underlying haemodynamic process responsible for the development of cardiomyopathy in the previous pregnancy.[13] Unfortunately, there is no consensus on appropriate advice regarding the advisability of future pregnancy after a single episode of peripartum cardiomyopathy.[14] However, the evidence that a persistent reduction in ventricular function can occur with a subsequent pregnancy should be shared with the women and her family at the time of prepregnancy counselling,[10,15] and they should be advised to give serious consideration to the option of avoiding additional pregnancies.

Connective tissue disorders and bicuspid aortic valve

Marfan syndrome is one of the most common hereditary connective tissue disorders and is associated with an abnormal gene for fibrillin located on chromosome 15.[16-18] Marfan syndrome can be associated with many cardiovascular complications, including aortic dilatation, dissection and rupture. Pregnancy increases the risk of dissection, particularly when there is a family history of aortic dissection, and some women may have significant acceleration of aortic dilatation with or without aortic regurgitation.[19] The exact mechanism is unclear, although the hyperdynamic circulation and increase in volume load associated with pregnancy might contribute. The published data, however, represent a bias towards reporting the complications of pregnancy, since the uncomplicated cases tend not to be reported. Those women with mild aortic root dilatation prepregnancy (less than 40 mm) sometimes have no increase in the rate of deterioration when compared with women with Marfan syndrome who have never been pregnant.[19,20] This is somewhat unpredictable, however, and even women with a normal aortic size can develop dissection.[21] This means that during pregnancy close surveillance is necessary, even in women with no previous cardiovascular problems. The prophylactic use of beta-adrenergic receptor blockade may be beneficial but this is unproven as there have been no large prospective randomised trials. Some patients with Marfan syndrome also have mitral valve prolapse and varying degrees of mitral regurgitation: this too may progress with the volume load of pregnancy, but long-term data are lacking. Certainly, the possibility of progression of both valvular and aortic complications should be discussed with the prospective mother at the time of preconception counselling.

Structural abnormalities of the great arterial walls in patients with congenital heart disease are an increasing focus of attention.[22-25] The association of bicuspid aortic valve with aortic medial abnormalities has been known for decades, and the loss of smooth muscle cells and degeneration of the elastic medial fibres ? so-called 'cystic medial necrosis' ? in some ways resembles the histological appearance of Marfan syndrome.[24,26,27] The presence of a bicuspid aortic valve is associated with aortic dilatation even in the setting of a functionally normal aortic valve.[28,29] A bicuspid aortic valve increases the propensity to aneurysm formation and increases the risk of dissection at least nine-fold.[30]

While bicuspid aortic valves have not been found to be associated with any specific chromosomal abnormality, patients have been shown to have significantly less fibrillin-1 in their aortic media than their counterparts with tricuspid aortic valves.[27] Whether pregnancy causes further aortic dilatation in women who already have a dilated aortic root is uncertain, but oestrogen has been shown to inhibit collagen and elastin deposition in the aorta, and progestogen has been reported to accelerate deposition of non-collagenous proteins in the aortas of rats.[31] In addition, it has been reported that pregnancy may be accompanied by fragmentation of elastic fibres, a decrease in mucopolysaccharides and an increase in smooth muscle.[23] Whether these gestational changes are additive to the underlying histological abnormality is uncertain. Ageing and the presence of systemic hypertension can produce similar histological abnormalities.[32]

Because of these concerns, the same recommendations as for Marfan syndrome are often applied to women with bicuspid aortic valve and aortic dilatation at the time of prepregnancy counselling. Thus, women who have an aortic root dimension greater than 40 mm should be informed of the potential for further aortic dilatation, aneurysm formation or even dissection, although this is based more on general principles rather than on the evidence of published data. Women with coarctation of the aorta (a common association of bicuspid aortic valve) are also known to have an aortopathy,[23,24,33] and they too may experience further aortic dilatation during pregnancy. However, there have been no reports of sequential imaging studies and long-term outcome data are also lacking.

Tissue valve prostheses

Some authors have reported that pregnancy accelerates structural tissue valve degeneration, although the exact mechanism is unclear.[34-37] Sbarouni and Oakley[38] reported that 35% of 49 tissue prostheses degenerated significantly during pregnancy or shortly afterwards. Other authors, however, have failed to confirm these findings.[39,40] Jamieson et al.[41] reviewed the outcomes of 237 women with 255 tissue prostheses to see whether pregnancy resulted in structural valve deterioration. Fifty-three women had a pregnancy and 202 were never pregnant. The freedom from structural valve deterioration at 10 years for the non-pregnant group was 54% versus 45% for the pregnant group (p = not significant).

Thus, the issue remains controversial. It is possible that the appearance of accelerated valve degeneration simply reflects the accepted more rapid degeneration of tissue prostheses in younger age groups.[42] Nonetheless, all patients with tissue prostheses must accept that, for the long-term, a repeat valve replacement is inevitable and this imposes an additional risk at the time of re-operation. This risk may be relatively low in contemporary surgical series, but in earlier reports the mortality was between 3.8% and 8.8%.[36,41] It is important, therefore, to discuss these issues in detail with the woman at the time of implantation of the tissue prosthesis, and include the possibility that pregnancy might accelerate degeneration of the valve. The facts that a re-operation is associated with a higher risk than the first surgery, and that if a mother dies at re-operation her baby would be left without a biological mother, should be acknowledged.[43]

Conclusions

The provision of appropriate counselling to women with cardiac disease about their long-term outcomes following pregnancy is problematic. Few or no evidence-based guidelines are available, and most published data involve small cohort studies or isolated case reports. In some cases of cardiac disease with subclinical or mild cardiac dysfunction, particularly in the setting of AV valve regurgitation, there is some evidence that ventricular function and/or AV valve regurgitation worsens and does not return to the prepregnant state. There is no consensus, but some evidence suggests that tissue valve prostheses may degenerate more rapidly during pregnancy. Women with Marfan syndrome and those with aortic dilatation secondary to bicuspid valve have an inherent vulnerability to aortic dilatation and may experience more rapid dilatation or even dissection during pregnancy.

There are, however, many uncertainties about all of these issues since only small cohort studies have been published and there are no large prospective multicentre randomised trials that include serial echocardiographic monitoring. This emphasizes the need for future multicentre research initiatives to answer prospectively the many questions that still remain.

References

1. Lund CJ, Donovan JC. Blood volume during pregnancy. Significance of plasma and red cell volumes. *Am J Obstet Gynecol* 1967;98:394–403.
2. Chesley LC. Plasma and red cell volumes during pregnancy. *Am J Obstet Gynecol* 1972;112:440–50
3. Ueland K. Maternal cardiovascular dynamics. VII. Intrapartum blood volume changes. *Am J Obstet Gynecol* 1976;126:671–7.
4. Robson SC, Hunter S, Boys RJ, Dunlop W. Serial study of factors influencing changes in cardiac output during human pregnancy. *Am J Physiol.* 1989;256(4 Pt 2):H1060–5.
5. Mabie WC, DiSessa TG, Crocker LG, Sibai BM, Arheart KL. A longitudinal study of cardiac output in normal human pregnancy. *Am J Obstet Gynecol* 1994;170:849–56.
6. Clark SL, Cotton DB, Lee W, Bishop C, Hill T, Southwick J, et al. Central hemodynamic assessment of normal term pregnancy. *Am J Obstet Gynecol.* 1989;161(6 Pt 1):1439–42.
7. Katz R, Karliner JS, Resnik R. Effects of a natural volume overload state (pregnancy) on left ventricular performance in normal human subjects. *Circulation* 1978;58(3 Pt 1):434–41.
8. Capeless EL, Clapp JF. Cardiovascular changes in early phase of pregnancy. *Am J Obstet Gynecol.* 1989;161(6 Pt 1):1449–53.
9. Guedes A, Mercier LA, Leduc L, Berube L, Marcotte F, Dore A. Impact of pregnancy on the systemic right ventricle after a Mustard operation for transposition of the great arteries. *J Am Coll Cardiol* 2004;44:433–7.
10. Elkayam U. Pregnant again after peripartum cardiomyopathy: to be or not to be? *Eur Heart J* 2002;23:753–6.

11. Heider AL, Kuller JA, Strauss RA, Wells SR. Peripartum cardiomyopathy: a review of the literature. *Obstet Gynecol Surv* 1999;54:526–31.

12. Elkayam U, Akhter MW, Singh H, Khan S, Bitar F, Hameed A, *et al*. Pregnancy-associated cardiomyopathy: clinical characteristics and a comparison between early and late presentation. *Circulation* 2005;111:2050–5.

13. Lampert MB, Weinert L, Hibbard J, Korcarz C, Lindheimer M, Lang RM. Contractile reserve in patients with peripartum cardiomyopathy and recovered left ventricular function. *Am J Obstet Gynecol*. 1997;176(1 Pt 1):189–95.

14. Pearson GD, Veille JC, Rahimtoola S, Hsia J, Oakley CM, Hosenpud JD, *et al*. Peripartum cardiomyopathy: National Heart, Lung, and Blood Institute and Office of Rare Diseases (National Institutes of Health) workshop recommendations and review. *JAMA* 2000;283:1183–8.

15. Elkayam U, Tummala PP, Rao K, Akhter MW, Karaalp IS, Wani OR, *et al*. Maternal and fetal outcomes of subsequent pregnancies in women with peripartum cardiomyopathy. *N Engl J Med* 2001;344:1567–71. Erratum in: *N Engl J Med* 2001;345:552.

16. Milewicz DM, Pyeritz RE, Crawford ES, Byers PH. Marfan syndrome: defective synthesis, secretion, and extracellular matrix formation of fibrillin by cultured dermal fibroblasts. *J Clin Invest* 1992;89:79–86.

17. Milewicz DM, Grossfield J, Cao SN, Kielty C, Covitz W, Jewett T. A mutation in FBN1 disrupts profibrillin processing and results in isolated skeletal features of the Marfan syndrome. *J Clin Invest* 1995;95:2373–8.

18. Dietz HC, Cutting GR, Pyeritz RE, Maslen CL, Sakai LY, Corson GM, *et al*. Marfan syndrome caused by a recurrent *de novo* missense mutation in the fibrillin gene. *Nature* 1991;352:337–9.

19. Rossiter JP, Repke JT, Morales AJ, Murphy EA, Pyeritz RE. A prospective longitudinal evaluation of pregnancy in the Marfan syndrome. *Am J Obstet Gynecol* 1995;173:1599–606.

20. Pyeritz RE. Maternal and fetal complications of pregnancy in the Marfan syndrome. *Am J Med* 1981;71:784–90.

21. Lipscomb KJ, Smith JC, Clarke B, Donnai P, Harris R. Outcome of pregnancy in women with Marfan's syndrome. *Br J Obstet Gynaecol* 1997;104:201–6.

22. Dodds GA 3rd, Warnes CA, Danielson GK. Aortic valve replacement after repair of pulmonary atresia and ventricular septal defect or tetralogy of Fallot. *J Thorac Cardiovasc Surg* 1997;113:736–41.

23. Niwa K, Perloff JK, Bhuta SM, Laks H, Drinkwater DC, Child JS, *et al*. Structural abnormalities of great arterial walls in congenital heart disease: light and electron microscopic analyses. *Circulation* 2001;103:393–400.

24. Warnes CA. Bicuspid aortic valve and coarctation: two villains part of a diffuse problem. *Heart* 2003;89:965–6.

25. Warnes CA, Child JS. Aortic root dilatation after repair of tetralogy of Fallot: pathology from the past? *Circulation* 2002;106:1310–11.

26. de Sa M, Moshkovitz Y, Butany J, David TE. Histologic abnormalities of the ascending aorta and pulmonary trunk in patients with bicuspid aortic valve disease: clinical relevance to the Ross procedure. *J Thorac Cardiovasc Surg* 1999;118:588–94.

27. Fedak PW, Verma S, David TE, Leask RL, Weisel RD, Butany J. Clinical and pathophysiological implications of a bicuspid aortic valve. *Circulation* 2002;106:900–4.

28. Nistri S, Sorbo MD, Marin M, Palisi M, Scognamiglio R, Thiene G. Aortic root dilatation in young men with normally functioning bicuspid aortic valves. *Heart* 1999;82:19–22.

29. Sabet HY, Edwards WD, Tazelaar HD, Daly RC. Congenitally bicuspid aortic valves: a surgical pathology study of 542 cases (1991 through 1996) and a literature review of 2,715 additional cases. *Mayo Clin Proc* 1999;74:14–26.

30. Edwards WD, Leaf DS, Edwards JE. Dissecting aortic aneurysm associated with congenital bicuspid aortic valve. *Circulation* 1978;57:1022–5.

31. Wolinsky H. Effects of estrogen and progestogen treatment on the response of the aorta of male rats to hypertension. Morphological and chemical studies. *Circ Res* 1972;30:341–9.

32. Carlson RG, Lillehei CW, Edwards JE. Cystic medial necrosis of the ascending aorta in relation to age and hypertension. *Am J Cardiol* 1970;25:411–15.

33. Isner JM, Donaldson RF, Fulton D, Bhan I, Payne DD, Cleveland RJ. Cystic medial necrosis in coarctation of the aorta: a potential factor contributing to adverse consequences observed after percutaneous balloon angioplasty of coarctation sites. *Circulation* 1987;75:689–95.

34. Born D, Martinez EE, Almeida PA, Santos DV, Carvalho AC, Moron AF, et al. Pregnancy in patients with prosthetic heart valves: the effects of anticoagulation on mother, fetus, and neonate. *Am Heart J* 1992;124:413–17.

35. Bortolotti U, Milano A, Mazzucco A, Valfre C, Russo R, Valente M, et al. Pregnancy in patients with a porcine valve bioprosthesis. *Am J Cardiol* 1982;50:1051–4.

36. Badduke BR, Jamieson WR, Miyagishima RT, Munro AI, Gerein AN, MacNab J, et al. Pregnancy and childbearing in a population with biologic valvular prostheses. *J Thorac Cardiovasc Surg* 1991;102:179–86.

37. Sadler L, McCowan L, White H, Stewart A, Bracken M, North R. Pregnancy outcomes and cardiac complications in women with mechanical, bioprosthetic and homograft valves. *BJOG* 2000;107:245–53.

38. Sbarouni E, Oakley CM. Outcome of pregnancy in women with valve prostheses. *Br Heart J* 1994;71:196–201.

39. North RA, Sadler L, Stewart AW, McCowan LM, Kerr AR, White HD. Long-term survival and valve-related complications in young women with cardiac valve replacements. *Circulation* 1999;99:2669–76.

40. Salazar E, Espinola N, Roman L, Casanova JM. Effect of pregnancy on the duration of bovine pericardial bioprostheses. *Am Heart J.* 1999;137(4 Pt 1):714–20.

41. Jamieson WR, Miller DC, Akins CW, Munro AI, Glower DD, Moore KA, et al. Pregnancy and bioprostheses: influence on structural valve deterioration. *Ann Thorac Surg* 1995;60(2 Suppl):S282–6; discussion S287.

42. Yun KL, Miller DC, Moore KA, Mitchell RS, Oyer PE, Stinson EB, et al. Durability of the Hancock MO bioprosthesis compared with standard aortic valve bioprostheses. *Ann Thorac Surg* 1995;60(2 Suppl):S221–8.

43. Hung L, Rahimtoola SH. Prosthetic heart valves and pregnancy. *Circulation* 2003;107:1240–6.

Chapter 24

Consensus views arising from the 51st Study Group: Heart Disease and Pregnancy

Overarching consensus views

General

1. There should be an agreed national registry for the collection of data on pregnancy in women with heart disease. These data should be collected centrally to produce a data set that would enable a more detailed analysis of risk factors for poor pregnancy and long-term outcomes (including maternal survival and infant disability). This would greatly improve the counselling information available for women.
2. There should be recognised networks for the provision of care for women with heart disease and appropriate referral links should be established. These will need to be specifically funded as the detailed care these women need cannot be provided from routine obstetric and cardiac resources.

Preconception

3. A proactive approach to preconception counselling should be started in adolescence (at age 12–15 years, depending on individual maturity) and this should include advice on safe and effective contraception. Proper advice should be given at the appropriate age and not delayed until transfer to the adult cardiological services.
4. All women of reproductive age with congenital or acquired heart disease should have access to specialised multidisciplinary preconception counselling so as to empower them to make choices about pregnancy.
5. All women with significant heart disease should be reviewed regularly to ensure that there has been a recent assessment prior to pregnancy.
6. Women with heart disease are often at increased risk when assisted conception is undertaken. The advice of the multidisciplinary team should be sought before any such treatment is commenced.

7. In counselling women about motherhood, alternatives to the woman carrying the baby herself can be considered (for example surrogacy or adoption).

8. All clinicians should be aware, and should educate others, that the majority of pregnant women who die of heart disease have not previously been identified as 'at risk'.

Antenatal care

9. Once they are pregnant, all women with heart disease should be assessed clinically as soon as possible by a multidisciplinary team ('the specialist high-risk obstetric team') and appropriate investigations (such as echocardiography and magnetic resonance imaging) undertaken. Direct self-referral should be allowed, to avoid any bureaucratic delays. The core members of the multi-disciplinary team should be obstetricians, cardiologists and anaesthetists but midwives (as many women with mild or moderately severe heart disease will have carefully monitored normal births), neonatologists (some women will deliver growth-restricted or preterm infants) and intensivists (some women will need intensive care) should also be involved in care when appropriate.

10. Following multidisciplinary assessment, appropriate care can be arranged at a district general hospital or tertiary unit (where the multidisciplinary team is based), according to the complexity of the heart disease, the risk assessment and the locally available facilities and expertise. (A tertiary unit can be defined as a hospital (or group of hospitals) able to provide combined obstetric, cardiological and surgical expertise in the care of women with heart disease.)

11. All pregnant women with heart disease should undergo risk stratification by the multidisciplinary team to determine the frequency and content of antenatal care.

12. Immigrants to the UK (or to other developed countries) who have not had childhood health screening are a high-risk group for undiagnosed heart disease, and any cardiovascular or respiratory symptoms should lead to careful clinical and echocardiographic assessment, with consideration of additional imaging as appropriate.

13. Women with congenital heart disease are at a relatively increased risk of having a baby affected with congenital heart disease and should be offered fetal echocardiography, performed by a fully trained fetal cardiologist.

14. There is an urgent need to develop more specialist high-risk obstetric units with appropriate multidisciplinary teams.

15. Any tertiary centre caring for pregnant women with heart disease should have facilities for prolonged high-level maternal surveillance within the obstetric unit. There should also be direct access to adult critical care facilities.

Intrapartum care

16. Management of intrapartum care should be supervised by a team experienced in the care of women with heart disease (obstetrician, anaesthetist and midwife), with a cardiologist readily available.

17. A clear plan for management of labour and the puerperium in women with heart disease should be established in advance, be well documented and be distributed widely (including to the woman herself) so that all personnel likely to be involved in the woman's intrapartum and postpartum care are fully informed.

18.   The main objective of management should be to minimise any additional load on the cardiovascular system from delivery and the puerperium. This is usually best achieved by aiming for spontaneous onset of labour, providing effective pain relief with low-dose regional analgesia and, if necessary, assisting vaginal delivery with instruments such as the ventouse or forceps, limiting or even avoiding active maternal bearing down ('pushing').

19.   Vaginal delivery is the preferred mode of delivery over caesarean section for most women with heart disease – whether congenital or acquired – unless obstetric or specific cardiac considerations determine otherwise.

20.   Induction of labour may be appropriate, to optimise the timing of delivery in relation to anticoagulation and the availability of specific medical staff or because of deteriorating maternal cardiac function. However, it should be recognised that induction of labour before 41 weeks of gestation, especially in nulliparous women with an unfavourable cervix, increases the likelihood of caesarean section.

Postpartum care

21.   High-level maternal surveillance is required until the main haemodynamic challenges following delivery have passed. For particularly unstable cardiac conditions (such as pulmonary hypertension or cardiomyopathy), such surveillance may be required for up to 2 weeks. Multidisciplinary surveillance should be maintained until it is judged the woman is well enough to leave hospital. Multidisciplinary follow-up assessment should take place, as a minimum, at 6 weeks after delivery (and in cases where there are continuing concerns, at 6 months), beyond which time the woman should return to her periodic cardiac outpatient care.

Additional consensus views

General

22.   If any pregnant or postpartum woman has unexpected and persistent dyspnoea or is noted to be unusually tachypnoeic or tachycardic, and pulmonary embolus has been excluded, she may have peripartum cardiomyopathy and should be investigated further by a cardiologist, and usually by echocardiography.

Preconception

23.   Any cardiac surgical interventions in women of childbearing age should take into account the effect they may have on pregnancy. For example, because of the risks associated with prosthetic mechanical valves in pregnancy, consideration should be given to using tissue valves for valve replacement.

24.   Preconception assessment and risk stratification for women with pre-existing heart disease can be refined by cardiopulmonary exercise testing (including maximum oxygen uptake).

25.   Contraceptive choice for women with heart disease should be tailored to the particular patient, taking into account any increased risks of thrombosis or infection associated with the various contraceptive methods and their interaction with the various heart lesions.

26.   A key requirement for contraception is efficacy. Unlike healthy women who use contraception for family spacing, the consequences of contraceptive failure can be fatal for women with severe heart disease. Subdermal progestogen implants (such as Implanon®) and progestogen-loaded intrauterine devices (such as Mirena®) are the most efficacious and are also the safest methods for most women with significant heart disease.

27.   In the event of unprotected sexual intercourse, women with heart disease should be aware that emergency contraception that is known to be safe for women with heart disease is available. Urgent access to termination of pregnancy should be readily available.

Antenatal

28.   Levels of mitral and aortic stenosis that are not problematic in non-pregnant women may be poorly tolerated in pregnancy. Reduction of heart rate is often the key to successful management, especially in stenosis of the mitral valve. Beta blockers are useful in this context.

29.   Cardiac surgery during pregnancy should only be considered for women who are refractory to medical treatment or when there is no catheter-based interventional alternative. Percutaneous catheter interventions are safe and effective in the treatment of coronary disease and mitral and pulmonary valve stenosis. In contrast, balloon dilatation for aortic valve disease should only be considered for highly selected cases as it carries a higher risk and a lower success rate. Such interventions in pregnancy should only be performed by experienced operators and radiation exposure should be minimised. If cardiac surgery requiring the use of cardiopulmonary bypass does need to be performed, consideration should be given to early delivery of the fetus if it is viable. If cardiopulmonary bypass is necessary, the deep hypothermia and low perfusion pressure associated with the standard techniques carries a 30% risk of fetal mortality. In the interests of the fetus, if possible, hypothermia should be avoided and perfusion pressures kept as high as possible. With these adjustments, fetal mortality can be as low as 10%.

30.   In pregnancy, if there is clinical evidence of acute coronary insufficiency or myocardial infarction, coronary angiography is appropriate. The radiation exposure of the fetus is not sufficient to contraindicate this essential diagnostic procedure. The first choice for treatment of acute coronary syndrome in pregnancy is percutaneous catheter intervention.

31.   Only centres with experienced teams and expertise in pregnancy and heart disease should carry out such surgical or catheter-based procedures, except in situations where transfer to such a centre would entail a greater risk.

32.   Women with pulmonary arterial hypertension – irrespective of aetiology – should be advised of the very high risks of pregnancy (about 30–50% mortality) and be given clear advice about contraception. For some of these women, pulmonary arterial vasodilator therapy during pregnancy and the puerperium may improve the chances of maternal survival.

33.   Tertiary units should offer a hotel facility to enable women who live some distance from the hospital to stay on site, to avoid (a) a delay in receiving appropriate care when they go into labour and (b) the need to induce labour solely to avoid this risk.

34.   Screening efficiency would be improved if fetal cardiac ultrasound screening

were offered on the basis of a nuchal translucency thickness exceeding 3.5 cm, as well as on the basis of family or personal history.

35. Audited training programmes in fetal cardiac scanning for ultrasonographers are advised in order to improve detection rates of fetal heart disease at the 20 week anomaly scan.

36. The threshold for starting thromboprophylaxis should be lower for pregnant women with heart disease than for the same conditions in non-pregnant women.

37. Thrombolysis may cause bleeding from the placental site but should be given in women with life-threatening thromboembolic disease or acute coronary insufficiency.

38. There is currently no ideal regimen of anticoagulation in women with mechanical heart valves in pregnancy. Women should be offered a choice between the higher rates of fetal loss associated with the use of warfarin and the higher risk of maternal valve thrombosis with subcutaneous heparin.

39. Low-dose aspirin (75–150 mg daily) is a safe and possibly effective adjunct to low molecular weight heparin in pregnant women with mechanical heart valves or an otherwise increased risk of intracardiac thrombosis.

40. In pregnant women with mechanical heart valves who elect to use subcutaneous heparin, the dose of low molecular weight heparin should be at therapeutic levels and guided by monitoring of antifactor Xa activity at least monthly. We suggest a peak (3–4 hour post-dose) level of at least 1.0 iu/ml and a trough level of at least 0.5 iu/ml. It might be possible to reduce the risk of valve thrombosis (currently estimated to be about 10%) by using higher doses but this remains speculative.

41. In women on beta blockers (for example for the treatment of systemic hypertension or to reduce the risk of arrhythmia) there is a small increased risk of intrauterine growth restriction and fetal growth should thus be monitored regularly, using ultrasound measurement of fetal abdominal circumference, if there is any clinical suspicion of poor growth.

42. All pregnant women whose condition places them at risk of aortopathy (such as those with repaired coarctation, Marfan syndrome or aortopathy associated with bicuspid aortic valve) should be made aware of the symptoms of acute dissection and be advised to seek urgent help if they experience any of them.

43. Every attempt should be made to establish the details of the cardiac diagnoses and any previous cardiac surgical or catheter-based procedures before or at preconception counselling, as this will enhance opportunities for optimising cardiac status during pregnancy.

44. When planning care, specific instructions should be recorded regarding intra-partum antibiotic prophylaxis. There is currently no evidence that prophylactic antibiotics are necessary to prevent endocarditis in an uncomplicated vaginal delivery. However, prophylactic antibiotics should be given in all cases of operative delivery and to women at increased risk, such as those with mechanical valves or a history of previous endocarditis. Prophylactic antibiotic cover should also be given before any intervention likely to be associated with significant or recurrent bacteraemia. The possibility of endocarditis should also be considered in any woman with a cardiac defect who has positive blood cultures.

45. Pregnant women with previous Kawasaki disease and coronary artery aneurysm (with or without coronary artery stenosis) should be given antiplate-let and/or anticoagulant thromboprophylaxis.

46. Timely restoration of sinus rhythm is strongly advisable in pregnant women with tachyarrhythmias and underlying heart disease. Direct current (DC) cardioversion is safe, although attention should be paid to airway management because of the risk of aspiration/regurgitation of gastric contents, and care should be taken to avoid the supine position with its accompanying risk of aortocaval compression. Careful fetal monitoring is also advisable.

Intrapartum

47. Care should be delivered by designated professionals as part of the multidisciplinary team.
48. With any surgical intervention, meticulous attention must be paid to haemostasis to avoid haemorrhage, which can cause marked cardiovascular instability in pregnant women with reduced cardiac reserve.
49. In the management of the third stage of labour in women with heart disease, bolus doses of oxytocin can cause severe hypotension and should thus be avoided. Low-dose oxytocin infusions are safer and may be equally effective. Ergometrine is best avoided in most cases as it can cause acute hypertension. Misoprostol may be safer but it can cause problems such as hyperthermia and data are still limited in this population. It should be used only if the benefits outweigh any potential risks. At caesarean section, uterine compression sutures may be effective in controlling uterine haemorrhage due to atony, and may allow the avoidance of any uterotonic agent.
50. Regional or general anaesthesia for caesarean section should be used in such a way as to optimise cardiovascular stability and should only be given by anaesthetists experienced in their use in pregnant women with heart disease.
51. In all high-risk pregnancy centres, guidelines should be in place (and regularly rehearsed) for dealing with cardiac arrest. Regular staff attendance at adult and neonatal resuscitation courses should be mandatory. All equipment, including bleep systems, should be serviced and checked regularly to ensure operational efficiency.

Puerperium

52. Angiotensin-converting enzyme (ACE) inhibitors are safe to use in breast-feeding mothers. This knowledge should be more widely disseminated and appreciated.
53. Because of the increased risk of postpartum haemorrhage in women with heart disease who are anticoagulated, the introduction or reintroduction of warfarin should be delayed until at least 2 days postpartum. Meticulous monitoring of anticoagulation is essential.

Appendix A

New York Heart Association classification of cardiovascular disease

Table A.1. New York Heart Association classification of cardiovascular disease

Class	Description
I	Patients who are not limited by cardiac disease in their physical activity. Ordinary physical activity does not precipitate the occurrence of symptoms such as fatigue, palpitations, dyspnoea and angina.
II	Patients in whom the cardiac disease causes a slight limitation in physical activity. These patients are comfortable at rest, but ordinary physical activity will precipitate symptoms.
III	Patients in whom the cardiac disease results in a marked limitation of physical activity. They are comfortable at rest, but less than ordinary physical activity will precipitate symptoms.
IV	Patients in whom the cardiac disease results in the inability to carry on physical activity without discomfort. Symptoms may be present even at rest, and discomfort is increased by any physical activity.

Index

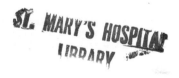